TOXIC SHOT

Facing the Dangers of the COVID "Vaccines"

Byram Bridle, PhD & Harvey Risch, MD, PhD

With Matt Bain, MD, Steven Hatfill, MD, MMed, Peter McCullough, MD, MPH, Jane Orient, MD, Jessica Rose, PhD, Josh Stirling, MBA, James Thorp, MD, Kelly Victory, MD, Naomi Wolf, PhD, Martin Wucher, DDS

Foreword by Sen. Ron Johnson

Toxic Shot:
Facing the Dangers of the COVID "Vaccines"
© 2024 by Byram Bridle and Harvey Risch
All Rights Reserved

NIV: All Scripture quotations, unless otherwise indicated, are taken from the Holy Bible, New International Version®, NIV®. Copyright ©1973, 1978, 1984, 2011 by Biblica, Inc.™ Used by permission of Zondervan. All rights reserved worldwide. www.zondervan.com. The "NIV" and "New International Version" are trademarks registered in the United States Patent and Trademark Office by Biblica, Inc.™

This book contains advice and information relating to health care. It should be used to supplement rather than replace the advice of your doctor or another trained health professional. You are advised to consult your health professional with regard to matters related to your health, and in particular regarding matters that may require diagnosis or medical attention. All efforts have been made to assure the accuracy of the information in this book as of the date of publication. The publisher and the author disclaim liability for any medical outcomes that may occur as a result of applying the methods suggested in this book.

This is a work of nonfiction. All people, locations, events, and situations are portrayed to the best of the author's memory.

No part of this book may be reproduced, stored in a retrieval system, or transmitted by any means without the written permission of the author and publisher.

Published in the United States of America
1 2 3 4 5 6 7 8 9 10

IN MEMORIAM

Dr. Ramin Oskoui

Dr. Vladimir "Zev" Zelenko

Courage in standing for the truth in times of deceit

זכרונם לברכה

Be not afraid

TABLE OF CONTENTS

Foreword by Senator Ron Johnson 7

Introduction: An Urgent Call 15

Chapter 1: The COVID-19 modRNA Shots Are Not Real Vaccines
by Byram W. Bridle, PhD 27

Chapter 2: A Government Prototype Rushed to Market without Adequate Testing
by Harvey Risch, MD, PhD 39

Chapter 3: Introduction to *The Pfizer Papers*: Pfizer's Crimes Against Humanity
by Naomi Wolf, PhD 48

Chapter 4: The Spike Protein Is Harmful by Itself
by Martin Wucher, DDS 58

Chapter 5: Debunking CDC's Bad Science
by Steven J. Hatfill, MD, MSc, MMed 67

Chapter 6: Safety Signals from the Vaccine Adverse Event Reporting System (VAERS)
by Jessica Rose, PhD 92

Chapter 7: Immunological Harms of the modRNA "Vaccines"
by Byram W. Bridle, PhD 106

Chapter 8: Cardiac and Cardiovascular Damage from the modRNA "Vaccines"
by Dr. Peter A. McCullough, MD, MPH 118

Chapter 9: Neurological Injuries from the modRNA "Vaccines"
by Matt Bain, MD 128

Chapter 10: Cancer Risks of the modRNA COVID-19 "Vaccines"
by Jane Orient, MD 149

Chapter 11: COVID-19 "Vaccine" Effects on Women of
    Reproductive Age and Pregnancy
    by James A. Thorp, MD 163

Chapter 12: Risks to Children
    by Kelly Victory, MD 187

Chapter 13: "Vaccine" Mortality Insights from Autopsy Reports
    *by Peter A. McCullough, MD, MPH, and
    Harvey Risch, MD, PhD, et al.* 203

Chapter 14: "All Hands on Deck"—The Catastrophe of
    US Longevity, and What We Can Do about It
    by Josh Stirling, MBA 211

Endnotes 228
Acknowledgments 305
About the Authors 307

FOREWORD

By Senator Ron Johnson

The images and news coming out of China, Italy, and New York City in the first three months of 2020 were undoubtedly alarming: photos of first responders and health professionals in biohazard suits and reports of COVID-19 hotspots and deaths dominated news cycles. Was this new virus as deadly as Ebola, with a 40 percent case fatality rate (CFR)?[1] Or MERS, with a 36 percent CFR?[2] Or the original SARS-CoV-1 strain, which triggered a global outbreak in 2003, with a 9.6 percent CFR?[3]

Then on March 17, 2020, in an article published in *STAT News*, Stanford professor Dr. John Ioannidis analyzed the data from the *Diamond Princess* cruise ship that was quarantined due to a COVID outbreak. From that data, Dr. Ioannidis projected an infection fatality rate (IFR) for SARS-CoV-2 of 0.125 percent, with a predicted case fatality rate somewhere between 0.05 percent and 1 percent.[4] (For perspective, an average flu season has an IFR of approximately 0.1 percent.[5]) By April 2020, Oxford's Centre for Evidence-Based Medicine was also predicting an IFR well below 1 percent—probably no worse than double a bad flu season.[6]

Dr. Ioannidis's analysis has stood the test of time. An October 2022 study by Dr. Ioannidis and others, based on pre-vaccination seroprevalence data, calculated a median COVID IFR for ages under seventy of 0.095 percent, and possibly as low as 0.07 percent.[7]

I wasn't immune to the fear sweeping the country, but those two early predictions provided valuable perspective, eased my concerns, and made me highly skeptical of the scaremongering and draconian responses that would dominate the next two years. Unfortunately, far too many in power found it useful to stoke fear in service of their own interests and agendas.

In March 2020, as lockdowns loomed, I publicly stated that we tragically lose tens of thousands of people in traffic fatalities each year, but we don't shut down our highways.[8] From the White House podium, Anthony

Fauci said that comment was "totally way out."[9] Actually, my comment was an apt analogy. There was no way we could shut down our entire economy to "slow the spread"—the collateral damage to society would simply be too great. We had to continue on with our lives. In a recent and very limited mea culpa, former NIH director Dr. Francis Collins admitted, "If you're a public-health person, you attach a zero value to whether this actually totally disrupts people's lives, ruins the economy, and has many kids kept out of school in a way that they never quite recovered"—all of which amounted to "another mistake we made."[10]

Federal workers, like other white-collar office workers, could "work" from home. But blue-collar workers had to go in to work to keep our economy operating, and they did. The inequity of the shutdowns didn't end with the disparity between blue- and white-collar workers. Small Main Street businesses were shut down by government edict, and many went bankrupt, wiping out the lifetime savings of their owners. But big-box stores and tech giants *not only stayed open, they thrived* as their smaller competitors were destroyed. Oxfam reported that billionaires worldwide increased their wealth by $3.9 trillion between March 18 and December 31, 2020.[11]

I have labeled those who imposed pandemic tyranny on society the "COVID Cartel": the Biden administration, federal health agencies, Big Pharma, the mainstream media, and big tech, including social media giants. Their assaults on freedom have been breathtaking: mask mandates, forced lockdowns, mandating "vaccines" that failed to stop infection or transmission, suppression and censorship of the truth, withholding information or outright lying to the public, and vilifying and destroying the careers of doctors and others who disagreed with the Cartel.

Ever since emails of Anthony Fauci and others became available through a Freedom of Information Act (FOIA) request, it's been obvious there was an immediate attempt to cover up our government's funding of dangerous biological research that might have helped create the coronavirus. We may never definitively know the pandemic's origin, but the concerted and coordinated effort to label as a "conspiracy theory" any talk of the virus being man-made was just the first in a long line of falsehoods pushed by the COVID Cartel.

Public health authorities also told us the shot's lab-modified mRNA (modRNA) would stay in the arm muscle, even though it was encapsulated in lipid nanoparticles (LNPs) designed to permeate difficult-to-permeate barriers—like the blood-brain or placenta barriers. Japanese health officials released Pfizer's biodistribution study of the LNPs in rats, showing they spread all over the body and concentrated in the liver, spleen, adrenal glands, and ovaries.[12] Why was this important information, together with adverse events that occurred during the trials, hidden from the public? *The fact that both the Food and Drug Administration (FDA) and Pfizer fought to keep the trial data bottled up for seventy-five years speaks volumes about their lack of honesty and transparency.*[13]

So much of what the COVID Cartel was saying and doing simply made no sense. Haven't we always believed that early disease detection enables early treatment and produces better outcomes? Why was that fundamental tenet of medicine not only ignored but sabotaged? Why were frontline doctors, who had the courage and compassion to treat COVID patients from the start of the pandemic, censored, vilified, and subjected to fierce professional retribution? How could health officials deny the effectiveness of our natural immune system when approximately 40 percent of people testing positive for COVID were asymptomatic?[14]

The National Institutes of Health (NIH) guideline for COVID, if you tested positive, was simply to go home and isolate yourself. In other words, *do nothing* and hope you don't get so sick you require hospitalization. Far too often, stories of COVID hospitalizations were horrific. Patients lost their freedom. Family members couldn't comfort dying loved ones. Patient and family member requests to administer multidrug protocols using cheap, widely available, FDA-approved generic drugs were rejected in favor of highly expensive Remdesivir and ventilators with a depressingly low rate of success. As of this writing, affluent America, with only 4 percent of the world's population, accounts for 16 percent of COVID deaths globally.[15]

I don't know how anyone could review the results of our response to COVID and conclude it was anything but a miserable failure. The *human toll* of the economic devastation caused by futile, purposeless shutdowns is incalculable. Hundreds of thousands of innocent people were condemned to death by the false discrediting of early treatment, sabotaged with shoddy science to ensure the modRNA products—which failed to qualify as real "vaccines" by any historic standard (chapter 1)—would obtain emergency use authorization (EUA): *by law, regulators can only grant an EUA if they believe there are no other effective treatments.* In the US alone, estimates of the *economic cost* of our response will top $14 trillion by the end of 2023.[16]

The COVID Cartel is still denying the deaths and disabilities caused by the experimental gene therapy pushed on billions of people globally, but they are all too real. With the long-term impacts still unknown, I fear serious health issues will surface and linger far into the future.

The liability protection granted to vaccine manufacturers in the National Childhood Vaccine Injury Act of 1986 eliminated an important control over vaccine quality and safety.[17] It has also incentivized an explosion in new vaccines, including the COVID "vaccine." Although the title of the bill would make most people think the law heightens awareness of vaccine injuries and provides just compensation to those who suffer from them, nothing could be further from the truth. As of January 2024, *only ten individuals have successfully obtained compensation for COVID "vaccine" injuries*, their combined payouts a measly $36,945—more of an insult than just compensation.[18] This area of law will need to be updated as "vaccine" injuries mount to a level that cannot be denied.

By the time the COVID "vaccines" obtained their EUAs, the Cartel was firmly in control of the narrative. Phrases such as "follow the science," "safe and effective," "no one is safe until everyone is safe," "nobody will be safe [unless] everybody is vaccinated," and "this is a pandemic of the unvaccinated" were used ad nauseam to bludgeon the public into submission.[19]

A few months into the "vaccine" rollout, the FDA and the Centers for Disease Control and Prevention (CDC) began to undermine and denigrate their own Vaccine Adverse Event Reporting System (VAERS), the safety surveillance system they had just touted prior to granting an EUA to the COVID vaccines.[20] In an attempt to marginalize VAERS information, so-called "fact-checkers" pointed out that anyone could file a report, suggesting that anti-vaccine activists might game the system by filing false reports.[21]

Denigrating and dismissing VAERS represented a break with all established precedent for vaccine safety monitoring. In 1976, the swine flu vaccine program was terminated after approximately 400–500 cases of Guillain-Barré syndrome and several dozen deaths were associated with the vaccine.[22] By the end of April 2021, just four months into the COVID vaccine rollout, VAERS was already reporting 2,926 deaths worldwide within thirty days of vaccination, with 46.1 percent of those deaths occurring on day zero, one, or two following vaccination.[23] When I asked then-NIH director Francis Collins about what VAERS was showing at that point in time, he acknowledged six deaths had been attributed to the Johnson & Johnson "vaccine," but as to the other 2,920 deaths reported on VAERS, he callously stated, "Senator, people die."

That breezy attitude pretty well sums up our federal health agencies' stance on modRNA "vaccine" injuries and deaths. As a result of that indifference and lack of acknowledgment, those who have been injured by these products are largely ignored and do not receive effective treatment. Again, *current compensation for "vaccine" injuries is woefully inadequate.*

As of December 29, 2023, VAERS showed 1,621,120 adverse events and 36,986 deaths reported worldwide associated with the COVID "vaccines." Roughly 9,030 (24.4 percent) of those deaths occurred within two days of "vaccination."[24] VAERS data might not prove causation, but that correlation between death and "vaccination" should certainly concern federal health officials and lead to robust investigation.

But it hasn't. Why not?

Federal health officials have not only ignored VAERS, they've also attempted to bury the results of V-Safe, a safety surveillance system specifically set up for the COVID-19 "vaccines" (chapter 5). It took attorney Aaron Siri, working on behalf of the Informed Consent Action Network (ICAN), over two years to pry the V-Safe data out of the iron grip of the CDC. Here is what CDC was hiding: of the 10 million individuals that voluntarily registered and submitted data to V-Safe, 782,913 (7.7 percent) had symptoms or health conditions requiring medical attention, emergency room intervention, and/or hospitalization following their COVID-19 "vaccination." Over 25 percent reported those symptoms or health conditions rendered them unable to work or do normal daily activities. These shocking results, presented in further detail by Dr. Hatfill in chapter 5, were kept hidden from the public for over two years, and even now have still not been widely reported.[25]

A poll taken in March 2023 by Rasmussen Reports showed that 11 percent of American adults said a member of their household died from COVID-19, *but an almost equal percentage—10 percent—said a member of their household died as a result of COVID-19 "vaccine" side effects.*[26] Over the last three years, the number of sudden deaths of sports figures, famous personalities, and other young healthy people has been impossible not to notice. Global data on excess deaths by country, highlighted by Josh Stirling in chapter 14, are becoming harder and harder to ignore. But even as the COVID Cartel downplays this reality and continues to push booster shots, the American public is rapidly losing faith in them. The low uptake of the fall 2023 COVID-19 "booster" by children (4.9 percent) and adults (13.9 percent)—as of November 13, 2023—is testament to this fact.

As long as I can remember, those faced with a serious medical condition are advised to seek a second, and possibly even a third, opinion. Once again, that basic tenet of medicine has been violated. Throughout the pandemic, the COVID Cartel presented its views as definitive and inarguable—only their narrative was allowed. Anything contrary to its edicts was labeled dangerous "misinformation."

As a US senator, I worked to expose the insanity of our COVID response with hearings in 2020—when I was chairman of the Senate Committee on Homeland Security and Governmental Affairs—and public events in 2021 and 2022, after we lost the majority. In May 2020, my hearing featured Dr. John Ioannidis testifying about COVID fatality rates and Dr. Pierre Kory testifying about the use of corticosteroids in hospital treatment.[27] In November and December 2020 hearings on early treatment, doctors like Peter McCullough, George Fareed, and Pierre Kory testified about their successful multidrug protocols using safe, generic drugs like hydroxychloroquine and ivermectin.[28] In an egregious display of COVID Cartel censorship, Dr. Kory's powerful opening statement was taken down after receiving more than eight million views on YouTube.

My first public event after Republicans lost the majority was in Milwaukee, in June 2021, where five "vaccine"-injured individuals told their stories.[29] In November 2021, I held another event on "vaccine" injuries in Washington, DC, that included medical experts and the "vaccine"-injured.[30] On January 24, 2022, I hosted a five-hour-long public event in DC titled COVID-19: A Second Opinion.[31] That event was organized around Dr. McCullough's four pillars of pandemic response: 1) limiting the spread, 2) early treatment, 3) hospital treatment, and 4) vaccination.[32] It has been viewed online over seven million times, demonstrating the public's desire for more and better information.

Finally, on December 7, 2022, I assembled many of the same experts from the Second Opinion event to talk about COVID "vaccines"—what they are, how they work, and how they could cause injury.[33] For each of my last three public events, I invited the head or representatives of federal health agencies and "vaccine" manufacturers. Not only did they not attend, most of them did not even show the courtesy of declining the invitation. Although there have been repeated offers to openly discuss "vaccine" efficacy and safety—most famously the $2.6 million offered by Joe Rogan and others to "vaccine" advocate Peter Hotez—representatives of the COVID Cartel have simply refused to engage in public debate.[34]

Federal health agencies have also refused to be transparent. To date, I have written over sixty oversight letters asking for information the American people have a right to know. I think it's accurate to say *the agencies have stonewalled me and the American public.* I also continue to be amazed and disheartened that so few in Congress—and throughout the medical establishment—show any interest in conducting oversight of our response to COVID and, in particular, asking questions about COVID "vaccine" development, emergency use authorizations and approvals, and the reality of COVID "vaccine" injuries.

As disappointed as I am with my congressional colleagues' lack of curiosity regarding our failed response to COVID, I am far more grateful to those health-care workers, journalists, attorneys, and others who have had the open minds and courage to challenge the COVID Cartel and its narrative. Many of those brave individuals have contributed to this book, and many more continue to work tirelessly behind the scenes to uncover and expose the truth.

This task will not be easy. The COVID Cartel will never admit they were wrong, simply because the body count from their corrupt actions is too high. And considering who the members of the COVID Cartel are, they will use all the awesome power at their disposal to frustrate every effort to expose them and prove them wrong.

But once someone's eyes have been opened to the truth, it is almost impossible to close them. As more and more people become aware of what has happened, and is still happening, I have to believe truth has the power to overcome lies. This book will help open people's hearts and minds, and I am sincerely grateful to the authors and contributors.

INTRODUCTION

AN URGENT CALL

The COVID-19 pandemic triggered an unprecedented public health response, culminating in the introduction of experimental injections using lab-modified messenger mRNA (modRNA), manufactured by Fosun-Pfizer-BioNTech and Moderna. The "Operation Warp Speed" deployment of the modRNA shots in less than a year—based on prototype technology funded over the previous decade by the US Department of Defense—was hailed as a "scientific miracle."

The experimental "vaccines"—which do not stop infection or transmission of the virus and therefore *fail to qualify as real vaccines*—offered vulnerable individuals a few months' protection against severe COVID-19 illness. But they are deeply flawed, flatly contradicting claims they are "safe and effective." In addition to failing to stop infection and transmission, they carry *real risks*, which must be weighed carefully against the risks of COVID-19—particularly in the case of healthy young people, for whom the disease poses minimal threat.

Over three years into the mass "vaccination" campaign, data on injuries and deaths caused by the modRNA products are incomplete, reflecting a notable lack of due diligence on the part of public health authorities. However, the information that does exist indicates that for millions of healthy people, forced to get the shots under the false pretext of "stopping the pandemic," they are not merely useless but also damaging—in some cases, deadly.

In 2021–2022 the United States, Europe, Canada, Australia, Japan, and South Korea *all saw excess mortality not associated with COVID-19*, while preterm births, stillbirths, and maternal mortality increased in 2021, followed by an *unprecedented plunge in birth rates* in 2022. As of this writing, no plausible alternative explanation has been offered besides the experimental product rollout. Researchers have demonstrated multiple mechanisms of harm from the "vaccines," centering on the encoded spike protein, highly toxic in its own right, but also point to the well-established inflammatory properties of the lipid nanoparticle (LNP) delivery system. Yet the modRNA shots are still being marketed as "safe and effective."

With no long-term safety data and no way to predict lasting impacts on fertility or child development, we are likely entering a painful period of discovery, in which we only gradually learn the full effects of these experimental therapies. But we already have more than enough evidence of harm to make the correct course crystal clear: *the modRNA products must be withdrawn immediately*. Continuing to pretend the "vaccines" are safe and effective, when compelling evidence says they are not, is fatal folly. Adding them to the childhood vaccination schedule, and forcing shots on healthy young people as a requirement to work or attend college, is monstrous.

We must follow the example of peer countries, by halting the modRNA mass injection program before even more damage is done. The modRNA experimental shots must be removed from the childhood vaccination schedule immediately. Causal mechanisms of "vaccine" damage must be transparently investigated, and compensation paid to "vaccine"-injured people or their surviving family members. Development of modRNA therapies for other human uses, and even veterinary applications, must be paused. We make this call in the name of objective science and humanity.

IMPORTANT TERMINOLOGY

In the medical world, names and terms convey vital information about the nature of a product that helps patients and medical professionals weigh its risks and benefits, facilitating informed consent. Two terms used by this book's coauthors deserve particular attention when considering the experimental COVID-19 shots:

- As noted above, "modRNA" stands for "nucleoside modified messenger RNA"—used throughout FDA documents concerning the Pfizer and Moderna products. The authors use the term to emphasize that the laboratory-modified modRNA used in the "vaccines" differs from naturally occurring mRNA (messenger RNA) in multiple ways that could affect the safety and efficacy of these products (for example, the substitution of artificial pseudouridine for uridine has been shown to suppress innate immune function).[35]

- "Pro-vaccine." Unlike conventional vaccines, modRNA products do not contain the target antigens. Rather, they contain the *genetic instructions* that a patient's body reads to produce the target spike protein antigen. This resembles pro-drugs—molecules that lack the desired pharmacologic action until the body converts them to an active form (here, "pro" indicates a precursor, requiring further action by our bodies to become effective).[36] Some authors use "pro-vaccine"[37] to signify this important distinction, which has regulatory consequences.

However, contributors to this book refer to the modRNA shots with a variety of terms, all reflecting their unanimous rejection of the official claim the experimental modRNA injections are "vaccines"—*a deception so bold, public health authorities tried to change the definition of the word* vaccine *to conceal their falsehoods* (chapter 1).

BOOK OUTLINE

This book documents a range of harms inflicted by the modRNA "vaccines"—which, as noted, fail to meet the basic definition of a real vaccine for reasons set forth in chapter 1 (please see below for full titles and details). Chapters 2 through 5 deal with key regulatory lapses by the Food and Drug Administration (FDA) and Centers for Disease Control and Prevention (CDC), before, during, and after issuance of emergency use authorizations (EUAs) for the experimental injections; this second edition includes a new chapter 3 by DailyClout founder Naomi Wolf, recounting the pioneering crowd-sourced effort to analyze Pfizer documents released under FOIA and previewing some of their shocking findings, presented in full in *The Pfizer Papers: Pfizer's Crimes Against Humanity* (Skyhorse, Fall 2024).[38] Chapter 6 presents an overview of the record-breaking numbers of "vaccine" injuries and deaths with the COVID-19 shots that have been recorded by the Vaccine Adverse Event Reporting System (VAERS). Chapters 7 through 13 take a closer look at some of the most common kinds of "vaccine" injuries—covering immunological, cardiological, neurological, carcinogenic (cancer-causing), reproductive, and pediatric harms. Finally, chapter 14 documents massive increases in non-COVID mortality and disability from 2021 to 2023, concluding with a proposal for health insurers and others stakeholders to carry out mass screening as a first step toward treatment and compensation for the "vaccine"-injured or their surviving family members.

Below is a quick summary of each chapter (please see "About the Authors" at the end of the book for biographical information about the coauthors).

Chapter 1: The COVID-19 modRNA Shots Are Not Real Vaccines

Dr. Byram Bridle highlights crucial distinctions between real vaccines and the experimental COVID-19 shots, which fail to qualify as true vaccines on multiple counts. The most important is their failure to stop infection or transmission—the central purpose of real vaccines and the rationale presented by public health authorities to justify mass "vaccination."

Chapter 2: A Government Prototype Rushed to Market without Adequate Testing

Dr. Harvey Risch examines the "vaccine" testing and manufacturing agreements signed by Pfizer and Moderna with the Pentagon in the spring of 2020, showing how their unusual terms appear to have freed the "vaccine"-makers from responsibility to conduct clinical trials with official oversight. The chapter then reviews some of FDA's previous regulatory lapses, and their disastrous impact on public health.

Chapter 3: Introduction to *The Pfizer Papers: Pfizer's Crimes Against Humanity*

Dr. Naomi Wolf, founder and CEO of DailyClout, gives a preview of the shocking findings from their groundbreaking, crowd-sourced analysis of COVID "vaccine" dangers, based on internal documents which the FDA tried to keep secret for 75 years, but was later forced to divulge under a court order. These damning data, drawn from Pfizer's own clinical trial and post-marketing safety tracking, are presented in full in the forthcoming DailyClout book, *The Pfizer Papers: Pfizer's Crimes Against Humanity* (Skyhorse, Fall 2024).[39]

Chapter 4: The Spike Protein Is Harmful by Itself

Dr. Martin Wucher focuses on one of FDA's most serious lapses: neglecting to study the spike protein encoded by the modRNA shots. Originally part of the outer coat of the COVID-19 virus, where it functions as a "key" to "unlock" (infect) cells, spike proteins are also produced in large amounts by the modRNA products, triggering a short-lived immune response in the form of antibodies. However, FDA *failed to consider the possibility the spike protein might be harmful by itself.* Dr. Wucher explores the growing body of evidence that the spike protein is highly pathogenic, causing harms on its own, independent of the rest of the COVID-19 virus—requiring immediate withdrawal of the shots.

Chapter 5: Debunking CDC's Bad Science

FDA's failure to ensure adequate testing was compounded by the Centers for Disease Control and Prevention (CDC), whose public health policies appear intended to obscure, rather than clarify, the key issues of "vaccine" efficacy and safety. Following a comprehensive accounting of the agency's scientific and regulatory failures from 2020 to 2023, Dr. Steven Hatfill shows that CDC and its Big Tech partners used advanced data-mining technology from the Census Bureau to monitor and censor the daily communications of Americans who were trying to share dissenting views about COVID-19—abrogating their right to free speech in *a constitutional betrayal of the people it was meant to serve.*

Chapter 6: Safety Signals from the Vaccine Adverse Event Reporting System (VAERS)

FDA, Department of Health and Human Services (HHS), and CDC created and implemented VAERS in 1990 to receive reports of adverse events associated with, and potentially caused by, biological products such as vaccines. Dr. Jessica Rose uses VAERS data to demonstrate that—despite the admitted limitations of the system—the sheer numbers, range, and rates of occurrence of adverse events associated with the COVID-19 injectable products—including deaths—are *wholly unprecedented,* demanding the immediate withdrawal of the COVID-19 injectable products.

Chapter 7: Immunological Harms of the modRNA "Vaccines"

Returning to the issue of "vaccine" damage to immune function, Dr. Bridle presents public health data clearly pointing to immune harms, including an apparent *increase in likelihood of infection among the "vaccinated."* Dr. Bridle reviews some likely mechanisms of immune harm from the modRNA products, before presenting yet more evidence that public health authorities have been actively suppressing negative information about this critical issue.

Chapter 8: Cardiac and Cardiovascular Damage from the modRNA "Vaccines"

Dr. Peter McCullough takes a closer look at the true incidence and severity of two of the most serious complications of the modRNA "vaccines": myocarditis (inflammation of the heart muscle) and blood clots. After presenting evidence that public health authorities are underestimating their true prevalence, Dr. McCullough outlines short-, mid-, and long-term health consequences, including sudden death from heart failure—*especially among young men*.

Chapter 9: Neurological Injuries from the modRNA "Vaccines"

After explaining how his own initial enthusiasm for COVID-19 "vaccination" led to treating neurological injuries from the modRNA "vaccines," Dr. Matt Bain reviews over a dozen categories of common neurological injury likely resulting from modRNA "vaccination": acute transverse myelitis, acute disseminated encephalomyelitis, stroke, small-fiber neuropathy, Guillain-Barré syndrome, Bell's palsy, and myasthenia gravis, among others. Dr. Bain concludes with an overview of some promising treatments for "vaccine" injuries.

Chapter 10: Cancer Risks of the modRNA "Vaccines"

Dr. Jane Orient emphasizes that any discussion of potential cancer risks must start with the fact that *cancer is both poorly understood and extraordinarily complex* in terms of underlying factors, triggers, and timing. Noting widespread social media reports of sudden, fast-developing cancers after "vaccination," Dr. Orient acknowledges plausible hypotheses about potential causal mechanisms. However, she reiterates that, because of the huge scale of the problem, the very long time frame, and the many unknowns, *the highest priority must be a concerted, well-resourced national post-"vaccination" cancer surveillance effort,* as well as urgent study of the causal mechanisms behind "vaccination"-related cancers.

Chapter 11: COVID-19 "Vaccine" Effects on Women of Reproductive Age and Pregnancy

Dr. James Thorp reviewed ultrasound images from 27,000 pregnant women from 2020 to 2023, putting him in a unique position to directly observe the physiological impact of the modRNA "vaccines" on the health of pregnant women and their fetuses. His chapter reviews the well-documented adverse effects of the COVID-19 experimental gene therapies on women's fertility, fetal viability and pregnancy, live births, and maternal health, and also exposes deliberate deceptions in the campaign to persuade the public that the modRNA shots were safe, effective, and necessary in pregnancy.

Chapter 12: Risks to Children

Dr. Kelly Victory addresses one of the central issues in the COVID-19 "vaccine" debate: the necessity and safety of "vaccination" in children. Taking the foundational ethical principles of medicine as her touchstone—with particular focus on the need for healthcare professionals to be transparent in presenting cost-benefit risk analyses to the parents of young children—Dr. Victory debunks all rationales offered for childhood "vaccination" and highlights *even higher rates of certain adverse events among children.*

Chapter 13: "Vaccine" Mortality Insights from Autopsy Reports

Drs. McCullough and Risch and their collaborators explore possible causal links between the COVID-19 "vaccines" and deaths, using autopsy and postmortem data. Clustering of harms in certain organ systems, close resemblance to post-"vaccination" deaths reported through pharmaco-vigilance systems, and consistency with likely mechanisms of harm described elsewhere, all strongly suggest that *COVID-19 "vaccines" were the main or contributing cause of death in most cases.* Circulating spike protein, produced uncontrollably throughout the body by the experimental shots, is likely the main mechanism of harm.

Chapter 14: "All Hands on Deck"—The Catastrophe of US Longevity and What We Can Do about It

Veteran insurance executive and entrepreneur Josh Stirling analyzes official data to reveal shocking, unexplained increases in death and disability among working-age Americans, from 2021 onward. From 2021 to 2023, Stirling notes around 600,000 excess deaths *not due to COVID-19*, as well as over two million newly disabled Americans, concentrated in demographic groups typically at low risk of disability. Pointing to a systemic cause, Stirling proposes large-scale screening with cheap, easily performed blood tests, to identify members of the population who have been exposed to known pathogenic agents.

A NOTE TO READERS

The dangers of the modRNA shots present an emerging area of knowledge beyond the scope of a single volume. We are only beginning to understand some of the ways the experimental modRNA products inflict harms on our bodies, uncovering fresh questions that will take decades of research to answer. Therefore, this book cannot present a definitive, exhaustive treatment of this critical subject. Among other limitations, this book neglects many kinds of common injury already linked to the modRNA "vaccines" by compelling evidence, or deals with them only briefly—including skin rashes, loss or impairment of vision, and tinnitus or ringing in the ears. Injuries not discussed here *may still be valid complaints deserving follow-up and, if appropriate, compensation for the "vaccine"-injured.* We strongly recommend reviewing the evidence of "vaccine" injuries drawn from Pfizer's own post-market safety monitoring, analyzed in the January 2023 DailyClout book *Pfizer Documents Analysis Reports*, and a follow-up volume, *The Pfizer Papers: Pfizer's Crimes against Humanity*, due out in Fall 2024.[40] As noted, some topline details of their explosive findings are presented in broad overview by DailyClout founder and CEO Naomi Wolf, PhD, in chapter 3.

This book does not address the potential for "shedding," or spreading of modRNA or the resulting spike protein between people through ordinary social contact. However, "vaccine" modRNA has been found in maternal breast milk up to forty-five hours after injection, raising the possibility of transmission to nursing infants. There is also evidence of shedding via exocrine secretions, suggesting modRNA can spread through saliva, sweat, and sexual contact.[41] We also do not address new research showing potentially dangerous DNA contaminants in modRNA shots.[42] We encourage readers to continue to monitor scientific research, as further evidence of modRNA "vaccine" harms is likely to come to light in the years and decades to come.

This book plainly contradicts official claims that the modRNA shots are "safe and effective." *Explicitly, this means we believe support for the modRNA "vaccines" is based on low-quality research or mischaracterization of findings presented without key context.* While this book will deal with *some* of the most important errors and misrepresentations, the sheer volume of flawed research makes it impossible to refute *every* piece of bad science cited by "vaccine" backers. Here we refer the reader to comments made by Dr. Marcia Angell, a highly respected physician, author,[43] and longtime editor of the *New England Journal of Medicine (NEJM)* in 2009:

> It is simply no longer possible to believe much of the clinical research that is published, or to rely on the judgment of trusted physicians or authoritative medical guidelines. I take no pleasure in the conclusion, which I reached slowly and reluctantly over my two decades as an editor of *The New England Journal of Medicine*.... No one knows the total amount provided by drug companies to physicians, but I estimate from the annual reports of the top 9 U.S.-based drug companies that it comes to tens of billions of dollars a year in North America alone. By such means, the pharmaceutical industry has gained enormous control over how doctors evaluate and use its own products. Its extensive ties to physicians, particularly senior faculty at prestigious medical schools, affect the results of research, the way medicine is practiced, and even the definition of what constitutes a disease.[44]

Instead of attempting to debunk all the errors and deceptions falsely presented as "the science," we urge the reader to demand an official response to the evidence of harms presented here, all drawn from peer-reviewed research published in reputable scientific journals. Failure to do so on the part of public health authorities *can only be interpreted as a concession that the harms are real.*

Purported "experts" will accuse the authors of this book of spreading "misinformation," despite the massive primary scientific data supporting our claims. All too often, claims of misinformation have simply been window dressing for censorship and suppression of free speech. It is a crucial tenet of scientific discourse that anyone deemed to be disseminating misinformation should be engaged publicly in professional debate, to definitively demonstrate their scientific errors. Would-be accusers are also admonished that "not turning up to the discussion at all seems to result in the worst effect."[45]

Before this book is labeled "misinformation," the authors demand a public debate.

Drs. McCullough, Risch, and Thorp are affiliated with, and receive salary support and/or hold equity positions, in The Wellness Company, Boca Raton, Florida. Josh Stirling is the founder and president of the nonprofit Insurance Collaboration to Save Lives. Dr. Bridle is a cofounder and the chief operating officer of ImmunoCeutica. *Neither these companies, nor any other corporate interest, had any role in funding, analysis, or publication of this book.*

The authors vouch for their chapters alone, although they may refer to other chapters for corroboration or additional detail. They hold a range of opinions about many COVID-19–related subjects, expressed here or elsewhere, none of which should be interpreted as the view of the group. Some authors believe there are promising treatments for "vaccine" injuries, but *we wish to emphasize that no healthy person should receive an modRNA injection in the mistaken belief "vaccine" injuries are not an issue of concern, or that they are easily treated.*

The authors are unanimous that the COVID-19 infection itself could always be effectively treated with safe, widely available generic drugs with abundant scientific support.[46] However, *even when effective early treatment was denied,* the risk posed by COVID-19 to healthy young people remained vanishingly small due to the strength of their natural immune response—making a universal "vaccination" campaign unnecessary and inappropriate.

Due to the urgency of this subject, this book attempts to reach as wide an audience as possible, including medical professionals. Some authors have included technical discussions of medical issues in hopes of aiding other clinicians. *However, no content in this book is intended as medical advice to the reader.* Nothing printed here can serve as a substitute for diagnosis, treatment, or advice from a licensed medical professional. Any treatment you undertake should be discussed with a licensed medical professional. Never disregard or delay seeking medical advice because of anything you read in this book. If you are having a medical emergency, call 911 or go to the nearest emergency room immediately. No physician-patient relationship is created through this book, and none of the authors make any representations, express or implied, with respect to this book's content or its use.

This second edition (September 2024) includes a new chapter 3 by Naomi Wolf, PhD, as well as a number of minor corrections and clarifications throughout the text and endnotes.

CHAPTER 1

THE COVID-19 MODRNA SHOTS ARE NOT REAL VACCINES

By Byram W. Bridle, PhD

Any criticisms of the COVID-19 modRNA "vaccines" are immediately labeled "misinformation" and critics dismissed as "anti-vaxxers," but the authors of this book firmly reject these insulting and defamatory labels. As doctors and scientists, parents and friends, we have received standard vaccines, presented our children for vaccination, and encouraged patients and loved ones to receive appropriate vaccines and boosters as recommended.

However, it is crucial to distinguish between *real vaccines* and the experimental modRNA products, which fail to meet the basic definition of what a vaccine should be—in purpose or function. Before detailing the risks of the modRNA products, it's important to address the questions: What makes a good vaccine? And how do the modRNA products, as marketed, *already fall short of these long-accepted standards?*

The following pages will show that the modRNA shots *fail to qualify as true vaccines* because they:

1. Do not confer immunity to COVID-19;
2. Generate the wrong type of immune response, targeting the wrong part of the body, raising autoimmune risks;
3. Do not stop transmission of COVID-19;
4. Contain known toxic chemical components that make repeated doses highly unsafe;
5. Expose recipients to many of the harms of COVID-19 itself, via the toxic spike protein;

6. Are driving the emergence of variants that evade the "vaccines," and
7. Appear to be making "vaccinated" individuals *more likely to contract COVID-19*.

WHAT DOES A REAL VACCINE DO?

According to all historic scientific and regulatory precedents, a proposed vaccine must satisfy certain conditions and possess key attributes, without which it cannot qualify as a true vaccine. As detailed later in this chapter, US public health authorities tried to change the technical definition of a vaccine in 2021, by removing any references to "immunity," but this sort of dishonest gambit makes no difference.[47] The criteria of a real vaccine are based on guidelines, institutional wisdom, and best practices accumulated over decades of collective scientific effort. They are not "up for debate" or revision, though federal bureaucrats may flatter themselves otherwise. From a scientific, medical, and ethical viewpoint, any deviation from these standards is immediately disqualifying. This is not a matter of choice or convenience. It is central to ensuring vaccine safety and efficacy.

Above all, a real vaccine is one that confers immunity in someone with a mature, healthy immune system. This means the person can clear an infection by the causative agent of a disease, prior to the onset of signs and symptoms of illness. It also means that the pathogen cannot replicate inside a person sufficiently to transmit a threshold dose that will make someone else sick.

Historically, the goal of vaccination has been to try to achieve one of two types of immunity. The first is *sterilizing immunity*, whereby a person's cells never even get infected with a virus. Theoretically, this can be achieved by activating components of the immune system, including antibodies—special molecules created by our immune system to stick to viruses, or other disease-causing microbes like bacteria, disabling them—to intercept the virus before it can ever even enter a cell. But sterilizing immunity is very difficult to achieve. A second, more reasonable goal is *near-sterilizing immunity*. In this case, some individual virus particles (virions) can evade the first line of defenses that neutralize a virus while it is outside a cell. So, some cells *do* get infected. However, other weapons of the immune system, such as T cells, can kill the infected cells before they can produce enough new viruses that can replicate out of control, causing and spreading disease.

The definition thus far is based solely on the *efficacy* of a vaccine (its ability to induce immunity). The second, and equally important, criterion is *safety*. A vaccine should never impose risks that are equal to, or exceed, the risks of natural infection. In fact, vaccine-induced side effects *should be much rarer and more tolerable* than harms from infection, simply because vaccines are administered to many healthy people who might not even get infected. It makes no sense to expose someone to potentially serious harms from vaccination to "protect" them against a disease that poses no real threat to them.

A real vaccine can clearly be a useful tool for promoting public health. Specifically, it can "trick" the body into thinking it is infected with a virus, without experiencing the full extent of the disease. It is important to note that some side effects of real vaccines are normal and unavoidable, just as with natural infection. Soreness, temporary fevers, and general malaise (feeling unwell) are common by-products of a robust immune response, whether induced by natural infection or by vaccination. Again, however, a real vaccine *will never expose a person to the direct damage caused by the pathogen itself.* As such, real vaccines can be great tools for helping a population achieve what is known as "herd immunity." To understand this concept, we first need to know what "immunity" means.

IMMUNITY AND HERD IMMUNITY

According to the CDC, "immunity" is defined as "protection from an infectious disease. If you are immune to a disease, you can be exposed to it without becoming infected."[48] But a point of clarification is required: *complete* protection from infection, basically corresponding to "sterilizing immunity," is almost impossible to achieve. So, we must modify this definition to indicate that a state of immunity protects against "productive infection"—one that allows a virus to replicate out of control, causing and spreading disease. Preventing a *productive* infection, as opposed to completely blocking infection, is a much more reasonable goal for vaccine development, because it still stops infection and transmission—a goal corresponding to "near-sterilizing immunity."

The concept of "herd immunity" means a virus will stop spreading once *most* people develop immune responses that simultaneously protect against disease and transmission of the pathogen causing disease.[49] This does not require *every* person to become immune, just a majority, and near-sterilizing immunity is sufficient. There are two ways for people to gain near-sterilizing immunity to a viral infection like SARS-CoV-2—allowing herd immunity: (1) natural immunity, resulting from becoming infected with the virus and recovering through our own immune response,[50] and (2) vaccination with a vaccine that has undergone properly conducted preclinical studies and the full suite of clinical trials, with excellent short-to-long-term safety profiles.

NATURALLY ACQUIRED IMMUNITY IS THE GOLD STANDARD FOR REAL VACCINES

Traditional vaccine technologies include using whole, inactivated viruses that can no longer replicate in cells; attenuated viruses, weakened so they can no longer cause disease; or pieces of a virus (subunits) mixed with an "adjuvant"—a material that helps boost the immune response. Whatever the means, however, *a real vaccine always simulates the gold standard of natural infection*, triggering an appropriate, enduring immune response without causing disease. According to this long-accepted standard, if the person is subsequently exposed to the virus, their immune system should successfully recognize the threat for years to come, due to "immunological memory." This vaccine-primed immune response will be faster and more robust, and the virus more likely cleared before symptomatic disease, than among unvaccinated individuals.

Above all, the numerous shortcomings of the modRNA shots—compared to a real vaccine (*Fig. 1*)—reflect their failure to mimic or recapitulate natural immunity in any meaningful way. Contrary to official statements downplaying "natural immunity" acquired from the body's organic immune response, research conducted early in the mass "vaccination" program showed that unvaccinated individuals who are infected, and recover through their own natural immune response, display both superior protection against repeated infection, and lower rates of transmission to others, than "vaccinated" individuals.[51]

The experimental modRNA jabs fell short in every way.

ELEMENTS OF NATURAL IMMUNITY

A real vaccine typically works in *several different ways*, mirroring natural immunity. An effective immune response against viral infection is usually dominated by T cells, which can detect and kill virus-infected cells in the body. This prevents infected cells from serving as virus production factories and protects uninfected cells. Viruses also trigger relatively low-magnitude antibody responses. Antibodies are most effective against pathogens that live outside cells, like bacteria. But our immune system makes some antibodies against viruses, because viruses spend a short period of their life cycle outside cells, in transit from an infected cell to a new cell, giving the immune system a chance to disable them with antibodies.

Although natural antibodies against viruses are produced in relatively small numbers, there are certain specific subtypes that are ideal for neutralizing a virus. These antibodies are custom-made to "grab" the virus and prevent it from infecting a cell, clearing the virus from the body without harm, using only a relatively small number of targeted antibodies. This is important because producing too many antibodies can trigger harmful autoimmune reactions.

In short, a real antiviral vaccine will recapitulate natural immunity by generating lots of T cells that can recognize when the target virus is inside infected cells, as well as targeted antibodies that can prevent the virus from entering other cells in the first place. To effectively recapitulate natural immunity, these T cells and antibodies should be concentrated where the virus enters the body—in the case of SARS-CoV-2, the respiratory tract. In stark contrast, the modRNA "vaccines" produce antibodies in the blood, far from the natural site of infection.

Figure 1

Real Vaccine vs. modRNA "Vaccines": What Are the Key Differences?

Real Vaccine	modRNA Products
Enables both antibody and T cell responses at the site of infection (for COVID-19, respiratory tissues) including memory cells for long-term immunity	Emphasize antibody responses in the blood (not the site of infection) keyed to a single component of COVID-19 variants that are now extinct
Targets several different parts of the virus, for wide, durable immune response to future strains	Target one part of the virus, the spike protein, which mutates rapidly, making jabs obsolete
Enables immune cells to produce small numbers of highly targeted, effective antibodies	Tell cells to produce large numbers of antibodies targeting a single antigen, with autoimmune risks
Never exposes recipient to ill effects of the pathogen targeted by the vaccine, or comparable harms	Distribute toxic spike proteins uncontrollably throughout the body, inflicting range of harms
Confers lasting immunity, making repeated boosters unnecessary (lessening exposure to vaccine harms)	Have negative efficacy by 6 months, requiring boosters (exposing recipients to vaccine harms)
Prevents productive infection and therefore also transmission, helping achieve herd immunity	Don't prevent infection or transmission, enabling evolution of variants that evade the vaccines

A real vaccine will also trigger a strong *innate immune* response. An *innate* response is one that uses immunological weapons that can be brought into the fight against a virus much faster than it takes to generate T cell and antibody responses, including white blood cells such as macrophages and natural killer cells. In this case, an innate immune response precedes T cell and antibody responses. An innate immune response of sufficient magnitude and quality can stop a viral infection without the need for T cells and antibodies.

As noted, natural antibody responses against viruses are usually of low magnitude, only employing *certain subtypes of antibodies*. Although most antibodies are specific to a particular virus, some can cross-react with (recognize) components of a person's own body, risking an autoimmune reaction, where the immune system attacks the person's own body. This is why the immune system typically only generates the type and quantity of antibodies that it needs, so that too many antibodies don't spill over into unwanted autoimmune damage. The immune system also uses qualitatively ideal virus-specific antibodies that are custom-made to disable a particular virus—neutralizing in nature. Inducing the wrong types of antibodies, like those used against bacteria that live outside cells, can make matters worse through a mechanism known as antibody-dependent enhancement of disease. For example, the wrong types of antibodies can promote viral entry into a cell instead of neutralizing it, making infection more likely.

This is one of several ways in which natural immunity resulting from COVID-19 infection—producing a relatively small number of various antibodies, targeting many different parts of the virus—is stronger and more enduring than the modRNA injections, which *focus on just one highly mutable component*: the spike protein, from a strain of the virus that has already vanished, replaced by variants with different spike proteins.

To cite yet another example, the modRNA shots were administered into the shoulder muscle, tricking the body into thinking there is a systemic infection, with an immune response emphasizing antibodies in the blood. However, SARS-CoV-2 infects the respiratory system via abundant mucosal surfaces. The best way to induce an immune response at a mucosal surface is to vaccinate by a mucosal route, such as intranasally or by inhalation. Antibodies in the blood can never prevent infection or transmission of a virus that targets the nasal passages and lungs. One can only assume that tests administering the "vaccines" directly to the respiratory system failed either due to a lack of efficacy, safety issues, or both.

THE MODRNA "VACCINES" DO NOT STOP INFECTION OR TRANSMISSION

Above all, the most important thing a real vaccine must do is prevent productive infection—the ability to pass the infection to others—thereby stopping the spread of an infectious disease. *But the modRNA "vaccines" have no impact on infection or transmission*, negating the only argument for forcing healthy young people, or anyone else at low risk of severe disease, to get "vaccinated." In fact, as new viral variants emerge, there is evidence the "vaccines" are making people *more likely to get infected*, via several well-known immune processes (chapter 7).

It must be emphasized: claims that mass "vaccination" would lower transmission of COVID-19 enough to "end the pandemic" were *never* supported.[52] In October 2022, Pfizer's president of international markets, Janine Small, told the European Parliament's Special Committee on the COVID Pandemic that the company never studied whether its "vaccine" prevented transmission before seeking emergency use authorization (EUA) in December 2020.[53]

Pfizer's clinical phase III study, carried out in the second half of 2020, only examined rates of symptomatic infection in "vaccinated" individuals, not their ability to pass the virus to others, and did not measure asymptomatic infections (occurring without symptoms) in "vaccinated" subjects.[54] The Pfizer study, as well as a CDC study conducted from December 2020 to March 2021, showed absolute reductions of only 0.84-0.88 percent (less than 1 percent) in symptomatic infection but again did not address asymptomatic infection or transmission.[55]

Reduction in symptomatic infection *may* have caused a short-lived reduction in transmission of the original COVID-19 strain, but this was never measured. As new variants emerged, the ability of the "vaccines" to stop symptomatic infection dwindled rapidly, along with their more ambiguous impact on transmission—developments predicted by scientists but widely ignored.[56]

By the time the results of the CDC study were publicized in late March 2021, the "wild type" (original) COVID-19 strain had already been mostly replaced in the US by the new alpha variant (first identified in the United Kingdom[57]). The Pfizer modRNA "vaccine" showed a roughly 50 percent reduction in transmission of alpha twelve weeks after "vaccination," compared to unvaccinated individuals—barely meeting the traditional standard for vaccine efficacy.[58] In the face of the delta variant, which became dominant in the United States in the second half of June 2021, the Pfizer "vaccine" produced no real difference in transmission at twelve weeks.[59]

Thus, by the time the Pfizer "vaccine" was made widely available to American adults in May 2021, its ability to stop transmission was quickly headed to zero at three months postvaccination, as reflected in outbreaks among groups of mostly "vaccinated" individuals throughout the summer of 2021.[60] In August 2021, CDC director Rochelle Walensky finally admitted the modRNA "vaccines" did not prevent transmission, even as institutions including colleges and universities moved to mandate vaccination on the assumption that they did.[61]

It is hardly surprising modRNA injections have had no lasting impact on COVID-19 transmission.[62] In fact, as new variants continue to emerge, modRNA "vaccination" appears to be *making infection more likely*: a 2022 Cleveland Clinic study of COVID-19 infection in 52,000 individuals—broken down by "vaccination" status—found the more shots individuals got, the more likely they were to become diagnosed with COVID-19.[63] The immune science behind this trend will be discussed in greater depth in chapter 7, but clearly "vaccines" that produce *higher rates of infection* cannot possibly "end a pandemic."

CDC TRIED TO REDEFINE "VACCINE"

Prior to 2014, CDC defined a vaccine as: "Injection of a killed or weakened infectious organism in order to prevent the disease."[64] In 2015, in response to new vaccine technologies such as "subunit" vaccines, CDC updated the definition to: "A product that stimulates a person's immune system to produce immunity to a specific disease, protecting the person from that disease."[65] Combined with CDC's definition of immunity, this meant that something could only be called a vaccine if it protected people from acquiring and spreading a disease. This is also the classical definition used in immunology textbooks. *Most importantly, it is the definition most people assume when they hear the term "vaccine," with implications for informed consent.*

Indeed, the *original* goal for the modRNA shots—produced at "warp speed"—was to *prevent* COVID-19 disease: the initial report on Pfizer-BioNTech's clinical trial stated, "The first primary end point was the efficacy of BNT162b2 against confirmed Covid-19."[66] This was reiterated in the initial contract made between Pfizer and the United States' Department of Defense, where the stated goal was to manufacture a "mRNA-based coronavirus vaccine aimed at preventing COVID-19 infection."[67]

When failure to prevent infection and transmission could no longer be denied, CDC simply "moved the goalposts," redefining a "vaccine" on its website as: "A preparation that is used to stimulate the body's immune response against diseases."[68] Importantly, this change removed the term "immunity" from the definition. In a letter dated August 23, 2021—responding to a citizen petition demanding proof of efficacy against transmission—FDA appeared to invoke the new definition, noting, "a vaccine can meet the EUA standard without any evidence that the vaccine prevents infection or transmission. To that end, there is no requirement that the clinical trials supporting a vaccine's licensure or authorization be designed to determine whether the vaccine prevents infection of a pathogen or transmission of that pathogen to others."[69]

CDC's new definition—omitting immunity—allows novel products that fail to prevent infection and transmission to be recategorized as "vaccines." Remarkably, according to the new definition, things like yogurt and sauerkraut could be considered "vaccines" by virtue of their ability to stimulate beneficial immune responses.[70] As such, the wording change attempts to fundamentally alter the functional definition of a vaccine. But the real, long-established meaning cannot be changed by simple bureaucratic fiat. *The COVID-19 jabs fail to meet the traditional and textbook definitions of vaccines, which is what most people have in mind when giving consent.*

THE MODRNA SHOTS ARE "LEAKY VACCINES"

A "leaky vaccine," such as the modRNA injections, doesn't produce true immunity in the recipient. Someone who receives a "leaky vaccine" is not protected against productive infection, meaning the individual can also pass their infection to others. When this occurs in "vaccinated" individuals, they are known as "breakthrough infections."

Breakthrough COVID-19 infections among the "vaccinated" have been much more common than repeat infections in people with natural acquired immunity, rendering nonsensical any mandated shots for people who already had COVID-19.[71] However, the problem with "leaky vaccines" goes well beyond this. Indeed, they can even promote the emergence of variants of the viruses that they were originally designed to protect against.[72]

Biologists have long known that application of nonlethal selective pressure to a biological entity that is capable of mutating will lead to emergence of variants that can escape the selective pressure: examples include the emergence of chemotherapy-resistant cancers, in cell biology, and the rise of antibiotic-resistant bacteria through the inconsistent application or misuse of the drugs.

The same principle applies to vaccines and viruses. If a "vaccine" fails to confer sterilizing or near-sterilizing immunity on an individual who then gets sick, that person may become a reservoir that selects for a variant that can escape the nonlethal immune response trained by the vaccine.[73] A clear sign of this happening is variants with changes concentrated in the antigen targeted by the vaccine. In the case of the COVID-19 jabs, the immune responses they induced manifestly failed to confer true immunity against SARS-CoV-2, a virus very prone to mutation. The result was a dramatic increase in the emergence of variants of SARS-CoV-2 that coincided with the public rollout of the COVID-19 injections. *Notably, most of the mutations accumulated in the spike protein, the precise structure targeted by the modRNA and adenovector shots.*

BOOSTERS SHOULD HAVE BEEN RULED OUT BY KNOWN TOXICITY OF LNPS

The decision to misrepresent the modRNA injections as real vaccines was likely a ploy, at least in part, to sidestep a key issue: the firmly established toxicity of the lipid nanoparticle (LNP) delivery system. Peer-reviewed scientific publications have highlighted serious safety issues related to the administration of lipid nanoparticles used to deliver modRNAs. These issues include toxicity in the lungs, the liver, systemic toxicity, and even destruction of the very cells the immune system needs to function.[74]

Ironically, this toxicity is exactly why Moderna and Pfizer strategically focused on LNPs as vaccine technologies. Assuming they would be producing a real vaccine, both companies also assumed only one dose would be required in a person's lifetime and baselessly extended this model to the modRNA "vaccines." This was of critical importance *because it was already well-known that repeated administration of LNPs is toxic.*[75] Thus, any mass vaccination strategy that even potentially contemplated boosters should have been immediately disavowed.

This was openly discussed in the news media prior to the declared COVID-19 pandemic, only to be forgotten when it mattered most. One 2016 article about Moderna stated:

> In nature, mRNA molecules function like recipe books, directing cellular machinery to make specific proteins. Moderna believes it can play that system to its advantage by using synthetic mRNA to compel cells to produce whichever proteins it chooses. In effect, the mRNA would turn cells into tiny drug factories. It's highly risky. Big pharma companies had tried similar work and abandoned it because it's exceedingly hard to get RNA into cells without triggering nasty side effects.[76]

The article continued:

> Delivery—actually getting RNA into cells—has long bedeviled the whole field. On their own, RNA molecules have a hard time reaching their targets. They work better if they're wrapped up in a delivery mechanism, such as nanoparticles made of lipids. But those nanoparticles can lead to dangerous side effects, especially if a patient has to take repeated doses over months or years. Novartis abandoned the related realm of RNA interference over concerns about toxicity, as did Merck and Roche.

The reason LNPs were rejected as a delivery mechanism for chemotherapy was the need for multiple doses, judged too risky due to LNPs' toxicity. Yet *billions of people have now been given multiple doses of lipid nanoparticle-encased modRNA shots.*

CONCLUSION

If the modRNA injections simply didn't work, we might ask, what was the harm in trying? In fact, the harms were substantial, including keying recipients' immune response to an extinct virus and speeding the emergence of variants. Along with the many other risks addressed in this book, these facts leave responsible public health authorities no alternative but to withdraw these inadequately tested experimental therapies from the market entirely.

Looking ahead, if public confidence in vaccines is to be restored, we must have a new infusion of rigor and objectivity in vaccine studies, including long-term active safety monitoring with proper control groups studied in parallel for the duration of any experiment. Some approved vaccines may need to be reviewed, and possibly withdrawn. All studies should be conducted by researchers without conflicts of interest and monitored by agencies committed to the public good—*not handmaidens of Big Pharma*.

Until that time, we need a global moratorium on modRNA "vaccines," whose development has clearly outpaced the "speed of science." Uncontrolled biodistribution and LNP toxicity present massive obstacles—to cite just two issues with no clear means of resolution. The sad reality is that the incessant "safe and effective" mantra was a falsehood, and a seemingly deliberate one at that. Trust, lost in the blink of an eye, requires a long demonstration of consistent integrity to restore.

CHAPTER 2

A GOVERNMENT PROTOTYPE RUSHED TO MARKET WITHOUT ADEQUATE TESTING

By Harvey Risch, MD, PhD

As reflected in Pfizer's failure to measure transmission, the COVID-19 modRNA products don't just differ from ordinary vaccines in the way they work but also in the absence of normal testing. This chapter will show that—contrary to official claims of rigorous review—*the modRNA "vaccines" were rushed into service after inadequate clinical trials, conducted without formal oversight, and despite clear signs of lack of safety.*

The modRNA injections' exemption from standard testing reflects the fact that they are not a normal medical product, but rather a long-term project of the US government and its corporate partners, pursued with a determination that seems to have overwhelmed all other considerations, including safety.

Civilian interest in mRNA vaccines dates back several decades, with growing involvement by the US military from 2011 onward. Following foundational research in the 1970s and 1980s, the first attempts—in the 1990s and early 2000s—to create murine (mouse) mRNA vaccines for cancer and influenza failed due to rapid decay of mRNA molecules and harmful inflammatory reactions in the animal subjects. But in 2005 researchers discovered that substituting certain man-made nucleic acids enabled lab-modified mRNA (modRNA) to evade destruction by the immune system, allowing it to penetrate cells to initiate protein synthesis.[77] This technical breakthrough attracted the attention of investors, who funded biotech start-ups like BioNTech (2008) and Moderna (2010) to bring modRNA products to market.[78]

In 2011 the Pentagon office in charge of future technology, the Defense Advanced Research Projects Administration (DARPA), began funding research into "gene-encoded vaccines" using DNA or modRNA through its Autonomous Diagnostics to Enable Prevention and Therapeutics (ADEPT) program—in part to defend against possible use of viruses as bioweapons. With participants including Moderna, ADEPT was followed in 2016 by DARPA's Pandemic Prevention Platform (P3), which aimed "to develop an integrated end-to-end platform that uses nucleic acid sequences to halt the spread of viral infections in sixty days or less." Pfizer also received funding from DARPA to research modRNA vaccines.[79] From 2016 onward, additional funding for modRNA vaccine research came from the Biomedical Advanced Research and Development Authority (BARDA) and the National Institutes of Health (NIH).[80] In 2019, shortly before COVID-19 emerged, NIH entered into a research and profit-sharing agreement with Moderna to codevelop coronavirus vaccines.[81]

DOD-PFIZER OTA

Because the modRNA "vaccines" developed under Operation Warp Speed involved technology created by DARPA, BARDA, and NIH—with NIH eventually acknowledged as part owner of the Moderna "vaccine"—they were legally designated as government prototypes for "medical countermeasures" (MCMs).[82] Intriguingly, both the Pfizer and Moderna contracts with the Department of Defense for "vaccine" manufacturing include a number of items redacted on the grounds that their public disclosure "would impair the application of state-of-the-art technology within a U.S. weapon system."[83]

Since the modRNA shots were *military prototypes rather than traditional vaccines*, the Department of Defense commissioned the Pfizer "vaccine" through an open-ended other transaction agreement, issued under the department's other transaction authority (OTA). An OTA is not a contract but rather a "contractual instrument" for emergency procurement from "non-traditional" military contractors, suspending most rules for federal procurement.[84]

The terms of the OTA with Pfizer effectively made the company responsible for policing itself and freed it from usual standards and regulations, including government oversight of clinical trials.[85] Pfizer agreed to "meet the necessary FDA requirements for conducting ongoing and planned clinical trials," but it appears this was just a promise, with no provision for enforcement.

Pfizer confirmed this legal loophole in its argument against whistleblower Brook Jackson's lawsuit, which alleged that the company's clinical trials didn't follow usual standards for testing new medical treatments. In an April 2022 court filing, Pfizer's attorneys noted that the statement of work (SOW) in Pfizer's OTA with the Department of Defense didn't require compliance with normal clinical testing guidelines:

> Because of pandemic-related exigencies, the agreement was not a standard federal procurement contract, but rather a "prototype" agreement.... Such agreements are executed under DoD's Other Transaction Authority ("OTA") and, as a statutory matter, are not subject to the Federal Acquisition Regulation ("FAR"), which is the primary regulation otherwise used by Government agencies in their acquisition of supplies and services with appropriated funds.... The SOW describes a "large scale vaccine manufacturing demonstration" that imposes no requirements relating to Good Clinical Practices ("GCP") or related FDA regulations.... It states explicitly that Pfizer's "clinical trials" are "out-of-scope," "not related" to the agreement, and that the relevant studies were undertaken at Pfizer's expense "without the use of Government funding...." Again, Relator's allegation that the SOW somehow tied payment to Pfizer's compliance with every particular of the clinical protocol or related FDA regulations...is mistaken and refuted by the SOW itself.[86]

Pfizer's lawyers noted that "neither the 'Pfizer-DoD contract' referenced in the complaint, nor the invoices submitted under that agreement, make any mention of the FDA clinical trial regulations...." In a separate filing supporting Pfizer in October 2022, Department of Justice lawyers also emphasized that the OTA didn't require Pfizer to meet normal clinical trial standards:

> The complaint does not identify any provision in the SOW for the Project Agreement between Pfizer and the Army that

conditioned Government payment for the vaccine on Pfizer's compliance with the clinical trial protocol or regulations. The SOW, which is attached to the complaint, further specifies that the Army did not regulate the conduct of the clinical trial.[87]

BARDA/DOD-MODERNA CONTRACTS

Meanwhile, BARDA and the Department of Defense commissioned the Moderna vaccine under two separate Federal Acquisition Regulation (FAR) contracts: the first for "vaccine" and the second for "vaccine manufacturing," whose provisions also appear to have rendered any requirement for standard clinical testing practically unenforceable. *Like the Pfizer OTA, the seeming lack of oversight in the Moderna contracts presumably reflects the fact that the modRNA "vaccines" are military prototypes for "medical countermeasures."*

Large portions of the contracts remain undisclosed, but enough information is visible to suggest they exempted Moderna from normal clinical testing standards. The portion of the contract with BARDA that covers clinical studies is heavily redacted, but the unredacted section headings cover only a fraction of the clinical categories usually required for vaccine approval. The statement of work specifies just one of multiple, standard investigations required by global guidelines for vaccine development: "Good Laboratory Practice," addressing reproductive toxicity in rats (uncovering fetal rib malformations—detailed in chapter 11).[88] Again like Pfizer's OTA, while the publicly visible portions of the BARDA contract state that Moderna's clinical studies should comply with FDA standards, they don't include any provisions for enforcing these requirements, such as making payment conditional on compliance.[89]

Pfizer and Moderna were further shielded from liability by pandemic emergency rules issued by the federal government. Under the terms of the state of emergency declared in March 2020, the use of any new agent or treatment is deemed not to be a "clinical trial," meaning individuals injected with the modRNA product aren't legally entitled to a guarantee that the "vaccines" work, or to informed consent about side effects.[90] The emergency declaration and emergency use authorizations (EUAs) for the modRNA "vaccines" also shield the "vaccine" makers from any legal liability for "vaccine" side effects including injury and death, *and even prevent victims from suing the "vaccine"-makers for willful wrongdoing, unless the federal government sues them successfully first.*[91]

TOXIC SHOT

PFIZER WHISTLEBLOWER ALLEGATIONS

The OTA may have freed Pfizer from legal responsibility for conducting standard clinical trials, but Brook Jackson's allegations are disturbing all the same.

In fall 2020 Ms. Jackson was employed as a regional director by Ventavia, a Pfizer subcontractor conducting clinical trials, with responsibility for overseeing modRNA "vaccine" trials at several sites in Texas. After witnessing what she described as major deviations from clinical trial standards, on September 25, 2020, she reported the alleged errors to FDA with a phone call and email. Ventavia fired her a few hours later.

According to an investigative report published by the *British Medical Journal* (*BMJ*) in November 2021, Ms. Jackson—who had over fifteen years of experience in clinical research management and had never previously been fired from a job—alleged that Ventavia

> ...falsified data, unblinded patients, employed inadequately trained vaccinators, and was slow to follow up on adverse events reported in Pfizer's pivotal phase III trial. Staff who conducted quality control checks were overwhelmed by the volume of problems they were finding. After repeatedly notifying Ventavia of these problems, the regional director, Brook Jackson, emailed a complaint to the US Food and Drug Administration (FDA). Ventavia fired her later the same day.[92]

Ms. Jackson provided the *BMJ* with internal company documents, photos, audio recordings, and emails, including records of meetings about apparent deviations such as "falsifying data." According to the *BMJ* investigation, an anonymous employee confided, "I don't think it was good clean data. It's a crazy mess," but according to Jackson, employees who reported deviations from protocol were "targeted" by management. One former executive later admitted privately that "everything that you complained about was spot on."

Yet FDA staff never inspected any of the Ventavia sites following Ms. Jackson's complaint. In fact, the agency only inspected 9 of a total of 153 testing sites involved in the broader Pfizer clinical trial, and just 10 of 99 Moderna sites.

Ms. Jackson's allegations are echoed by bizarre errors in other clinical studies for Pfizer, including the trial submitted to FDA to obtain emergency use authorization for the modRNA "vaccine" for children ages twelve to fifteen. In one case a healthy twelve-year-old girl, Maddie de Garay, suffered a severe adverse reaction to the Pfizer "vaccine." According to her mother, she can "barely see, suffers from tinnitus, mobility issues, vomiting, blood in her urine, numbness in her body, and has at least ten to twenty seizures a day."[93]

After her mother reported these injuries to her doctors, they diagnosed de Garay with anxiety and a rubber allergy. In the clinical trial results submitted to FDA, *Pfizer classified de Garay's symptoms as "neuralgia" and "abdominal discomfort."* Media reports about clinical trials from abroad provide examples of similar omissions and misclassifications.[94]

While lack of FDA oversight may have allowed Pfizer to cover up adverse effects from the modRNA "vaccines," one result is harder to explain away: the number of deaths following "vaccination." The total number of deaths from all causes in the "vaccinated" test group was *higher than the unvaccinated control group* over the six-month trial period, with twenty-one deaths among "vaccinated" subjects compared to seventeen deaths among unvaccinated subjects. Pfizer dismissed the test group deaths as unrelated to the "vaccine" but offered scant explanation.[95] As small as these numbers are, the twenty-one and seventeen deaths don't even reflect a 35 percent drop in mortality—far below the traditional 50 percent minimum standard assumed with real vaccines.

FDA responded to these concerns by restating its confidence in the integrity of the Pfizer phase III trial data. But the terms of the OTA, effectively freeing Pfizer from FDA oversight, undermine this confidence. The question becomes all the more urgent in light of FDA's culture of conflicts of interest (COIs), reflected in its *history of disastrous regulatory failures*.

FDA'S RECORD OF NEGLIGENCE

Following public criticism of FDA's slow review of potential treatments for HIV/AIDS in the 1980s, in 1992 Congress passed the Prescription Drug Use Fee Act (PDUFA), which increased the agency's funding by making drugmakers pay for technical review of new drugs. Under this arrangement, the pharmaceutical industry currently contributes nearly half (45 percent) of FDA's annual budget, raising concerns that pharmaceutical companies have too much influence over the agency tasked with overseeing them.[96]

One study found that "drugs approved by the FDA after the passage of PDUFA were more likely to be withdrawn from the market or receive a black box warning than medications approved prior to its enactment (26.7 per 100 drugs vs 21.2 per 100 drugs at up to 16 years of follow-up)."[97] Medical ethicists have argued that industry funding of FDA reviews "systematically slants important policy choices"; for example, by leading to underfunding of post-approval safety monitoring, which tends to run counter to drugmakers' commercial interests.[98]

Critics also warn of ethical conflicts arising from the "revolving door" between FDA and the pharmaceutical industry, in which FDA employees who review successful clinical trials for drugmakers leave the agency for high-paying jobs with those same companies.[99] Former FDA commissioner Scott Gottlieb's move to join Pfizer's board of directors in 2019—prompting Sen. Elizabeth Warren to condemn "revolving door influence-peddling"—was just one high-profile example.[100] In 2016 researchers tracked the employment of former FDA reviewers for hematology and oncology drugs who left the agency between 2001 and 2010, to find 57 percent of them worked or consulted for pharmaceutical companies.[101] The dependence of reviewers on drugmakers for their future livelihoods creates an incentive to "go easy" on those companies.

Ethical concerns extend to "independent" physician reviewers who serve on FDA advisory committees as external experts. Skirting required disclosure of conflicts of interest (COI), independent experts often receive large payments from pharmaceutical companies *after* voting to approve drugs—a clear COI that has sparked a great deal of criticism but no regulatory reform.[102] An investigation of drug approvals from 2013 to 2016 found that 40 out of 107 physician advisors "received more than $10,000 in post hoc earnings or research support from the makers of drugs that the panels voted to approve, or from competing firms," including 26 who received more than $100,000 and 7 who received $1 million or more.[103]

Ethicists warn the vast potential for COI inherent in this system, defined by a patron-client relationship between the pharmaceutical industry and its regulator, raises serious questions about official oversight and review of clinical trials.[104] In October 2020, *Science* magazine reviewed over 1,600 official inspection and enforcement documents from 2009 to 2019 and concluded, "FDA oversight of clinical trials is lax, slow moving, and secretive."[105] FDA often failed to enforce corrective measures in cases where companies had broken the law, including dangerous practices, fraud, and corrupt or simply falsified clinical trial data.

Recent years offer numerous examples of basic failures in FDA's oversight and review of clinical trials. The list of drugs approved after *compromised or negative studies* includes:

- Propulsid, a drug to increase stomach motility, was approved in 1993 despite clinical trial data showing the drug caused heart rate and rhythm disorders in 2.4 percent of 1,993 subjects. In the face of mounting evidence that Propulsid was dangerous, FDA allowed it to remain on the market for several more years, during which it was prescribed "off label" to children. The drug was blamed for 302 deaths before it was finally withdrawn in 1999.[106]

- Vioxx, a painkiller, received FDA approval in 1999, after inadequate clinical trials with incomplete data on cardiac effects. FDA allowed the drug to remain on the market despite "many warning signs" that it increased the risk of myocardial infarction. Merck voluntarily withdrew Vioxx in 2004 amid allegations of up to 30,000 deaths among people with heart conditions.[107]

- Flibanserin (Addyi), a drug to treat low libido in women, was rejected twice by FDA due to safety concerns and low efficacy but finally received approval in 2015 after the drug's new owner persuaded FDA to accept a different metric for efficacy. The drug remains on the market despite low efficacy, helping only 8 percent to 13 percent of subjects, and safety issues including potentially fatal interactions with alcohol and commonly used antibiotic and antifungal medications.[108]

- Eteplirsen, a drug to treat Duchenne muscular dystrophy—an inherited muscle-wasting disease—received FDA approval in 2015 after a clinical trial with just twelve subjects, which showed the drug increased the level of a key protein, dystrophin, by just 0.9 percent of the normal level, using a dubious measurement technique. The approval by FDA higher-ups triggered public criticism by the head reviewer and prompted senior scientists to quit in protest.[109]

- Aduhelm (aducanumab), an Alzheimer's drug, received FDA approval in June 2021, setting off a storm of criticism by experts noting the clinical trial showed no efficacy and potential brain bleeding. Major health-care providers and payers—including Medicare and the US Department of Veterans Affairs—declined to offer Aduhelm infusions, and in December 2022 a congressional report raised "serious concerns about FDA's lapses in protocol."[110]

Even more troubling are FDA's failures during the ongoing epidemic of opioid addiction, which has killed over one million Americans since the turn of the century. It has been fueled, in part, by FDA's hands-off stance toward opioid manufacturers like Purdue Pharma and its permissive approval process for new opioid medications. Many of these fatal decisions were made on the watch of former FDA acting commissioner Janet Woodcock, who—as director of FDA's Center for Drug Evaluation and Research—oversaw the 1995 approval of Purdue's OxyContin, one of the most powerful opioid medications ever created.

On January 27, 2021, a coalition of twenty-eight public health groups and opioid crisis organizations sent a letter to the Biden administration protesting Woodcock's appointment as acting commissioner, noting that "as the Director of the FDA's Center for Drug Evaluation and Research (CDER) for more than 25 years, Dr. Woodcock presided over one of the worst regulatory agency failures in U.S. history."[111]

The opioid catastrophe, resulting from FDA negligence with no means of redress, illustrates a crucial statutory problem: in addition to not prioritizing drug safety, FDA is the *final, ultimate authority* in making food, drug, vaccine, medical device, and other regulatory decisions. FDA regulatory approval decisions are viewed by physicians, pharmacists, and other clinicians as beyond argument—and indeed they are, in the sense that the agency operates without supervision or accountability, besides a passive and uninformed Congress.

FDA's disastrous history of approving ineffective and harmful treatments, while ignoring massive mortality resulting from its own lax oversight, would be more than enough reason to question its authorizations of the COVID-19 modRNA "vaccines," even under conditions of normal regulatory review. Considering the broad statutory exemptions from oversight granted under the terms of the Pfizer OTA and Moderna's BARDA contract and the lower evidentiary requirement for EUA ("reasonable to believe...may be effective"; Project BioShield Act of 2004, Pub. L. No. 108-276, § 4(a), 118 Stat. 855), it is fair to ask whether the "vaccine" makers were held to any standards of accountability whatsoever.

CHAPTER 3

INTRODUCTION TO *THE PFIZER PAPERS:* PFIZER'S CRIMES AGAINST HUMANITY

By Naomi Wolf, PhD

Acknowledgment: We are grateful to the DailyClout for permission to excerpt the following Introduction to The Pfizer Papers: Pfizer's Crimes Against Humanity *(Skyhorse, Fall 2024),*[112] *whose findings are cited by authors throughout this volume. Any use of "book," "volume," or the like in the following text are in reference to* The Pfizer Papers.

You are about to embark as a reader on a journey through an extraordinary story—one whose elements almost defy belief.

The Pfizer Papers is the result of a group of strangers—ordinary people with extraordinary skills, located in different places around the world, with different backgrounds and interests—who all came together, for no money or professional recompense at all; out of the goodness of their hearts, and motivated by love for true medicine and true science—to undertake a rigorous, painfully detailed, and complex research project, which spanned the years 2022 to the present, and which continues to this day.

The material they read through and analyzed involved 450,000 pages of documents, all written in extremely dense, technical language.

This far-flung, relentlessly pursued research project—under the leadership of DailyClout's COO, the remarkably gifted project director Amy Kelly—brought one of the largest and most corrupt institutions in the world, Pfizer, to its knees. This project, pursued by 3,250 strangers who worked virtually and became friends and colleagues, drove a global pharmaceutical behemoth to lose billions of dollars in revenue. It balked the plans of the most powerful politicians on earth. It bypassed the censorship of the most powerful tech companies on earth.

This is the ultimate David and Goliath story.

The story began when lawyer Aaron Siri successfully sued the Food and Drug Administration, to compel them to release "The Pfizer Documents." These are Pfizer's internal documents—as noted above, 450,000 pages in number—that detail the clinical trials Pfizer conducted in relation to its COVID mRNA injection. These trials were undertaken to secure the ultimate prize for a pharmaceutical company, the "EUA," or Emergency Use Authorization from the FDA. The FDA awarded EUA for ages 16+ to Pfizer in December 2020. The "pandemic," of course (a crisis in public health that a book of mine, *The Bodies of Others*, confirmed, involved hyped and manipulated "infections" data and skewed mortality documentation) became the pretext for the "urgency" that led the FDA to bestow EUA on Pfizer's (and Moderna's) novel drug. The EUA is the hall pass, essentially, allowing Pfizer to race right to market with a not-fully-tested product.

The Pfizer Papers also contains documentation of what happened in "post-marketing," meaning in the three months, December 2020 to February 2021, as the vaccine was rolled out upon the public. All leading spokespeople, and bought off media, called the injection "safe and effective," reading from what was a centralized script.

Many people who took this injection, as it was launched in 2020–2021–2022 and to the present, did not realize that normal testing for safety of a new vaccine—testing that typically takes ten to twelve years—had simply been bypassed via the mechanisms of a "state of emergency" and the FDA's "Emergency Use Authorization." They did not understand that the real "testing" was in fact Pfizer and the FDA observing whatever was happening to them and their loved ones, after these citizens rolled up their sleeves and submitted to the shot. As we can never forget, many millions of these people who submitted to the injection were "mandated" to take it, facing the threat of job loss, suspension of their education, or loss of their military positions if they refused; in some US states and overseas countries, people also faced the suspension of their rights to take transportation, cross borders, go to school or college, receive certain medical procedures, or enter buildings such as churches and synagogues, restaurants and gyms—if they refused.

The FDA asked the judge in the Aaron Siri lawsuit to withhold the release of the Pfizer documents for seventy-five years. Why would a government agency wish to conceal certain material until the present generation, those affected by what is in these documents, is dead and gone? There can be no good answer to that question.

Fortunately for history, and fortunately for millions of people whose lives were saved by this decision, the judge refused the FDA's request, and compelled the release of the documents; a tranche of 55,000 pages per month.

When I heard about this, though, I was concerned as a journalist. I knew that no reporter had the bandwidth to go through material of this volume. I also understood that virtually no reporter had the training or skill sets required to understand the multidimensional, technically highly specialized language of the reports. In order to understand the reports, one would need a background in immunology; statistics; biostatistics; pathology; oncology; sports medicine; obstetrics; neurology; cardiology; pharmacology; cellular biology; chemistry; and many other specialties. In addition to doctors and scientists, in order to understand what was really happening in the Pfizer documents, you would also need people deeply knowledgeable about government and pharmaceutical industry regulatory processes; you would need people who understood the FDA approval process; you would need medical fraud specialists; and eventually, in order to understand what crimes were committed in the Papers, you would need lawyers.

I was worried that without people with all of those skill sets reading through the documents, their volume and complexity would lead them to vanish down "the memory hole."

Enter Steve Bannon, the former Naval Officer, former Goldman Sachs investment banker, former advisor to President Trump, and current host of the most popular political podcast in America and one of the most listened-to worldwide, *WarRoom*.

He and I come from opposite ends of the political spectrum. I had been a lifelong Democrat, an advisor to President Bill Clinton's reelection campaign, and to Al Gore's presidential campaign. He, of course, is a staunch Republican-turned-MAGA. I had been deplatformed in June 2021, before the Pfizer documents came out, for the crime of warning that women were reporting menstrual dysregulation upon having received the mRNA injections. As a career-long writer on women's sexual and reproductive health issues, I knew that this was a serious danger signal and that this side effect would affect fertility. (Any eighth grader should be able to foresee that as well.) Upon my having posted this warning, I was banned from Twitter, Facebook, YouTube, and other platforms. I was attacked globally, all at once, as an "anti-vaxxer" and "conspiracy theorist"; and my life as a well-known, bestselling feminist author, within the legacy media, ended. No one in that world would talk to me anymore, publish my work, or return my calls. I was un-personed.

(It turned out, upon two successful lawsuits in 2023 by Missouri and Louisiana attorneys general, that it was actually the White House, the CDC, and senior leaders of other government agencies, including the Department of Homeland Security, that unlawfully pressured Twitter and Facebook to remove that cautionary tweet of mine, to shut me down, and to "BOLO" or Be On the Lookout for similar posts. This suppression is now the subject of a pending Supreme Court decision on whether or not it violated the First Amendment.)

In this dark time in my life, to my surprise, I received a text from Steve Bannon's producer, who invited me onto *WarRoom*. I brought forward my concerns about women's reproductive health in the wake of mRNA injection, and to my surprise he was respectful, thoughtful about the implications, and took the issue very seriously. I returned again and again, to bring that and other concerns that were emerging in relation to the mRNA injections to his audience. I was relieved to have a platform on which I could share these urgent warnings. At the same time, I was sad that the Left, which was supposed to champion feminism, seemed not to care at all about serious risks to women and unborn babies. I recognized the irony that a person whom I had been taught to believe was the Devil Incarnate, actually cared more about women and babies than did all of my right-on former colleagues, including the feminist health establishment, who had always spoken so loudly about women's wellbeing and women's rights.

Given my appearances on *WarRoom* leading up to 2022, it was natural that the subject of the Pfizer documents came up on that show when the documents were released. I shared my concern that they would be lost to history due to their volume and technical language. Bannon said something like, "Well, you will crowdsource a project to read through them."

I was taken aback, as I had zero skills related to, or knowledge about how possibly to do such a thing. I answered something like, "Of course."

So, my news and opinion platform DailyClout was deluged with offers from around the world, from *WarRoom* listeners with the skill sets needed, to decipher the Pfizer documents. I was terrified. It was chaos. I had excellent people on my team. But none of us knew how to manage or even organize the deluge of emails; we did not know how to evaluate the thousands of CVs; and even once we had "onboarded" these thousands of people, in different time zones, to "the project," our inboxes became even more terrifying, as it was literally impossible to organize 3,250 experts into an organization chart that could systematically work through these documents. Emails were getting tangled or went unanswered. People asked questions we could not answer. We had no idea what structure could allow such a huge number of disparate experts to work through the vast trove of material.

A few weeks in, as I was in despair, Bannon had me on again. He asked about the progress of the project, and I replied, more upbeat than I felt, that many people had joined us, and they were starting to read. "Of course, you will begin delivering reports," he prompted. "Of course," I answered, horrified at being in so far over my head.

I have never had a corporate job, so it had not even occurred to me that a series of reports was the format that the analyses of the documents should take.

Then something happened that I can only describe as providential. We put out a call to the volunteers for a project manager, and Amy Kelly reached out. Ms. Kelly is a Six Sigma-certified project manager, with extensive experience in telecommunications and tech project management. She is also a simply inexplicably effective leader. The day that she put her hand to the chaos in the inboxes, the waters were stilled. Peace and productivity prevailed. Ms. Kelly somehow effortlessly organized the volunteers into six working groups, with a supra-committee at the head of each, and the proper work began.

I can only explain the scope and smoothness and effectiveness of the work that followed, as occurring in a state of grace.

In the two years since Ms. Kelly and the volunteers have been working together, they have gone through 2,369 documents and data files totaling hundreds of thousands of pages and have issued almost one hundred reports. I taught the volunteers to write these in a language that everyone could understand—which I thought was very important to maximize their impact. And Amy Kelly meticulously revised almost all, and edited all, of them.

The first forty-six reports appeared in a self-published format that we put out. It was very important to us that they appear in a published form that was physical, and not just digital, as we wanted something that people could hand to their doctors, their loved ones, their congressional representatives.

These forty-six reports broke huge stories. We learned that Pfizer knew within three months after rollout in December 2020, that the vaccines did not work to stop COVID. Pfizer's language was "vaccine failure" and "failure of efficacy." One of the most common "adverse events" in the Pfizer documents is "COVID."

Pfizer knew that the vaccine materials—lipid nanoparticles, an industrial fat, coated in polyethylene glycol, a petroleum byproduct; mRNA; and spike protein—did not remain in the deltoid muscle, as claimed by all spokespeople. Rather, it dispersed throughout the body in forty-eight hours "like a shotgun blast," as one of the authors, Dr. Robert Chandler, put it; it crossed every membrane in the human body—including the blood-brain barrier—and accumulated in the liver, adrenals, spleen, brain, and, if one is a woman, in the ovaries. Dr. Chandler saw no mechanism whereby those materials leave the body, so every injection appears to pack more such materials into organs.

Pfizer hired 2,400 fulltime staffers to help process "the large increase of adverse event reports" being submitted to the company's Worldwide Safety database.

Pfizer knew by April 2021 that the injections damaged the hearts of young people.

Pfizer knew by February 28, 2021—just ninety days after the public rollout of their COVID vaccine—that its injection was linked to a myriad of adverse events. Far from being "chills," "fever," "fatigue," as the CDC and other authorities claimed were the most worrying side effects, the actual side effects were catastrophically serious.

These side effects included: death (which Pfizer does list as a "serious adverse event"). Indeed, over 1,233 deaths in first three months of the drug being publicly available.

Severe COVID-19; liver injury; neurological adverse events; facial paralysis; kidney injury; autoimmune diseases; chilblains (a localized form of vasculitis that affects the fingers and toes); multiple organ dysfunction syndrome (when more than one organ system is failing at once); the activation of dormant herpes zoster infections; skin and mucus membrane lesions; respiratory issues; damaged lung structure; respiratory failure; acute respiratory distress syndrome (a lung injury in which fluid leaks from the blood vessels into the lung tissue, causing stiffness which makes it harder to breathe and causes a reduction of oxygen and carbon dioxide exchange); and SARS (or SARS-CoV-1, which had not been seen in the world since 2004, but appears in the Pfizer documents as a side effect of the injections).

Thousands of people with arthritis-type joint pain, one of the most common side effect, were recorded. Other thousands with muscle pain, the second most common. Then, industrial-scale blood diseases: blood clots, lung clots, leg clots; thrombotic thrombocytopenia, a clotting disease of the blood vessels; vasculitis (the destruction of blood vessels via inflammation); astronomical rates of neurological disorders—dementias, tremors, Parkinson's, Alzheimer's, epilepsies. Horrific skin conditions. A florid plethora of cardiac issues; myocarditis, pericarditis, tachycardia, arrhythmia, and so on. Half of the serious adverse events related to the liver, including death, took place within seventy-two hours of the shot. Half of the strokes took place within forty-eight hours of injection.

But what really emerged from the first forty-six reports, was the fact that though COVID is ostensibly a respiratory disease, the papers did not focus on lungs or mucus membranes, but rather they center, creepily and consistently, on disrupting human reproduction.

By the time Pfizer's vaccine rolled out to the public, the pharmaceutical giant knew that they would be killing babies and significantly harming women and men's reproduction. The material in the documents makes it clear that damaging human's ability to reproduce and causing spontaneous abortions of babies is "not a bug, it is a feature."

Pfizer told vaccinated men to use two reliable forms of contraception or else to abstain from sex with childbearing-age women. In its protocol, the company defined "exposure" to the vaccine as including skin-to-skin contact, inhalation, and sexual contact. Pfizer mated vaccinated female rats and "untreated" male rats, and then examined those males, females, and their offspring for vaccine-related "toxicity." Based on just forty-four rats (and no humans), Pfizer declared no negative outcomes for ". . . mating performance, fertility, or any ovarian or uterine parameters . . . nor on embryo-fetal or postnatal survival, growth, or development," the implication being that its COVID vaccine was safe in pregnancy and did not harm babies. Pfizer knew that lipid nanoparticles have been known for years, to degrade sexual systems, and Amy Kelly in fact found nanoparticles, of which lipid nanoparticles are a subtype, pass through the blood-testis barrier and damage males' Sertoli cells, Leydig cells, and germ cells. Those are the factories of masculinity, affecting the hormones that turn boys at adolescence into men, with deep voices, broad shoulders, and the ability to father children. So, we have no idea if baby boys born to vaccinated moms, will turn into adults who are recognizably male and fertile. Pfizer enumerated the menstrual damages it knew it was causing to thousands of women, and the damage ranges from women bleeding every day, to having two periods a month, to no periods at all; to women hemorrhaging and passing tissue; to menopausal and post-menopausal women beginning to bleed again. Pfizer's scientists calmly observed and noted it all but did not tell women.

Babies suffered and died. In one section of the documents, over 80 percent of the pregnancies followed resulted in miscarriage or spontaneous abortion. In another section of the documents, two newborn babies died, and Pfizer described the cause of death as "maternal exposure" to the vaccine.

Pfizer knew that vaccine materials entered vaccinated moms' breast milk and poisoned babies. Four women's breast milk turned "blue-green." Pfizer produced a chart of sick babies, made ill from breastfeeding from vaccinated moms, with symptoms ranging from fever to edema (swollen flesh) to hives to vomiting. One poor baby had convulsions and was taken to the ER, where it died of multi-organ system failure.

In *The Pfizer Papers*, you'll find many more bombshell revelations, all published in the teeth of fierce censorship, as the most powerful forces in the world—including the White House, the staffers of the United States president himself; Dr. Rochelle Walensky of the CDC; the head of the FDA, Dr. Robert M Califf; Dr. Anthony Fauci; Twitter and Facebook; legacy media, including the *New York Times*, the BBC, the *Guardian* and NPR; OfCom, the British media regulatory agency; professional organizations such as the American College of Obstetricians and Gynecology, and the European Medicines Agency, the European equivalent of the FDA, and the Therapeutics Goods Administration, Australia's equivalent of the FDA—all sought to suppress the information that Amy Kelly, the research volunteers, and I brought to the world starting in 2022, and that you are about to absorb in the following pages.

Nonetheless, in spite of the most powerful censorship and retribution campaign launched in human history—made more powerful than past such campaigns by the amplifying effects of social media and AI—these volunteers' findings were not suppressed at last, and survived on alternative media, and on our site DailyClout.io; to be shared from mouth to mouth, saving millions of lives.

Fast forward to more recent events. What has the role of this information been in stopping this greatest crime ever committed against humanity?

The worst has happened. Disabilities are up by a million a month in the United States, according to former BlackRock hedge fund manager Edward Dowd. Excess deaths are way up in the US and Western Europe. Birth rates have plummeted, according to the mathematician Igor Chudov (and WarRoom/DailyClout Volunteer Researcher Dr. Robert Chandler) by 13–20 percent since 2021, based on government databases. Athletes are dropping dead. Turbo-cancers are on the rise. Conventional doctors may be "baffled" by all of this, but sadly, we, thanks to Amy Kelly and the volunteers, understand exactly what is happening.

Our relentless effort to get this information to the world, in an unimpeachable form, has finally paid off with results. The uptake for boosters is now 4 percent. Very few people "boosted" their children. Most colleges in the United States withdrew their vaccine "mandates." Pfizer's net revenue dropped in Q1 of 2024 to pre-2016 levels. OfCom, which had targeted Mark Steyn for "platforming" on his show my description of the reproductive and other harms in the Pfizer documents, is being sued by Steyn. The BBC had to report that vaccine injuries are real, as did the *New York Times*. AstraZeneca, a somewhat differently configured COVID vaccine in Europe, was withdrawn from the market in May 2024, following lawsuits involving thrombotic thrombocytopenia (a side effect about which our research volunteer Dr. Carol Taccetta had informed the FDA by letter in 2022), and the European Medicines Agency notably withdrew its EUA for AstraZeneca. Three days after we published our report showing that the FDA and CDC had received the eight-page "Pregnancy and Lactation Cumulative Review" confirming that Dr. Walensky knew about the lethality of the vaccine when she held her press conference telling pregnant women to get the injection, Dr. Walensky resigned.

TOXIC SHOT

It is difficult indeed to face this material in the roles that Amy Kelly and I play. No doubt for the volunteers, unearthing this criminal evidence is painful indeed. It may be hard to read some of what follows. As I have said elsewhere, seeing this material is like being among the Allied soldiers who first opened the gates of Auschwitz.

But the truth must be told.

Among other important reasons to tell these truths, people were injured and killed with a novel technology not deployed before in medicine; and these pages hold important clues as to the mechanisms of these injuries, and thus, they provide many signposts for physicians and scientists in the future, for treating the many injuries that these new mRNA technologies, injected into people's bodies, have brought about.

We must share the truth, as the truth saves and sustains; and eventually, the truth will heal.

CHAPTER 4

THE SPIKE PROTEIN IS HARMFUL BY ITSELF

By Martin Wucher, DDS

INTRODUCTION

Most cells and microbes, such as bacteria and viruses, have specific surface molecules that allow them to interact with their environment. In the case of COVID-19, the spike protein radiating from the virion (individual virus) functions like a key, unlocking a door on the surface of animal cells so the virus can insert its genetic material, hijack the cellular machinery, and compel the host cell to make more viruses.

The spike protein therefore functions as an "antigen": a foreign substance that triggers an immune response. Once immune cells identify the spike protein as part of a foreign pathogen, our bodies create "antibodies": complex molecules specifically designed to bind to the spike protein and disable the virus.

The modRNA "vaccines" are intended to accelerate our immune response to COVID-19 by using modRNA to deliver coded genetic instructions that force our cells to synthesize the spike protein. The spike protein, in turn, triggers the production of antibodies, training our immune system to recognize this part of the COVID-19 virus *before* we are infected. Unfortunately, this plan has a fatal flaw: as we will see, the "S1" tip of the spike protein is extremely toxic on its own, rendering the "vaccines" highly unsafe.

It is important to note that current research shows that not only the S1 protein but also the lab-modified modRNA and lipid nanoparticle technology used in the "vaccines" are also highly inflammatory (chapters 1, 5). Neither the S1 surface protein (the genetic component) nor the lipid vehicle has ever been used in human vaccinations before, and all should have been thoroughly researched and tested before mass application.[113]

SPIKE PROTEIN PERSISTENCE AND BIODISTRIBUTION

Among FDA's many lapses during the COVID-19 pandemic, perhaps the most devastating was failing to ensure that the spike protein—produced by the modRNA shots entering human cells—was safe before introducing it into billions of human beings around the world. This failure was compounded by FDA's inattention to the issue of biodistribution, meaning where the "vaccine" modRNA and spike protein go in the body. FDA has continued to neglect these issues, which were raised in an open letter delivered on June 1, 2021, signed by dozens of leading health experts, demanding the agency conduct and release the results of pharmacokinetic, biodistribution, and tissue-specific toxicity studies.[114]

Contrary to claims that the modRNA and encoded spike protein remain localized at the "vaccination" site in the upper arm, Pfizer's own biodistribution studies in animals—released after FOIA requests—have shown that "vaccine" components and modRNA travel throughout the body, accumulating in tissues *where they may remain for weeks or months*.[115]

Research published in November 2021 confirmed the spike protein produced by the "vaccines" persisted in human subjects for at least four months.[116] A study from July 2022 found modRNA from the "vaccines" circulating in the human body fifteen days after "vaccination," later extended to twenty-eight days in research published in January 2023.[117] The long persistence of both modRNA and the spike protein could play an important role in adverse events occurring months after "vaccination." Among other dangers, the modRNA's survival over twenty times longer than first claimed raises the possibility of uncontrolled production of spike protein.

FDA and the "vaccine" makers have yet to address a growing body of scientific evidence, including their own research, showing that the modRNA "vaccines" do not remain localized in the muscle where they are administered.

- Study 18530, conducted by Pfizer and released after a FOIA request, examined distribution of lipid nanoparticles (LNP) in rats following intramuscular injection. Within forty-eight hours, the LNPs accumulated in tissues and organ systems including liver, spleen, adrenal glands, bone marrow, lymph nodes, ovaries, and, to a smaller extent, testes.[118]

- Pfizer study 07302048, investigating biodistribution in mice, summarized by the European Medicines Authority (EMA), found distribution of a modRNA protein proxy to the lymph nodes and liver, lasting at least nine days after injection.[119] A separate EMA evaluation of the Moderna vaccine preclinical studies revealed that modRNA crossed the blood-brain barrier to penetrate neural tissues in rats.[120]

- Multiple Pfizer animal biodistribution studies released by Japanese health regulators showed that modRNA from vaccination left the injection site, entered the bloodstream, and accumulated in organs and tissues including the spleen, liver, adrenal glands, bone marrow, and ovaries.[121]

- Small amounts of modRNA have been found in breast milk of lactating mothers up to forty-five hours after "vaccination," raising the possibility of modRNA transmission to nursing infants.[122]

In view of the abundant evidence presented in the following sections of this chapter that the spike protein is harmful by itself, independent of the rest of the virus, this suggests that the modRNA "vaccines" are introducing a pathogenic (disease-causing) antigen into recipients in an uncontrolled and unpredictable fashion, causing injuries and mortality via a range of mechanisms. This constitutes a global medical emergency, requiring immediate withdrawal of the modRNA "vaccines."

WHAT IS THE SPIKE PROTEIN?

The wide distribution of "vaccine" modRNA and spike proteins throughout tissues and organs, and their persistence in human tissues for weeks and months respectively, is extremely concerning in light of accumulating evidence that the spike protein itself is a pathogen (causing disease). Before addressing specific mechanisms of harm, it is appropriate to conduct a quick overview of the spike protein, including its original purpose, function, and structure in the COVID-19 virus.

Each spike protein is a "trimer" composed of three "monomers," or bonded arms, which in turn consist of two subunits: the S1 glycoproteins at the end of the spike and the S2 stalks that connect the S1 tip to the rest of the virus.

COVID-19 Virion and Spike Protein

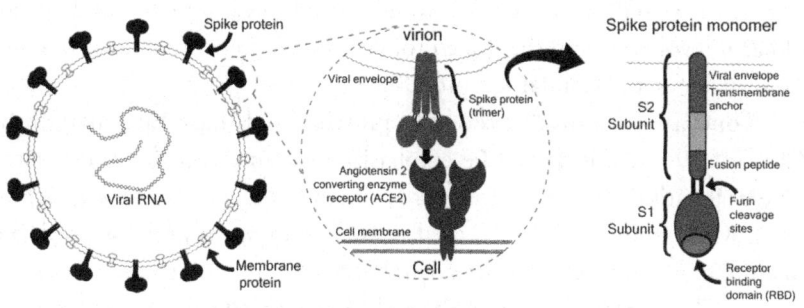

The S1 glycoprotein first gains access to the cell by bonding with an important protein in the target cell's membrane: angiotensin-converting enzyme 2 (ACE2), which plays a key role in a host of basic biological processes in human beings, helping our bodies carry out critical tasks. As its name indicates, ACE2 interacts with angiotensin 2, a vasoconstrictor (chemical that causes blood vessels to contract), to regulate the functioning of the heart and lungs.[123] ACE2 also helps regulate metabolism by controlling the functioning of mitochondria—the "powerhouses" of animal cells.

In coronaviruses, the S1 glycoprotein tip is connected to the S2 stalk by a "furin cleavage site" at the end of the S2 stalk. When the S1 glycoprotein tip bonds to ACE2 on the cell membrane, it triggers a change in the spike protein, opening the S2 cleaving site and splitting the S1 tip from the S2 stalk. The S2 stalk then interacts with an enzyme on the cell surface—transmembrane protease serine 2—leading to another cleaving of the entire S2 unit. Part of the S2 unit becomes a "fusion peptide," which allows the rest of the virus to fuse with the cell membrane and insert its genetic material for viral replication.

The COVID-19 virus is more infectious than other coronaviruses due to the presence of an extra furin cleavage site previously never seen in this class of coronaviruses.[124] The second cleavage site makes it easier for the spike protein to bind to the cell surface and insert its RNA for viral replication. (Some scientists have argued that the extra furin cleavage site could never have arisen in the virus through natural evolutionary processes, suggesting an artificial origin for COVID-19.)

THE SPIKE PROTEIN AS A PATHOGEN

Whatever the origins of the novel furin cleavage site, the spike protein's affinity for ACE2 likely explains much of the harm it causes to such a wide range of human cells—*but spike-ACE2 interactions are only part of the puzzle.* As we will see in the following research review, many mechanisms of harm revolve around the spike protein's interaction with a range of common enzymes and cellular receptors.

Contrary to claims that the spike protein is only harmful as part of the COVID-19 virus, it should be emphasized that most of the studies cited here deal with the effects of the spike protein *in isolation from the rest of the virus.* Most studies cited here used recombinant spike proteins produced in animal cell cultures, or "pseudoviral vectors" containing cloned versions of the spike protein—meaning the spike protein's effects occurred *without the rest of the COVID-19 virus.* Again, this is especially concerning when the encoding modRNA can persist for weeks, inducing cells to produce unknown amounts of spike protein. Regarding one of the most important modRNA "vaccine" harms, clinical research published in January 2023 showed that post-modRNA-"vaccination" myocarditis is strongly linked to the level of "free" spike protein in blood plasma (not attached to a virus or neutralized by an antibody)—confirming yet again that *the spike protein is dangerous by itself.*[125]

More research is needed, but there is already enough data on hand from laboratory and pathology studies to understand some ways the spike protein harms animal tissues. This list of studies showing multiple, overlapping mechanisms of harm is not intended to be exhaustive.

1. *Spike protein interactions with ACE2.* The spike protein's "stickiness" with ACE2 downregulates and suppresses production of the enzyme, leading to disruption of ACE2-regulated systems and harm in a wide range of cells.[126] The following studies, many dealing with overlapping systems and disease processes, demonstrate that the spike protein can inflict harms through multiple mechanisms involving ACE2.

    o A study by Salk Institute scientists published in March 2021 showed the spike protein damages endothelial tissue by lowering levels of ACE2, leading to fragmentation of mitochondria in endothelial cells and causing inflammation. Researchers noted that the process contributes to cardiovascular damage, specifically injuries to the lungs.[127]

- A study published in September 2020 showed that the spike protein binds to blood platelets via ACE2, leading to formation of blood clots.[128]

- A study published in May 2022 demonstrated that the spike protein's interaction with ACE2 disrupts the functioning of the "renin-angiotensin-aldosterone system" (RAS), a multiorgan system involving the kidneys that regulates blood volume, blood pressure, and electrolytes. The study found that by binding ACE2, the spike protein induces "a hyperinflammatory state in several organs, leading to lung injury, hematological alterations, and immunological dysregulation."[129]

- The spike protein suppresses immune responses by binding with ACE2 on important immune cells—the CD8+ cytotoxic T lymphocytes. This stops the T lymphocytes from forming a temporary junction with infected cells, called an "immunological synapse," preventing the T cells from identifying foreign antigens on an infected cell to trigger an immune response.[130]

- The spike protein initiates chemical signaling within cells that destabilizes and degrades ACE2 mRNA, causing ACE2 levels to fall and leading to the death of pulmonary (lung) artery endothelial cells in the lab.[131]

2. *Interactions with CD147.* The spike protein reacts with CD147, a glycoprotein found in the membranes of human white blood cells, platelets, and endothelial cells, which helps control cell proliferation and apoptosis (cell death), as well as inflammatory and immune functions.

- A study published in December 2021 demonstrated the spike protein disrupts human cardiac pericytes, which help protect heart cells, through an extracellular chemical signal triggered by the spike's interaction with CD147, resulting in inflammation of heart tissue and death of cardiac pericytes.[132]

○ Italian research published in February 2022 showed the spike protein interacted with CD147 to activate blood platelets, providing another mechanism for inflammation and blood clotting.[133]

3. *Interactions with toll-like receptors.* The spike protein interacts with toll-like receptors (TLRs), special pattern-recognizing proteins found in the membrane or within animal cells. A total of thirteen different toll-like receptors (TLRs 1–13) play an important role regulating countless physiological processes, but TLR4 and TLR2 seem especially reactive with the spike protein. Again, this review is simply intended to give some idea of the range of harms associated with the spike.

○ A Japanese study published in February 2021 showed the spike protein interacts with TLR4 on human and mouse macrophages, to activate the macrophages and "strongly provoke" increased cytokine production, leading to an inflammatory response.[134]

○ Research first publicized in July 2022 confirmed the spike protein interacted with TLR4 in cardiac muscle cells (myocytes), triggering inflammation leading to heart damage. The lead author explained, "Besides directly damaging the heart muscle cells, the spike protein itself is very inflammatory and may cause systemic inflammation that indirectly causes heart problems."[135]

○ In a December 2021 study, University of Texas researchers showed that the spike protein interacts with TLR2 to trigger an inflammatory response, signaling macrophages in humans and mice to increase production of inflammatory cytokines and chemokines. The authors noted an inflammatory response to the spike protein damaging lung epithelial cells.[136]

○ A study published in July 2022 found the spike protein interacted with TLR2 to promote blood clotting and

- inflammation by encouraging the formation of "neutrophil extracellular traps," tangles of fiber created by white blood cells to catch foreign pathogens, also leading to blood clots.[137]
  - An Italian study published in January 2023 demonstrated the spike protein's interaction with TLR4 on blood platelets resulted in thrombosis (blood clots).[138]
  - In February 2023, Brazilian researchers showed the spike protein's interaction with TLR4 resulted in neuroinflammation and cognitive dysfunction in mice, suggesting this may be one of the mechanisms behind the "brain fog" and memory losses associated with COVID-19 infection and "vaccination."[139]

4. *Other mechanisms of harm.* The spike protein also appears to cause harms independently of the processes involving ACE2, CD147, and TLRs outlined above. Once again, the list of mechanisms below should not be considered exhaustive.
   - A study published in December 2021 showed the spike protein binds and disables heparan sulfate, which normally regulates heparin, an important clotting factor, raising the risk of blood clots.[140]
   - A study from August 2021 demonstrated the spike protein interacts with fibrinogen, a protein that plays a key role in coagulation, to form blood clots that are especially resistant to anti-clotting factors. The authors note a potential connection to the formation of microclots, which have been found following both COVID infection and "vaccination."[141]
   - Research published in December 2022 showed the spike protein causes hemagglutination, or clumping of red blood cells, via electrostatic attraction between glycans (long carbohydrate molecules) on the tip of the spike and complementary glycoconjugates (carbohydrates bonded to lipids or proteins) on red blood cells.[142]

- Spike protein activated platelets via the C42b receptor, causing the platelets to interact with inflammatory monocytes that produced cytokines, possibly contributing to "cytokine storm"—the runaway immune reaction responsible for much COVID-19 mortality.[143]
- The spike protein causes "barrier dysfunction" in the lungs, leading to "vascular leakage" of fluids into the lungs, by stimulating endothelial and epithelial cells in the lungs to release chemical messengers called glycosaminoglycans, integrins, and TGF-β, according to multiple studies.[144]
- The spike protein has been shown to both cross the blood-brain barrier and disrupt its activity, and has been found in encephalitic lesions post-"vaccination," pointing to the likelihood of neurological harms.[145] Research showed the spike protein caused the death of neuronal cells in the brains of mice via an inflammatory reaction.[146]

The spike protein encoded in the modRNA "vaccines" clearly presents formidable pathogenic potential, but once again it should be emphasized that the spike protein is likely just one harmful part of the "vaccines." As noted in chapters 1 and 5, additional safety concerns surround the inflammatory properties of the lipid nanoparticles used to deliver the modRNA, as well as the lab-modified modRNA itself.

CHAPTER 5

DEBUNKING CDC'S BAD SCIENCE

By Steven J. Hatfill, MD, MSc, MMed

The 2020–2023 COVID-19 crisis saw many significant failures by the Centers for Disease Control and Prevention (CDC). First, it developed and released a faulty polymerase chain reaction (PCR) test, then failed to nationally reduce the cycle threshold (Ct) of the test—key to test accuracy—when it generated massive numbers of false positives.[147] Then, CDC used these ballooning false positives to support the false claim that significant asymptomatic COVID-19 transmission was occurring, setting the stage for "societal lockdowns." CDC also first ignored, then systematically misrepresented, studies showing the efficacy of early treatment for COVID-19 with safe, cost-effective generic drugs.[148]

Yet CDC's most tragic mistakes concern the experimental modRNA pseudo-vaccines. While the US market for these products has been dominated by two pharmaceutical manufacturers, Moderna and Pfizer-Biotech, the discussion of harms in this chapter holds true for all modRNA "vaccines" based on the genetic sequence of the COVID-19 viral spike protein—*and may also be relevant to the adenovector shots (J&J, AstraZeneca), which also encode the toxic spike protein* (chapters 4, 9, 13).

All the modRNA "vaccines" seem to feature extremely narrow safety margins: any incorrect dosing or faulty manufacturing, subzero storage, or product testing can lead to toxic effects. A portion of the modRNA shots' evident toxicity may also be due to incorrect administration—for example, mistaken intravenous versus intramuscular injection, reflecting CDC's recommendation against aspiration of the syringe plunger.[149] Some "vaccine" injuries also appear to be correlated with sloppy manufacturing practices, resulting in "hot lots" or bad batches of the experimental modRNA products—for example, containing hyperconcentrated lipid nanoparticles even more harmful than regular doses.[150]

However, it is an inescapable fact that *the spike protein produced by the modRNA shots is highly toxic on its own and in all contexts*, with potential for harm regardless of how it is delivered (chapter 4). By prompting recipients' cellular machinery to make large amounts of the spike protein, and distributing it uncontrollably throughout their bodies, the modRNA "vaccines" may have induced a transient immune response to the original COVID-19 strain (chapter 1)—but they also inflicted a wide range of damages to human health, including countless deaths.

From the start, CDC tried to cover up its failing mass-"vaccination" policy with faulty, misleading analysis and misstatements.[151] When this failed to staunch online discussion of "vaccine" injuries, CDC and its Big Tech partners resorted to using advanced data-mining technology from the Census Bureau to monitor and censor the daily communications of all Americans on social media. This is not speculation, but well-substantiated by FOIA-recovered documents brought to light by government watchdogs. These facts have received little to no coverage in the mainstream media, which—through their inaccurate, deceptive reporting; smearing early treatments; and promoting "vaccines"—have contributed to the preventable deaths of hundreds of thousands of Americans.

MULTIPLE SOURCES POINT TO WIDESPREAD HARMS: THE V-SAFE DATABASE

Millions of Americans have been injured, crippled, or killed by the modRNA "vaccines," mandated for healthy young adults despite a negative benefit-to-harm ratio demonstrated from the start. The figures regarding injection-related adverse events are shocking. Data from CDC's own V-safe safety-monitoring database, a mobile app introduced in December 2020 that uses text messaging and web surveys to follow up on post-vaccination adverse events, point to unacceptable rates of vaccine injury.

Considering the highly experimental nature of the modRNA COVID-19 "vaccines," a real-time vaccine adverse-event surveillance system was required. However, such a system was not readily available. In response, CDC contracted with Oracle to develop a near-real-time vaccine adverse-event monitoring system based on cell-phone messaging, called "V-safe."[152]

Anyone with access to a smartphone could register with V-safe and report post-"vaccination" side effects. The system was comprehensive, with post-"vaccination" reports to be made on V-safe at one, two, three, four, five, and six weeks after their immunization or booster injections, and then at three, six, and twelve months later. V-safe opened for registration on December 13, 2020, with "tick the box" answer choices designed to monitor side effects. It should be noted that, while the modRNA "vaccines" would soon be promoted for pregnant women, there was no effort by CDC to expand the existing pregnancy registry with any detailed obstetric/gynecological questions.

In 2020 and 2021 some 10.1 million people signed up for V-safe and began submitting post-vaccination health reports—but then something strange happened. In March 2022, CDC released *some* of this check-the-box data. However, for the section on "health impacts" (such as "sought medical care," "missed school or work," or "was unable to perform normal daily activities"), CDC only released data from the first week after "vaccination." This showed between 0.8 percent and 1 percent reporting needing medical care in the first seven days, depending on dose, brand, and recipient's age. Using this data, medical researchers published peer-reviewed studies demonstrating the supposed safety of the modRNA "vaccines."[153]

However, attorney Aaron Siri noticed that CDC's released V-safe data *failed to contain even a single study or report with health impact data further out than the first week.*[154] Despite numerous requests, the CDC refused to release any V-safe data past one week. In response, the nonprofit Informed Consent Action Network (ICAN) sued CDC and forced the release of all the raw data—comprising some 144 million real-time entries into the V-safe database.[155]

The data were alarming. Out of a total 10.1 million registered users, a total of 782,913 reported seeking medical care—most *after* the first week. This represented 7.7 percent of the registered V-safe users.[156] While 782,913 V-safe users submitted at least one report of seeking medical care, there were 2,108,022 total reports, indicating *many had to seek care repeatedly.* Most alarming was the increase in severe side effects as the post-"vaccination" interval increased. Within one week of individuals three years of age and older receiving the first dose of the Pfizer "vaccine," some 0.32 percent reported seeking medical care. However, this steadily increased to 6.93 percent by days thirty-six to forty-two. The peer-reviewed literature shows the same time-gap for the development of the most severe "vaccine" adverse events such as autoimmune arthritis, brain inflammation, prolonged myocarditis, nerve damage, or immune destruction of the body's circulating blood platelets and other clotting abnormalities. This was a clear danger sign.[157]

The 10.1 million registered V-safe users reported over 71 million symptoms, out of which over 4.1 million were categorized as severe enough to make normal daily activities difficult or impossible. Some 23.3 million symptoms were reported as moderate, with a limitation of normal daily activity. There were 4 million reports of joint pain, with 1.9 million reported as moderate *and 400,000 reported as severe.* While only 13,963 infants were in the V-safe database, over 33,000 symptoms were reported in this demographic alone. Independent polls and surveys also reveal an extraordinarily high prevalence of "vaccine" injuries.[158]

The simple fact is the United States has the world's highest number of nationally reported COVID-19 deaths at over 1.1 million, despite around 75 percent of the population reportedly receiving a COVID-19 "vaccine." This has been accompanied by an increase in all-cause US mortality in 2021–2022, *excluding* COVID-19 deaths, compared to the pre-pandemic average, alongside a reduction in average lifespan.[159]

COMING TO GRIPS WITH CDC'S FAILURES

A number of key issues and questions stand out, suggesting a pattern of systematic, seemingly deliberate negligence during the development, authorization, and mass administration of the experimental modRNA "vaccines":

1. Moderna apparently used data from a different product in its EUA application;
2. Failure to test modRNA "vaccines" on people who actually needed them;
3. Relative risk reduction vs. absolute risk reduction;
4. Manufacturer clinical trials did not support a mass modRNA "vaccination" program;
5. Animal testing was incomplete;
6. CDC ignored safety signals;
7. Threats to pregnancy;
8. Failure to implement a comprehensive national adverse-event surveillance system;

9. High mutation rate of the COVID-19 virus precluded effective mass "vaccination";
10. CDC failing to monitor and adjust "vaccine" benefit-to-harm ratios;
11. Abnormal "prion-like" amyloid proteins resulting from COVID-19 modRNA shots;
12. Immunity from COVID-19 infection is far superior to the short-lived modRNA shots;
13. Herd immunity and the "Minimal Infecting Human Dose$_{50}$";
14. CDC ignored FDA's own experts.

Even more disturbing than its scientific and administrative lapses is *CDC's active complicity in surveillance and censorship of public speech by ordinary Americans*—the closing subject of this chapter.

1. Moderna apparently used data from a different product in its modRNA "vaccine" emergency use authorization (EUA) application.

Documents obtained by a FOIA lawsuit disclosed that, in Moderna's rush to obtain market share, the animal and human trial testing of the company's experimental modRNA "vaccine" was hasty and perfunctory. The FOIA documents suggest that to save time and money, the pharmaceutical company "bootstrapped" its earlier existing pharmacokinetic studies—for a modRNA "vaccine" for a pathogen called cytomegalovirus (CMV)—*and expanded the data to include its proposed new vaccine for COVID-19.*

The FOIA-recovered document "Pharmacokinetics Written Summary" stated: "The results of a biodistribution study of mRNA-1647 [Cytomegalovirus mRNA vaccine] support the development of mRNA-1273 [COVID-19 vaccine]." This implies that Moderna was using its previous biodistribution study of the cytomegalovirus mRNA-1647 "vaccine" to shorten the FDA safety process for the COVID-19 "vaccine."

Ultimately, Moderna appeared to submit the data generated from its earlier studies on CMV, not COVID-19, in its application for emergency use authorization for the COVID injections. However, COVID-19 and CMV are two very different pathogens:

- Cytomegalovirus is a relatively slow-mutating DNA virus, while COVID-19 was caused by a rapidly mutating RNA virus.

- While the lipid (fatty content) mixture coating the modRNA nanoparticles were the same, unlike the cytomegalovirus "vaccine," the modRNA inside the COVID-19 "vaccine" coded for the highly active, toxic spike protein.[160]

2. The CDC never ensured that the modRNA "vaccines" were tested on the high-risk individuals (ostensibly) most likely to benefit from the experimental product.

Early in the pandemic, the CDC determined that physically fit, working-age adults generally experienced only limited illness from COVID-19, while children seemed to have a large degree of resistance, likely due to low levels of the ACE-2 viral receptors in their upper airways.[161] Pregnant women also did not seem to be at elevated risk for severe COVID-19.

The population groups most at risk for serious disease included the elderly, the obese, and the over-fifty population suffering from heart problems, diabetes, and other chronic diseases. These were the groups most likely to benefit from any COVID "vaccine," and these were the population groups that Moderna and the other clinical vaccine studies should have concentrated on. *Yet none of the rushed vaccine clinical trials enrolled these most-at-risk patients, and further, no clinical trials were designed to measure any "vaccine"-mediated reduction in serious outcomes such as hospitalization, intensive care, admission, or death*—thereby omitting both the patients and the metrics most relevant to efficacy.

The Moderna and the Pfizer phase III "vaccine" trials evaluated only mild COVID-19 disease. Because most COVID-19 infections were self-limited illness, hospitalizations and deaths were simply too uncommon in the studied test populations to yield any meaningful findings. An assessment of "vaccine" efficacy for preventing hospitalization and death would have required a much larger sample size and much longer clinical trial duration to collect this necessary data, including a range of vulnerable individuals.

3. Relative risk reduction vs. absolute risk reduction.

Vaccine efficacy is often described as the *relative risk reduction* (RRR) between two groups, one group that gets vaccinated and one group that does not. Far more important, however, is the *absolute risk reduction (ARR)*, which includes the likelihood of a particular outcome with COVID-19 (such as the risk of hospitalization, ICU admission, or death), compared to someone who is "unvaccinated."

For example, let's say that one hundred people are in an unvaccinated group, and five of them are hospitalized with COVID-19. The baseline risk for being hospitalized with COVID-19 is 5 percent in this control group. Now take a group of one hundred people and give them all an experimental COVID-19 "vaccine." Two months later, we find that only one out of these one hundred individuals has been hospitalized with the virus (meaning 5 percent of the unvaccinated became hospitalized, compared to only 1 percent of the vaccinated group).

The individual's RRR as a member of the vaccinated group is 80 percent (1 percent divided by the baseline risk of 5 percent = –0.8). However, the ARR of an individual in the vaccinated group is much lower, at just 4 percent (5 percent minus 1 percent = 4 percent). A claimed effective RRR of 80 percent certainly sounds impressive—much less so the ARR of 4 percent.

4. Manufacturer clinical trials did not support a mass modRNA "vaccination" program.

In 2022, a group of prominent clinical data scientists reanalyzed the released data on the placebo-controlled, phase III randomized clinical trials of both the Pfizer and Moderna modRNA COVID-19 "vaccines" in adults (Clinical Trials NCT04368728 and NCT04470427), following FOIA requests. This independent reanalysis of the manufacturers' original phase III clinical trial data demonstrated a *negative benefit-to-harm ratio* in individuals who took the Pfizer and Moderna modRNA COVID-19 pseudo-vaccines—*in short, the shots were hurting people.*[162]

Reanalyzed data from both the Moderna and Pfizer clinical trials show the modRNA "vaccines" carry a *higher risk* of post-"vaccination" hospitalization, serious disability, or a life-changing event *than the risk of naturally acquiring a COVID-19 infection and being hospitalized with it.* In short, taking an modRNA "vaccine" as an adult was more dangerous, on average, than having a COVID-19 infection and being admitted to the hospital.[163] Full transparency of the COVID-19 "vaccine" clinical trial data is needed to properly evaluate the many remaining questions, but three years after the rollout of the of modRNA COVID-19 "vaccines," participant-level data still remain largely inaccessible.

5. Animal testing was incomplete.

During development of any new drug or biological agent like the modRNA "vaccines," "pharmacokinetics" studies are necessary for FDA to properly outline the absorption, distribution, metabolism, and excretion of any drug or vaccine candidate.[164] However, it appears that no pharmacokinetic evaluations were performed by the manufacturer on Moderna's modRNA-1273 COVID "vaccine," according to 699 pages of records from the Department of Health and Human Services (HHS)—obtained in December 2022 following repeated FOIA requests and lawsuits by the nonprofit Judicial Watch in December 2022. This included some data submitted to FDA as part of Moderna's application for an emergency use authorization for its modRNA COVID-19 "vaccine."[165]

These records revealed that *no pharmacokinetic studies had been performed by the manufacturer on the actual Moderna modRNA-1273 COVID "vaccine."* There were no complete absorption studies, no metabolism study data, and apparently no excretion studies. Instead, Judicial Watch uncovered a document titled "Pharmacokinetics Written Summary." Marked "Confidential," the document revealed that the information it contained was related to Moderna's new modRNA-1273 COVID-19 "vaccine"—but as noted, much of the data in the document seems to have actually been derived from Moderna's ongoing study of another modRNA "vaccine," for a DNA virus called "Cytomegalovirus mRNA-1647."[166]

Moderna had contracted out the bioavailability studies for the "DNA cytomegalovirus modRNA-1647 experimental vaccine" preparation to the Charles River Laboratories in Montreal, Canada. The resulting study, "A Single Dose Intramuscular Injection Tissue Distribution Study of modRNA-1647 in Male Sprague-Dawley Rats," showed that the lipid nanoparticles of the modRNA-1647 "vaccine" traveled from the site of muscle injection to the lymph nodes and spleen and then into general circulation ("lipid nanoparticle dispersion").[167] An appendix reveals that, in addition to distributing to the lymph nodes and spleen, the modRNA particles also distributed to the bone marrow, brain, eyes, heart, liver, lungs, stomach, and testes.[168] Research conducted both before and during the pandemic has also raised concerns that the lipid nanoparticles, which deliver the "vaccine" modRNA into human cells, may also be toxic.[169]

6. CDC ignored safety signals.

Public health authorities have disregarded post-"vaccination" adverse-events reports on the Vaccine Adverse Event Reporting System (VAERS) on the grounds that, because anyone can submit a report to VAERS, there is no way to know if the reports are authentic. *However, a responsible public health program, animated by an abundance of caution, should consider the possibility that reports of adverse reactions might be true, not proceed on the assumption they are false.* Public health authorities have also failed to address the issue of "masking," in which injuries caused by the modRNA "vaccines" go unrecognized or are misdiagnosed due to complex factors such as the use of other medications or preexisting health conditions. FDA's own scientists warned that masking is likely leading to underreporting of adverse events from the modRNA "vaccines": "Due to vaccine novelty, and an unprecedented dynamic of reporting, statistical signals…related to…COVID-19 vaccines are more prone to masking and, therefore, to being undetected or delayed."[170]

- *Ignoring ischemic stroke safety signals.* FDA and CDC dismissed a clear safety signal for ischemic stroke (in which blood supply to a part of the brain is reduced, potentially resulting in brain damage) on the false grounds that the signal only appeared in VAERS. In fact, similar signals appeared in Cov19VaxKB, an independent database used by researchers associated with NIH, as well as a CDC analysis—released in July 2022 after an FOIA request.[171]

- *Ignoring cancer safety signals.* FDA turned a blind eye to safety signals from CDC analyses indicating an increased risk of various kinds of cancers, which were only disclosed to the public in January 2023 after an FOIA request. Cancer risks that might be associated with the modRNA "vaccines" include: colon cancer, metastatic breast cancer, chronic lymphocytic leukemia, B cell lymphoma, follicular lymphoma, and metastases to the liver, bone, central nervous system, and lymph nodes.[172] While no large-scale formal studies of potential modRNA-"vaccine"-induced cancers have been reported, the possibility of LINE-1 transposon activity involving the spike protein modRNA suggests one biochemical mechanism for oncogenic "vaccine" side effects.

7. Threats to pregnancy.

The documents retrieved via FOIA also included a Moderna-prepared report titled "Nonclinical Overview," submitted to FDA. This document reveals that a "statistically significant" number of rats born to pregnant mothers injected with the modRNA "vaccine" preparations were found to have skeletal malformations known as "wavy ribs" and "rib nodules."[173] FDA dismissed this animal data, saying that the skeletal anomalies were normal variations and not considered an "adverse event."

However, some scientists insist *any* chemical or "vaccine"-induced changes to the rat fetal skeleton should be considered a major safety signal. Molecular biologists warned that anything associated with an increase in mammalian anatomical variation might also perturb fetal development of humans, particularly with respect to developing structures and organs, with increased risk of miscarriages.[174]

These findings should have prompted an immediate halt to any consideration of "vaccinating" pregnant mothers until the potential risks were completely investigated for biodistribution of lipid nanoparticles and modRNA to and through the placenta and the fetus. Instead, Moderna, FDA, and CDC kept this data hidden from the public for months.

In January 2021, soon after the "vaccine" rollout commenced, CDC updated its website to claim that the modRNA "vaccines" were "unlikely to pose a specific risk for people who are pregnant." Yet there was no real data to support this claim. Over the following months a flurry of around one hundred peer-reviewed papers appeared on PubMed, the research repository of the National Library of Medicine at NIH, with the majority confidently claiming there were no risks to pregnant individuals taking the modRNA "vaccines."[175] Yet, as outlined in chapter 11, there are signs that a concerning number of women were experiencing gynecological and obstetric issues after their modRNA "vaccinations." Of particular concern was the incidence of miscarriages in "vaccinated" women compared to the baseline in the unvaccinated population.

Declining a chance to recruit an identical control cohort of unvaccinated pregnant women in the V-safe registry, CDC simply refused to release the full pregnancy data from its V-safe surveillance system.[176]

Following CDC in lockstep, the leaders of the professional societies such as the American College of Obstetricians and Gynecologists (ACOG) and the Society for Maternal-Fetal Medicine (SMFM) both advised that COVID-19 "vaccines" not be withheld from pregnant or lactating women.

Yet an eight-page FOIA-released Pfizer document, dated April 20, 2021, and marked *Confidential*, but later reported by TrialSiteNews and then analyzed in depth by WarRoom/DailyClout research volunteers, described the proactive tracking of 458 pregnant women and 215 lactating women from the time the modRNA "vaccines" were released until February 28, 2021. The Pfizer document, titled "Pregnancy and Lactation Cumulative Review. FDA- CBER-2021-5683-0779746," suggested a potential doubling of the back- ground miscarriage rate that would be consistent with active "vaccine" nanoparticles transferring through the placenta to the fetus.[177] A later 286-page "Pfizer Periodic Safety Update Report Number #1," covering December 19, 2021, to June 18, 2022, first reported by Children's Health Defense Europe and also analyzed by DailyClout examined a clinical trial (C4591001) covering 144 pregnancies. This data was also consistent with the idea of a transplacental passage of the modRNA nanoparticles from the "vaccine."[178]

From the beginning, CDC has encouraged pregnant mothers to take the modRNA "vaccine," as well as booster injections manufactured with the same basic formulation. Yet from a safety point of view alone, *the modRNA "vaccines" for COVID-19 should never have been given to any pregnant woman.*

8. The CDC failed to implement an accurate national adverse event (AE) surveillance board to monitor the experimental modRNA "vaccines."

Considering the highly experimental nature of the COVID-19 "vaccines," it was essential that an independent Data Safety Monitoring Board (DSMB) be established to review all aspects of pre-clinical-trial animal testing and all resulting human clinical trials, and to monitor continuing efficacy and safety signals that might appear during the mass "vaccination" program.

Independent DSMBs are responsible for reviewing clinical-study safety findings, related data, and measurements, and are typically required for any study involving new therapies, high-risk populations, or multisite studies, among other criteria.[179] The experimental modRNA products clearly met at least one, and perhaps all, of these conditions.

Instead, CDC created a watered-down Advisory Committee on Immunization Practices (ACIP), with input from the compromised FDA (chapters 2, 3), to monitor the data from its legacy Vaccine Adverse Event Reporting System (VAERS), with its known shortcomings (chapter 6),[180] and the untried V-safe monitoring system.

In short, there was little chance CDC would be able to accurately monitor the ongoing benefit/risk ratio of any new highly experimental mass-"vaccination" program with the necessary sensitivity—*it was flying blind*. This is especially troubling because a large body of pre-pandemic research showed that historically adverse events following vaccination tend to be *underreported* by a large margin (chapter 6), suggesting VAERS reports may be "just the tip of the iceberg."[181] CDC has ignored this long-established phenomenon, instead implying that existing adverse events might be fake reports or represent *over*reporting. However, FDA scientists have acknowledged that VAERS is mis- and underreported up to fourteen times for myocarditis based on analyses by FDA, the Israeli Ministry of Health, and Kaiser-Permanente.[182] These data also show that, despite mandatory reporting, the VAERS Under Reporting Factor (URF) for deaths associated with COVID-19 "vaccines" is about ten for a seven-day window and thirty-six for a forty-two-day window. Yet CDC refuses to "connect the dots" and admit that these URFs, when applied to VAERS data, point to massive mortality and injury rates associated with the COVID-19 modRNA "vaccines."

9. The high mutation rate of the COVID-19 virus precluded any successful mass vaccination program once a pandemic was underway.

The rapid mutation of the COVID-19 virus, giving rise to a succession of increasingly "vaccine"-resistant strains, was predicted by scientists before the experimental modRNA products were even introduced (chapter 1). In early December 2020, just as the global mass-"vaccination" program began, an unusual COVID-19 viral strain appeared in patient samples from Kent in the United Kingdom. This COVID-19 variant, designated B.1.1.7 Alpha, had acquired seventeen mutations, including eight in the gene encoding the spike protein on the viral coat. The Alpha variant was estimated to be 40 percent to 80 percent more transmissible than the original Wuhan strain, with most estimates occupying the middle to higher end of this range. This was confirmed by tissue culture and animal models.[183]

On February 2, 2021, Public Health England reported B.1.1.7 viruses with E484K mutations that were of concern. By the end of March 2021, the first wave of new viral evolution involving B.1.1.7 Alpha descendants was well underway. "Breakthrough" infections were soon documented in Israel, trumpeted as the most heavily "vaccinated" country on the planet, and infections in "vaccinated" individuals quickly became commonplace.[184]

In the second half of 2021, the Delta variant B.1.617.2 spread from India to over 179 other countries, amid warnings that it was "40-60% more transmissible than Alpha and almost twice as transmissible as the original Wuhan strain of SARS-CoV-2."[185] It would go on to generate more than twenty-eight distinct viral variants. On August 2, 2021, scientists warned that achieving herd immunity through modRNA "vaccination" might not be possible because the Delta variant was being transmitted by the previously "vaccinated" population.[186]

During this time, CDC continued to make false claims that "vaccines" and "boosters" were working by reducing the number of serious infections. However, a study by the Francis Crick Institute, published in *The Lancet*, indicated that individuals who were fully "vaccinated" and "boosted" with the Pfizer-BioNTech vaccine had, on average, more than five times *lower* levels of neutralizing antibodies against the Delta variant, compared to the original COVID-19 strain.[187]

In September 2021, "vaccinated" people made up 23 percent of coronavirus fatalities. By February 2022, they made up 41 percent of hospital admissions, and by August 2022, 58 percent of COVID-19 deaths were in "vaccinated" or "boosted" individuals, according to an analysis conducted for *The Health 202* by Cynthia Cox, vice-president with the Kaiser Family Foundation.[188]

Simply put, the mass "vaccination" program was a failure. By all rights, CDC should have gone back and reassessed the original clinical trials, reviewed the latest research (now including over three thousand papers showing the spike protein's toxicity), and, most importantly, reassessed the harm-to-benefit ratio of the modRNA "vaccines" for young adults, pregnant females, and children. *But CDC did none of these things.*

10. CDC failed to monitor and adjust vaccine benefit-to-harm ratios.

As the vaccine rollout descended into mandates and coercion, CDC conducted a type of analysis called "proportional reporting ratio" (PRR) to analyze and compare—from December 14, 2020, to July 29, 2022—the adverse event reports associated with the Moderna and Pfizer COVID-19 "vaccines," specifically weighing them against all reports lodged with all other non-COVID-19 vaccines. *But the results were so shocking that CDC refused to make the results public.*

However, lawsuits eventually brought some of this information out into the open. The results of these FOIA requests show thousands of adverse modRNA "vaccine" events that met the definition of "serious." These included life-threatening conditions such as blood clotting in the lungs, heart attacks, new onset liver cirrhosis, massive fatal clotting in the large venous sinuses of the brain, and permanent scar tissue formation in the hearts of some "vaccine" recipients.[189]

Because myocarditis (inflammation and scarring of the heart) was already definitely associated with the modRNA "vaccines," anything with a danger signal larger than myocarditis should have been investigated with the highest priority. The PRR results returned *more than five hundred types of adverse event*, with reporting rates higher than myocarditis—yet CDC never showed any concern to conduct these investigations in an urgent manner.

Throughout the pandemic, CDC officials made multiple false statements concerning the safety of the "vaccines." For example, on April 19, 2023, a leading CDC official stated to the CDC Advisory Committee on Immunization Practices (ACIP) that CDC had never detected a safety signal for ischemic stroke (sudden interrupted blood supply to the brain) due to the modRNA "vaccines."[190] In truth, the FOIA documents showed that ischemic stroke *was indeed identified as a safety signal* for the original Moderna and Pfizer products, detected by CDC as early as spring 2022 (see Item 6).

According to other FOIA documents, CDC also identified abnormal, chronic, ringing in the ears (tinnitus) as a safety signal in its analysis of VAERS. Many neurologists consider this a sign of possible brain inflammation (chapter 9).[191] CDC tried to minimize any notion that this was caused by the modRNA "vaccines." However, at the same time, tinnitus is listed as a potential side effect of Johnson & Johnson's adenovector "vaccine," and regulators in some countries have linked tinnitus to AstraZeneca's "vaccine," which also codes for the inflammatory spike protein. While the Moderna and Pfizer modRNA products are not formally linked with tinnitus, there seems to be a statistically significant association.[192] In fact, thousands of reports of tinnitus were submitted to VAERS after COVID-19 vaccination, and post-vaccination tinnitus has been widely discussed online.[193] CDC and peer agencies have further failed to perform proper causality and proportional reporting ratio assessments, comparing modRNA "vaccine" injuries with historic norms, or empirical Bayesian data analyses, as required as part of standard safety monitoring,[194] or they have failed to release the results of such analyses as are performed.

11. Abnormal "prion-like" amyloid proteins can be deposited in the brain as a result of COVID-19 modRNA "vaccination."

One of the most shocking "vaccine" side effects was the sudden post-"vaccination" formation of massive abnormal, rubbery blood clots in the extremities causing death or amputation. Upon later analysis it was found that the unusual consistency of these clots was due to an abnormal "amyloid" deposition of the spike protein.[195]

As early as March 2020, forward-looking scientists published a paper describing the potential for the COVID-19 viral spike protein to aggregate into "prion-like," insoluble deposits in human tissues (chapter 9).[196] Prions are proteins that, because of their structure, are sensitive to undergoing abnormal three-dimensional folding and protease cutting to form harmful, insoluble, tough, cellular fibrils that cause abnormal deposits and cell death in healthy tissue.[197] Different types of proteins may form different types of "prions," and collectively these are termed "amyloid." These different "amyloids" or "prions" can play devastating roles in human disease.

For example, an abnormal folding of the B-amyloid protein is implicated in Alzheimer's disease. The alpha-synuclein protein is another prion-like protein that can form the harmful amyloid deposits seen in the Parkinson's disease spectrum and its associated forms of dementia. The historical APrP protein is found as harmful amyloid deposits in both the classical and the variant forms of Creutzfeldt-Jakob disease.

These serious and always fatal disorders take months to years to develop and run a terminal course. Predictably, the presence of these sequences in the COVID-19 "vaccines" have led to discoveries of harmful insoluble amyloid spike protein deposits in the brains of patients that have suffered a "vaccination"-associated death.[198]

On April 5, 2023, a large group of German scientists published mouse models and human COVID-19 autopsy findings that show the accumulation of the COVID-19 virus spike protein in the bone marrow of the skull, the membranes surrounding the brain, and within the structure of the brain itself.[199] Using an established mouse model, the injection of the actual spike protein alone was enough to cause brain cell death.

In human autopsy cases, the deposition of spike protein in the skull, long after COVID-19 infection, suggests that the long-term persistence of this amyloid-like protein may also contribute to long-term neurological signs and symptoms. These studies also detected the biomarkers of neurodegeneration molecules associated with Alzheimer's disease, the Parkinson's disease spectrum, and dementia. It is imperative that CDC urgently examine the modRNA sequences in *the newly recommended variant "vaccines" and boosters* to determine if the amylogenic areas of the new synthetic modRNA for the spike protein are still present.[200]

12. Natural immunity from COVID-19 infection is far superior to the short-lived modRNA shots.

As explained in chapter 1, the human immune system's response to viral infection typically occurs in two closely coordinated stages.[201] The initial first response is performed by special circulating lymphocyte cells called "cytotoxic T cells," and it is the primary defense of the human body against any viral infection. *It does not need antibodies to function.* When activated, these cytotoxic T cells act like miniature sledgehammers to destroy all the infected cells in the body that have been hijacked by the virus to make new viral offspring. This cytotoxic "cell-killing" response may also damage the surrounding normal tissues as well. The process is called "cell-mediated immunity" and it is the primary defense against viruses. The purpose of this cell-mediated T cell response is to keep the infected individual alive long enough to allow a second, more precise component of the immune system to kick into gear.

Within five to seven days, the initial "sledgehammer" T cell response of "cell-mediated immunity" is followed by a more precise, selective *antibody response*. Antibodies are special proteins made by another type of specialized lymphocyte, called "B cells." The antibodies that B cells produce are tailor-made, acting like a military sniper's bullets as they circulate through bloodstream and tissues, precisely clearing any of the remaining viruses before they can attach to more normal cells to produce more virus. This second, antibody-enabled immune response is called "humoral immunity."

When the virus is finally cleared from the body, the antibody levels in the blood drop and eventually disappear. However, that is not the end of the story. After the two-part antiviral immune response is over and the patient has recovered, some of these activated T cells and B cells go into "early retirement" and remain dormant for years, simply waiting to see if the virus ever reappears. Now called "memory T cells," "memory B cells," and shorter-lived "plasma cells," these can reactivate to provide durable long-term immunity if the virus or its later variants ever appear in the body again.

Typically, the immune system responds to many different proteins that make up an invading virus, so if one of these proteins later mutates to become unrecognizable, *the immune system will still be able to recognize other proteins that haven't mutated*, offering continued protection against the new viral strain. In the case of COVID-19, our immune system naturally forms antibodies to other parts of the virus besides the spike protein, such as the central "nucleocapsid" structure enclosing the viral modRNA, which are much less prone to mutation than the spike protein. Therefore, healthy individuals who have recovered from a COVID-19 infection develop a long-term, durable immunity that can work against "variants" that might develop later, recognizing many different parts of the virus.[202] This is referred to as "natural immunity."

However, this was not the case with the modRNA "vaccines," which trained the immune system to recognize only a *single protein* from a single, extinct strain of the COVID-19 virus—the spike protein of the original Wuhan strain. This virus no longer existed in nature by fall 2020, having mutated and long since been replaced by multiple successive variants, with mutations concentrated in the spike protein.[203] In fact, there is concern that repeated exposure to the original spike protein of the early Wuhan strain, as encoded by the modRNA shots, may interfere with the body's ability to respond to newer variant COVID-19 viral strains, by keying antibody production to the first (now extinct) spike protein—a well-demonstrated principle of immunology dubbed "original antigenic sin" (chapters 1, 7).[204]

There are now at least 150 peer-reviewed scientific papers demonstrating that natural immunity from COVID-19 infection is superior to the

COVID-19 modRNA shots.²⁰⁵ All show that natural immunity provides a broader cross-reactive viral variant spectrum and a safer, higher, longer-lasting level of viral protection than the modRNA shots.²⁰⁶

Meanwhile, FDA has refused to engage with mounting evidence that the COVID-19 "vaccines" may be making recipients *more—not less—likely* to catch COVID-19, and may also increase their vulnerability to severe disease and death. Data showing negative vaccine efficacy are most concerning as they may indicate immune suppression, which causes other, unreported, short-term adverse effects (chapter 7).

- Data presented by a CDC official to FDA's VRBPAC meeting on June 14, 2022, showed no statistical effect of the Pfizer "vaccine" on the Omicron variant by three months, *with efficacy becoming negative (increasing chances of infection) by seven months.*²⁰⁷

- A Cleveland Clinic study of "vaccinated" health-care workers found "a possible association with more prior vaccine doses and higher risk of COVID-19." The authors found that the risk "of COVID-19 increased with time since the most recent prior COVID-19 episode and with the number of vaccine doses previously received."²⁰⁸

- Analysis of mortality data from the Israeli Ministry of Health, alongside "vaccination" data from the country's largest health-care provider, reveals an increase in the number of COVID-19 deaths in "vaccinated" subjects. This analysis of mass "vaccination" outcomes from December 2020 to May 2021 suggested that there may have been at that time 121–413 excess COVID-19 deaths per million recipients associated with "vaccination," which would equal about 25,000–85,000 deaths in the US during that time.²⁰⁹

- Results from Denmark from spring 2021 are consistent with the findings in the Israeli data. The Danish Statens Serum Institut tracked outcomes in high-priority "vaccination" groups and found negative "vaccine" efficacy in terms of preventing COVID-19 mortality, with *increased likelihood of COVID-19-related deaths with the second dose.*²¹⁰

13. Natural infection, herd immunity, and the "minimal infectious human dose$_{50}$"

During a pandemic, immune and nonimmune individuals may frequently become exposed to very low amounts of virus and develop asymptomatic infections—yet still develop a strong immune response. This is due to a concept called a "minimal infectious human dose$_{50}$."

COVID-19 is an airborne transmitted infection, subject to a variety of environmental factors, including the size of the aerosol particles, the concentration of the virus, aerosol distribution, exposure to sunlight or other sources of ultraviolet light, atmospheric moisture, ambient air temperature, and atmospheric oxygen levels. All these factors contribute to natural biological decay, at a measurable rate per minute, for any human pathogen released into the air.[211]

The ability of any airborne viral contagion to infect new subjects depends on the minimal aerosol dose of that virus required to initiate either a *clinical* (symptomatic, more transmissible) or *sub-clinical* (mild, less transmissible) infection. A common baseline to study viral transmission is the "minimal infectious human dose" required to transmit infection to 50 percent of the population ("minimal infectious human dose$_{50}$" or "HID$_{50}$"). Importantly, a dose below this benchmark may result in asymptomatic infection that is not strong enough to become symptomatic or transmissible to others—*yet is still strong enough to activate the human immune system and establish a robust, viable natural immunity*.[212]

Throughout the entire COVID-19 pandemic, CDC leadership has continued to ignore the large population of recovered, naturally immune individuals predicted by the minimal infectious human dose$_{50}$. Instead, CDC has focused exclusively, and wrongly, on circulating antibody levels to support the US mass "vaccination program," even though the presence of antibodies in "vaccine" recipients does not necessarily equate to actual immunity against viral infections (in part because the antibodies are already obsolete in the face of ever-evolving viral variants).[213] In short, CDC has refused to acknowledge that most Americans already had superior natural immunity to COVID-19, and therefore no need of "vaccines."

The body of scientific evidence demonstrating that COVID-19 infection generated strong, lasting natural immunity is indisputable.[214] *In all cases, the real hallmark of immunity is the presence of "memory lymphocytes,"* not *the prolonged presence of circulating antibodies*. By claiming that a high level of circulating antibodies was evidence of active immunity, *CDC was intentionally, and deceptively, trying to support the continued use of the modRNA "vaccines."*

- The "SIREN" study published in *The Lancet* addressed the relationships between seropositivity in people with previous COVID-19 infection and subsequent risk of severe disease and hospitalization over the subsequent seven to twelve months. Prior infection decreased the risk of symptomatic reinfection by 93 percent.[215]

- Real-world occupational data, in the form of a Cleveland Clinic study in 2021, showed that *not one* of its 1,359 previously infected but "unvaccinated" employees had a COVID-19 infection over the duration of the study. The article concluded that previously infected individuals were "unlikely to benefit from COVID-19 vaccination."[216]

- Research has demonstrated the presence of long-lived plasma cells in those who have recovered from COVID-19. This implies an enduring capacity to respond to new infection, perhaps lasting years, by mounting a rapid secondary immune response that features highly selective new IgG antibodies.[217]

By November 2021, it was clear that individuals who experienced natural infection were generating and maintaining large numbers of latent memory B cells and memory T cells in their bodies. Typically, these individuals were capable of mounting a secondary immune response whenever a new variant of the COVID-19 virus became the dominant circulating strain.[218]

Natural immunity was found to be long-lasting. A study funded by the National Institutes of Health (NIH), from the La Jolla Institute for Immunology, found "durable immune responses" in 95 percent of the two hundred participants up to *eight months* after infection.[219] One of the largest studies to date, published in *Science* in February 2021, found that although antibodies declined over eight months, memory B cells *increased over time*, and the half-life of memory CD8+ and CD4+ T cells suggested a steady presence of T cell–mediated immunity.[220]

In April 2021, CDC simply decided to stop collecting data on the overwhelming number of "breakthrough" infections following modRNA injection, unless reinfection required hospitalization.[221] Indeed, it did everything in its power to confuse the issue with an incessant barrage of very poorly written papers published in its own *Morbidity and Mortality Weekly Report Journal* (MMWR). In general, these faulty papers incorrectly attempted to equate the presence of circulating antibodies with proof of long-term modRNA "vaccine"-induced immunity. *In fact, this was likely due to the prolonged presence in the body of the modRNA*, constantly generating more copies of the toxic spike protein from the original Wuhan strain, driving the immune system to exhaustion.

One study, conducted with a small sample size in Kentucky, concluded that modRNA "vaccination" of previously infected individuals provided *twice the protection against reinfection*, compared to an individual with only natural immunity, in order to again justify recommending the shots for everyone, including recovered individuals. However, the control population of this study consisted of "unvaccinated" people *who had previously been hospitalized with COVID-19*—who were, by definition, at much higher risk of reinfection and negative COVID-19 outcomes due to major comorbidities like old age, obesity, and diabetes. Presenting the impact of the modRNA shots on this small cohort of individuals, already hospitalized once for COVID-19, as representative of the population at large was grossly deceptive, directly contradicting CDC's own 2022 statement that the modRNA "vaccines" did not prevent infection. Yet this paper was sadly typical of the CDC's "scientific" work during the pandemic.[222]

Meanwhile, the numbers of crippling adverse "vaccine" events and "vaccine"-associated deaths were becoming more difficult to minimize.[223] Worse still, another international survey found that people with a history of SARS-CoV-2 infection experienced greater rates of side effects after "vaccination."[224]

14. FDA and CDC ignored FDA's own experts' advice against bivalent boosters.

A number of high-profile FDA officials and advisors have publicly warned that bivalent "boosters" would have no impact on transmission and would offer vulnerable individuals transient protection at best, but the agencies show no sign of revising their booster guidance.

- Writing in *JAMA* on December 9, 2022, Dr. Peter Marks, director of FDA's Center for Biologics Evaluation and Research, noted modRNA shots' inability to confer lasting immunity or lower transmission: "Continuing along the current path of the generation and administration of variant-specific vaccine boosters is inadequate as a long-term strategy for addressing COVID-19 in populations globally.... Simply updating the existing vaccine constructs with new variant sequences or even making trivalent or quadrivalent vaccines covering several variants is not likely to provide the depth and breadth of protection needed to interrupt viral transmission during a prolonged period."[225]

- In January 2023, FDA Vaccines and Related Biological Products Advisory Committee (VRBPAC) member Dr. Paul Offit told *Time* magazine, "The experience of the past year has taught us that chasing these Omicron variants with a bivalent vaccine is a losing game."[226]

CDC BLOCKS FREEDOM OF SPEECH TO CONTROL THE MODRNA "VACCINE" NARRATIVE

CDC directly and intentionally suppressed the American right to "freedom of speech" by censoring and eventually "deplatforming" expert physicians and scientists trying to warn the public that mass "vaccination" was the wrong pandemic response.

After the United Kingdom's 2019 general elections were subjected to "disinformation" targeting social media by Russian intelligence among others, the British government facilitated the creation of a formal global media censorship program, bringing together a conglomerate of media companies to stop online platforms from spreading any content the government labeled "disinformation" or "misinformation."

To roll out this global censorship regime, the British Broadcasting Corporation (BBC) convened a closed-door assembly of publishers and global media platforms at a "Trusted News Summit," where the companies formed a global media alliance spanning printed media, social media, and the broadcast news, across international platforms. When established, this "collective" would eventually include BBC, the European Broadcasting Union (EBU), Google/YouTube, the Hindu, the *Wall Street Journal*, the *Financial Times, First Draft,* Facebook, and eventually CBC/Radio-Canada, Twitter, Microsoft, *Associated Press, Agence France-Presse, Reuters,* and the Reuters Institute for the Study of Journalism, and an association with the *New York Times.* The alliance also included a sudden new crop of "fact-checking" organizations—supposedly independent but supported by interested corporate and nonprofit donors.[227]

This new international organization, called the Trusted News Initiative (TNI), enabled its conglomerate partners to track "disinformation"—often simply meaning disapproved forms of dissent—around the world and alert each other to undesirable opinions on their various platforms. Of course, it would be the journalists and their views and political affiliations at TNI, and its "fact-checkers," who would decide what was "misinformation" and "disinformation."

On December 10, 2020, BBC announced that TNI would start to combat the spread of anti-"vaccine" "disinformation," quickly encompassing most critical views of the modRNA injections.[228] National experts speaking in favor of early drug treatments, and urging caution with an experimental mass "vaccination" program, suddenly found themselves censored and "deplatformed" off social media such as Twitter, Facebook, and Instagram.

On July 27, 2022, an organization called America First Legal (AFL) released the first set of documents obtained through its yearlong litigation against CDC and HHS. The recovered documents, part of broader internal document dump dubbed the "Twitter Papers," show CDC suppressing free speech with a program to actively scan and censor social media—in part to cover up its own pandemic mistakes.

The "Twitter Papers" revealed the explicit secret collusion between CDC and Big Tech companies—such as Meta/Facebook, Instagram and Google—to censor whatever US federal health authorities deemed COVID-19 "misinformation."[229] A second document release by AFL on September 6, 2022, showed that CDC identified specific posts made by individuals on the Facebook and Twitter platforms for removal or suppression. CDC had also apparently co-opted the Census Bureau's Trust and Safety Social Media Misinformation Team to carefully monitor social media platforms through round-the-clock, automated data-mining.[230] *Outrageously, CDC reminded tech companies that the Census Bureau was tracking these posts to ensure compliance with censorship demands.* The released documents also revealed that

Facebook created a new position of "misinformation manager" to censor free speech on behalf of the Biden administration.

AFL's fourth document release, also in December 2022, revealed that the Biden administration had clandestine access to a Twitter portal to secretly identify and censor dissenting views. Meanwhile Facebook sent written documents to CDC confirming that it had banned more than sixteen million pieces of content containing individual opinions or information the Biden administration wanted suppressed.

The once revered and trusted CDC had become nothing more than an unconstitutional conveyor of propaganda, emanating from the executive branch of the US government. A deliberate, controlled, deplatforming and censorship of noted scientists and medical experts was now underway against anyone who dared contradict the dysfunctional NIH, CDC, and FDA.

This represents a major challenge to the First Amendment that requires urgent legal redress. While leading doctors and scientists were trying (at risk to their own careers) to warn the public about the high risk and low benefit associated with the poorly FDA-reviewed modRNA products being passed off as "vaccines," the TNI treated their concerns as disinformation.

On November 3, 2022, a link was posted referencing an investigation from the highly respected *British Medical Journal* (BMJ) to a private Facebook group. The article reported on the poor practices that allegedly occurred in Pfizer's modRNA COVID-19 "vaccine" trial (chapters 2, 3).[231] In November 2022, a "fact-checking" company called Lead Stories, which was responsible for half of all of Facebook's "fact-checking" in 2021, questioned the integrity of the *BMJ* story. The article was then issued a "Missing Context" rating, created by Facebook "to deal with content that could mislead without additional context but which was otherwise true or real."

The *BMJ*'s editor in chief was direct in his reply, quoted in the journal's cited follow-up investigation, stating:

> We should all be very worried that Facebook's actions won't stop *The BMJ* doing what is right, but the real question is: why is Facebook acting in this way? What is driving its world view? Is it ideology? Is it commercial interests? Is it incompetence? Users should be worried that, despite presenting itself as a neutral social media platform, Facebook is trying to control how people think under the guise of "fact checking."

For three years, expert doctors and scientists have watched helplessly, as journalists with no training in medicine have disseminated one-sided propaganda that parrots the opinions of federal health agencies. This has quickly expanded to include media harassment, slander, and, for far too many devoted doctors and scientists, the destruction of their careers—all simply because they were trying to do the right thing for their patients and the general public.

FROM BEYOND REASON TO BEYOND CONTROL

On December 15, 2022, a fifth document release showed that for months, CDC had been pushing for the modRNA "vaccination" of children, despite overwhelming evidence this was not an age group with a significant COVID risk. There was also no evidence proving the modRNA shots' long-term safety or efficacy in children. CDC's own data showed that COVID was less prevalent in children under eighteen, with the percentage of cases significantly trailing the share of the population. Yet, in a briefing slide titled "Policy Considerations," CDC was considering how to inject children *when a parent was not present*.[232]

This was, quite simply, a federal agency out of control.

CHAPTER 6

SAFETY SIGNALS FROM THE VACCINE ADVERSE EVENT REPORTING SYSTEM (VAERS)

By Jessica Rose, PhD

Following the global rollout of the COVID-19 injectable products, millions of individuals reported adverse events (AEs) using pharmacovigilance databases such as the Vaccine Adverse Event Reporting System (VAERS) in the United States, the Yellowcard system in the United Kingdom, the European Union Drug Regulating Authorities (EUDRA) system in Europe, and the Database of Adverse Event Notifications (DAEN) in Australia.[233] These databases reveal the same patterns:

- Atypically high numbers of AEs, and
- A broader range of AEs reported when compared with historical ranges for *all vaccines combined.*

This chapter summarizes the VAERS domestic data up to the time of writing (spring 2023) and highlights the relevance of any excess in AE reporting, or increase in range, in pharmacovigilance settings. Pharmacovigilance is especially relevant in the context of the modified mRNA (modRNA) COVID-19 injectable products manufactured by Pfizer/BioNTech (BNT162b2/Comirnaty) and Moderna (mRNA-1273)[234] because these products involve two novel technologies: the lipid nanoparticles and the modified mRNA encapsulated therein, that have never before been injected into humans en-masse. Analysis suggests the COVID-19 injections are likely the cause of large numbers of serious AEs, including life-changing injuries and deaths.

This chapter addresses some of the most serious AE types associated with the COVID-19 injectable products—including myocarditis and neurological AEs. It must be emphasized that these products have been causally-connected to many other kinds of injuries, including autoimmune disorders (chapter 7) and harms to fertility and pregnancy (chapter 11), which are, however, not addressed in this chapter.[235]

PHARMACOVIGILANCE, DATA INTEGRITY, AND UNDERREPORTING

Pharmacovigilance (PV) is the process of collecting, monitoring, and evaluating AEs to reduce potential harm to the public by calculating risk versus benefit.[236] VAERS acts as a pharmacovigilance tool by serving as an early-warning risk signal detector.

The US Food and Drug Administration (FDA) and Centers for Disease Control and Prevention (CDC) created and implemented VAERS in 1990 to receive reports of AEs that may be associated with biological products such as vaccines. The National Childhood Vaccine Injury Act of 1986 (NCVIA) requires health-care providers and vaccine manufacturers to report AEs to Health and Human Services (HHS) following the administration of vaccines.[237] As a pharmacovigilance tool, the primary purpose of the database is to serve as a signaling system for AEs not detected during premarket testing, such as the Pfizer phase III clinical trial.

It is a federal offense (18 U.S. Code § 1001) to knowingly file a false VAERS report so it is unlikely that there are many reports in the system that are fraudulent.[238] On the contrary, underreporting of AEs is a known and serious disadvantage of VAERS and other pharmacovigilance systems as published by Lazarus et al. 2011.[239]

As a passive reporting system, health-care providers, patients, or family members can technically file a VAERS report. Filing a VAERS report usually involves use of the online system which requires the user to set aside approximately 30 minutes to successfully file a VAERS report due to the multi-page system. Once completed, the individual is provided with a temporary VAERS ID, and once the report is vetted, and if accepted, the temporary VAERS ID is converted to a permanent one for uploading to the front-end user-accessible system.

It is reasonable to assume that many people do not succeed in reaching the permanent VAERS ID status due to 'timing out' on the online system.

In addition, some individuals simply do not even try due to a lack of recognition of association an AE with injection—even when there is a causal connection—further contributing to underreporting of AEs.

Historically, public health authorities have dealt with established underreporting of AEs, and particularly serious adverse events (SAEs), by calculating an underreporting factor for pharmacovigilance data.[240] To calculate the underreporting factor (URF), officials take the number of AEs from the vaccine clinical trial and extrapolate those to the total number of doses delivered in the US during a mass vaccination campaign to calculate the expected number of SAEs (ESAEs). Then they divide the ESAE figure by the number of AE reports received through VAERS, yielding a ratio that is the URF.

Calculation of the underreporting factor for AEs associated with the Pfizer modified mRNA products can be done using the Phase III clinical trial data. According to the FDA Safety Overview of the Pfizer/BioNTech COVID-19 product (Study C4591001—refer to section 5.2.6 page 33), 0.7 percent of Pfizer/BioNTech COVID-19 product recipients suffered SAEs.[241] This figure serves as a benchmark to estimate SAE rates in the general population. As of August 10, 2021, 197,399,471 Pfizer/BioNTech COVID-19 product doses had been administered in the US. Therefore, the number of expected SAE occurrences in US recipients at that time should have been around 1.4 million SAEs, based on the reported rate from the Pfizer/BioNTech clinical trials. Next, this figure is compared to actual reporting of SAEs via the Vaccine Adverse Event Reporting System (VAERS) to estimate the underreporting factor (URF). At that time there were 43,948 VAERS reports of SAEs. Dividing the expected number of SAEs by the reported number yields an underreporting factor of 31, meaning for every SAE report received, roughly thirty more went unreported (a low figure by historic standards).[242]

As of February 10, 2023, approximately 69 percent of the population of the United States received two doses (people fully vaccinated) of the COVID-19 products, with 1,502,065 AEs reported into VAERS, combined domestic and foreign data sets (the system also accepts international reports). There were just shy of one million reports filed in the domestic data set alone on that date. Based on the US domestic data, and using the URF of 31 for all VAERS-classified SAEs, estimates as of mid-February 2023 are as follows: 508,214 dead, 2,341,430 hospitalizations, 3,440,411 ER visits, 433,690 life-threatening events, 502,572 disabled, and 13,485 birth defects.

Considering the magnitude, severity, and range of safety signals emanating from VAERS in the context of COVID-19 products, it is *outrageous* that CDC, HHS, and FDA are not using this pharmacovigilance tool, and not performing proper causality and proportional reporting ratio (PRR) assessments or empirical Bayesian data analyses, as part of standard safety monitoring.[243] As part of the VAERS *Standard Operating Procedures*, published on January 29, 2021, CDC and FDA committed to perform routine VAERS surveillance to identify potential emergent safety concerns in the context of COVID-19 injectable products.[244] These agencies own this data and are responsible for analyzing it as regulators of the safety of biological products, *but it appears they are simply not doing their duty.*

VAERS DOMESTIC DATA

As of February 10, 2023, a staggering number of individuals have reported multiple AEs—ranging from chills to death—to the VAERS domestic database, in the context of the Moderna, Pfizer (mono and bivalent), Janssen, and Novavax COVID-19 injectable products. The number of individuals assigned VAERS IDs on that date was just short of 1 million (918,988). Within this cohort, the percentage of SAEs as a share of AEs stood at 24 percent (366,496)—9 percent above the VAERS handbook standard of 15 percent for other vaccines (a 60 percent increase).[245] In short, many more individuals are dying, being hospitalized, and becoming debilitated than what has been traditionally reported in the context of VAERS.

The fact that the AE reports and SAE reports have reached such excessive numbers, without any consideration of withdrawal, is confounding and alarming. Historically, products have been suspended or withdrawn based on a modest number of safety signals detected in VAERS. For example, in 1998, a hepatitis B vaccine product was linked to multiple sclerosis, followed by suspension.[246] In 1998–1999, rotavirus vaccines licensed in the US were found to contain porcine circovirus (PCV) type 1, and suspended.[247] In 2008, a meningococcal vaccine was withdrawn on suspicion of causing Guillain-Barré syndrome (GBS), a type of paralysis.[248] In 2009, an increased risk of narcolepsy was found following vaccination with a monovalent H1N1 influenza vaccine in several European countries during the H1N1 influenza pandemic, followed by suspension.[249]

The safety signals addressed by CDC or FDA officials over the past two years, in the context of the COVID-19 injectable products, have been limited to a few select adverse-event types—including myocarditis, thrombocytopenia syndrome (TTS), anaphylaxis, Guillain-Barré syndrome, and death—and in each case CDC expressly claims on its website that each event is rare.[250] But this is contradicted by CDC's own evidence.

A COVID-19 "vaccine" safety update by the Advisory Committee on Immunization Practices (ACIP), on June 23, 2021, showed increased myocarditis and pericarditis reporting rates in VAERS.[251] Additional evidence of higher-than-normal reporting rates of myocarditis in VAERS comes from ACIP, in two reports presented on August 30 and October 21, 2021—both titled *Myopericarditis following COVID-19 Vaccination: Updates from the Vaccine Adverse Event Reporting System (VAERS)*. It is striking that both reports reveal more than one hundred times the background reporting rate for males in the twelve-to-fifteen age group.[252]

In spite of these reports—all made by members of CDC's COVID-19 Vaccine Task Force Vaccine Safety Team—AE occurrence has been continually downplayed, described as mild and transient in the case of myocarditis, in particular.[253] Despite mounting evidences of specific harms due to COVID-19 injection-induced myocarditis, in February 2023 ACIP voted to recommend that the modRNA COVID-19 injectable products be added to the immunization schedule for children and adolescents aged eighteen years or younger—a flagrant breach of scientific integrity and regulatory responsibility.[254]

VAERS DATA IN CONTEXT

Perhaps the most compelling evidence of harms from the COVID-19 injectable products can be seen when AE reporting frequency in the context of *only* COVID-19 injectable products is compared to past AE reporting frequencies *for all vaccines combined*. For example, if the ten-year average of the absolute number of death reports (156) for all vaccines combined is compared to the absolute number of death reports for the COVID-19 injectable products administered in the United States in 2021 (9,774), one observes a 6,165 percent increase in absolute death reports. The increase between the ten-year average for all vaccines combined and the three-year average is smaller (at 3,410 percent) but still staggering. When the data per year is normalized to the total number of AEs reported for each respective year, this percent increase between the ten- and three-year averages becomes a 369 percent increase.

Many COVID-19 "vaccine" advocates claim that the excessive reporting of AEs in VAERS, including deaths, simply reflects more shots administered. This is a false claim, as shown by VAERS reports. According to CDC, 193.8 million doses of flu vaccine had been distributed in the United States as of February 26, 2021, for the 2020–2021 flu season—"the highest number of doses in a single flu season."[255] Whereas 558 million doses of COVID-19 "vaccines" were administered in the United States from December 14, 2020, through March 21, 2022[256]—this is 462 days. A flu season is a year (365 days), so it is fair to assume that if 193.8 million doses of flu vaccine were administered in 365 days, then around 245 million doses would be administered in 462 days.

Adjusting for the length of time, there were 2.3 times more doses of COVID product administered than for the flu for the same period of 462 days. It would make sense then, that the rate of reporting in VAERS should be about twice for COVID than for flu, if the products' safety profiles were comparable. Twice as many doses, with a proportional number reporting, should equate to twice as many reports.

On March 25, 2022, according to the WONDER/CDC system, there were 1,696 different types of AEs and 45,650 total AEs reported to VAERS in the context of the fourteen variations of flu vaccines. By contrast there were 10,526 different types of AEs and 5,368,444 total AEs reported to VAERS, in the context of the three variations of the COVID-19 products used in the United States. Given that there were twice as many COVID shots as flu shots administered in the same timeframe, this yields 6.2 times as many types of AE types reported, and *117.6 times as many reports of AEs* in the context of the COVID shots. The massive number and variety of AE reports in the context of the COVID-19 shots therefore cannot simply be the result of more shots being administered.

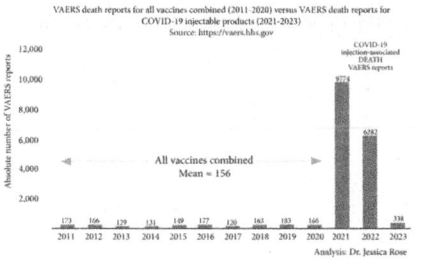 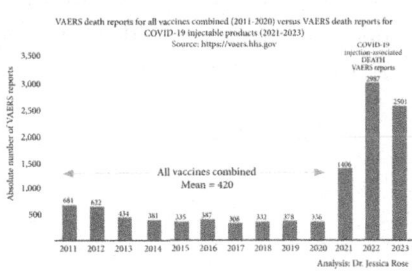

Figure 1: Absolute counts of death adverse event reports in VAERS as of February 10, 2023, for all vaccines combined (2011–2020) versus the COVID-19 products for 2021–2023 (left); normalized to total AE count per year (right).

It is important to note that not everyone who dies in the context of the COVID-19 shots dies immediately following injection. In many cases, for example, heart damage is incurred, and death may follow months or years later. (Note that if an individual with a myocarditis diagnosis does successfully file a VAERS report and subsequently dies, their VAERS report will very likely not be updated to reflect their death. This is just one of the ways that deaths, and many other AEs, are underreported.)

When the data is normalized to the total number of AE reports (Figure 1, right) the frequency of death occurrences in 2021 is higher than for the previous ten-year average. Perhaps even more significant, the frequency of death occurrences doubles in 2022. Since most of the first and second shots were administered in 2021, this is quite concerning and points to the likelihood that *delayed* deaths are occurring. HHS, CDC, and FDA's failure to act in the face of these excess deaths reports is an egregious dereliction of duty.

DEATH REPORTS

Death reports filed to VAERS as of February 10, 2023, tallied 16,394, representing 1.8 percent of all domestic AE reports. The distribution of reports is skewed heavily toward the elderly, but, again, it is not exclusive to the aged.[257]

Importantly, many death reports are clustered within the twenty-four-hour period following injection, a clear temporal signal confirming that the deaths were caused by the injections. The percentage is incrementally higher, depending on the dose: the higher the dose number, the higher the percentage of deaths in the twenty-four-hour window—as shown in Figure 2. This means that, with each successive dose, more people are dying faster after the injection. This indicates that the cumulative impacts of repeat dosing are negative, with people experiencing *more ill effects the more shots they receive.*

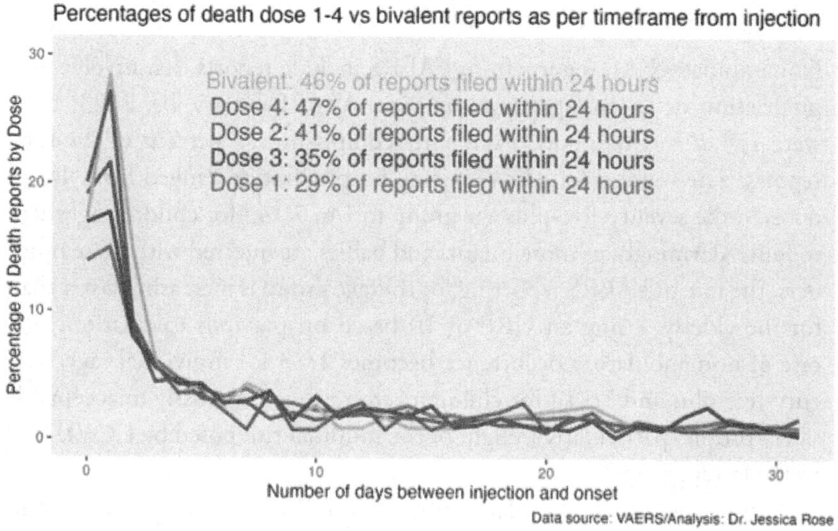
Percentages of death dose 1-4 vs bivalent reports as per timeframe from injection
Bivalent: 46% of reports filed within 24 hours
Dose 4: 47% of reports filed within 24 hours
Dose 2: 41% of reports filed within 24 hours
Dose 3: 35% of reports filed within 24 hours
Dose 1: 29% of reports filed within 24 hours
Percentage of Death reports by Dose
30
20
10
0
0
10
20
30
Number of days between injection and onset
Data source: VAERS/Analysis: Dr. Jessica Rose

Figure 2: Percentages of death reports made from the date of injection to death for doses 1–4 and for the bivalent product.

Dose response is a critical signal in the analysis of biological data with regard to causal assessments. It is, in fact, one of the Bradford Hill criteria, incepted by Sir Austin Bradford Hill in 1965. The Bradford Hill criteria include ten now widely-accepted criteria that, once satisfied, provide strong evidence of a causal relationship. VAERS data represents a data set that can be appraised for causal relationships between specific products and AEs using these criteria.[258] According to the Bradford Hill criterion Dose-Response, greater exposure leads to greater incidence of a given effect. This criterion is in accordance with published reports of immune system dysfunction, and reports of higher rates of COVID-19 associated hospitalization in injected individuals (chapters 1, 5, 7).

Considering that the SARS-CoV2 pathogen has not become more virulent and that, at its deadliest, it demonstrated an infection fatality rate was close to zero, it is unclear why public health authorities would continue to push administration of additional shots.[259] They are not required for acquired and sustained immunity—in fact, waning immunity has been reported, leading to "booster" requirements—and according to this and other data, the COVID-19 shots are inducing cumulative harms, some requiring hospitalization.[260]

NONAMBULATORY REPORTS

Nonambulatory AE reports from VAERS include reports that involve hospitalization or an emergency room visit. As of February 10, 2023, there were 154,204 nonambulatory reports comprising 17 percent of the total reports. The number of AEs requiring hospitalization ranged from 1/833 doses in the seventy-five-plus age group to 1 in 7,143 for children ages zero to four. Alarmingly, as more infants and babies are injected with these products, the rate of VAERS reporting for this age group is increasing faster than for the elderly. Using an URF of 10 based on previous calculations, the rate of nonambulatory occurrence becomes 1/83 for individuals ages seventy-five-plus and 1/714 for children zero to four—a grossly unacceptable safety profile, particularly in light of the minimal risk posed by COVID-19 to the latter group.

Safety signals arising in large numbers require assessment and immediate withdrawal of a product from the market if the product is determined to be the cause. In the case of SAEs like nonambulatory AEs (requiring an emergency room visit or hospitalization), these assessments should be automatic once even a hint of a signal of this type is detected.

NEUROLOGICAL REPORTS

There were 295,962 domestic neurological reports—including paralysis and white matter lesions—as of February 10, 2023, representing 32 percent of all US AE reports. The distribution of reports is clustered around the forty- to forty-nine-year-old age group, which is very concerning, since this cohort is not usually prone to these sorts of neurological issues.

It is also alarming that reports of neurological AEs to young children, including newborns, are being filed to VAERS at a rate of 1/6,250 for the zero-to-four age group. In the case of the forty-to-forty-nine age group, this rate is 1/746. This rate does not address underreporting, so if an URF of 31 is applied here, the rate of neurological AE occurrence becomes 1/24 for people in their forties. While this number is astonishingly high, it must be considered plausible in light of the sheer number and variety of neurological AEs reported, from paresthesia (sensations of numbness, burning, or prickling) to a feeling of being "electrified" (chapter 9).[261]

The signal of neurological harm generated from VAERS has been clear for two years, again requiring an immediate halt to the mass "vaccination" campaign.[262]

CARDIOVASCULAR REPORTS

US cardiovascular reports from VAERS, as of February 10, 2023, peaked at 232,526, representing 25 percent of all domestic AE reports. The distribution of normalized reports ranges from 1/962 doses in the seventy-five-plus age group to 1/8,264 doses in the zero-to-four age group.

Cardiovascular AEs can be very serious. Considering that they are frequently being reported in many young and healthy individuals (21 percent of reports are in individuals twenty-five to thirty-nine), this is extremely concerning and warrants immediate cessation of the modRNA products. Accounting for underreporting with an URF of 31, the rate of occurrence for cardiovascular AEs in individuals ages twenty-five to thirty-nine and older is *at least 1/40*. Soaring rates of myocarditis, in particular, have forced even CDC to acknowledge the trend, although it continues to dramatically underestimate the true incidence.[263]

A. Myocarditis

Myocarditis is inflammation of the myocardium (musculature) of the heart in the absence of ischemia (reduced blood flow and oxygen).[264] Although myocarditis is typically caused by viral infections, it can also result from exposure to toxic substances or immune reactions. Damaged muscle is prone to lethal cardiac arrythmias as well as cardiomyopathy, in which the walls of the heart stretch out, becoming thinner and weaker.[265]

The distribution of normalized reports of myocarditis is clustered around the forty- to forty-nine-year-old age group, but reports of myocarditis in younger age groups have frequently appeared since the beginning of the rollout of the COVID-19 modRNA shots. Incidence ranges from 1/538 doses for people in their forties to 1/5,347 doses for individuals ages five to eleven—markedly higher than CDC estimates. Due to the high number of reports among young people who are not at significant risk of severe COVID-19 disease, it is once again clear that an immediate halt to the rollout of the modRNA products is called for.

Another important finding from the VAERS data is a dose response observed in children, with more doses associated with higher rates of myocarditis. Figure 3 shows the myocarditis reports in VAERS as of March 2023, by age and dose. As noted, dose response is very important for establishing causality, showing that the injuries are in fact due to the "vaccines," not just coincidence. In this case, cumulative exposure to the shots in very young individuals leads to a multifold increase in reporting of AEs. This classic dose-response relationship leaves no doubt: *more shots result in more harm.*

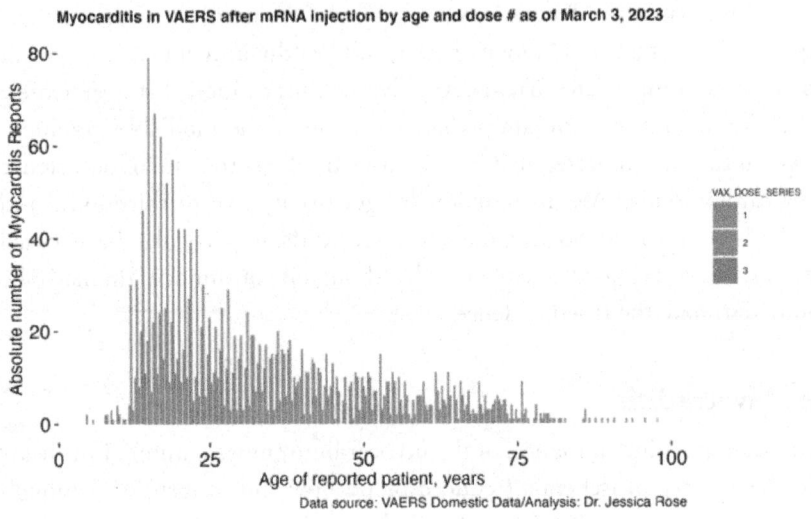

Figure 3: Absolute counts of myocarditis adverse event reports in VAERS as of March 2023, according to age and dose.

B. Cardiac amyloidosis

Cardiac amyloidosis, or "stiff heart" syndrome, is caused by deposits of abnormal proteins in the heart tissue, resulting in the heart no longer functioning properly due to the replacement of normal heart muscle tissue with amyloids. Cardiac amyloidosis is associated with thick heart walls and large atria. It can affect electrical conductivity, resulting in arrhythmias and heart block.[266]

A number of publications have reported that the spike protein of coronaviruses contains amyloidogenic peptides, which can cause cardiac amyloidosis.[267] This can lead to a range of diseases and conditions including heart failure, arrhythmias, orthostatic hypotension, syncope (loss of blood flow to the head, often leading to "passing out" or "fainting"), and pre-syncope.

A keyword search in VAERS for amyloids, fibrin, and syncope yields 23,195 reports. These reports cluster in young individuals—ages twelve to twenty-four. Accounting for underreporting with an URF of 31, this indicates a frequency of possible cardiac amyloidosis in 1/209 young adults ages eighteen to twenty-four. This is especially worrisome because cardiac amyloidosis is not a common diagnosis in this age group, or for injuries following injections, meaning they are unlikely to receive appropriate treatment. Some proportion of myocarditis diagnoses may actually be misdiagnoses of individuals suffering from cardiac amyloidosis.

ADVERSE EVENTS WITH BIVALENT PRODUCTS

Updated (bivalent) "boosters," which first became available on September 2, 2022, were associated with high-frequency reporting of AEs from the first week of the rollout. As of February 2023, there were 21,926 reports in VAERS made in connection with these shots, with 13 percent of the reports classified as serious adverse events (SAEs). Perhaps the most alarming trend in the data is the clustering of reports for children aged fifteen, as shown in Figure 4.

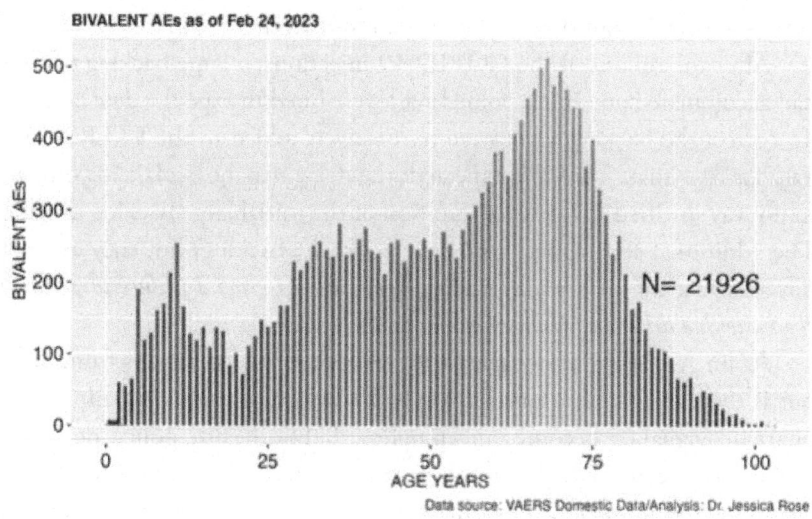

Figure 4: Distribution of VAERS reports in the context of the bivalent shots as of February 24, 2023.

Another important observation within the cohort of injected children under the age of nineteen is that half of the reports (51 percent) involve incorrect product administration either by dose, age, or product. These reports include frequent mentions of lack of dilution of product. *This means that hundreds, perhaps thousands, of children received undiluted products at concentrations not tested on children, with entirely unknown effects.*

DELAYS AND ABDICATIONS OF DUTY

VAERS is a functioning pharmacovigilance tool, but it is not being used as such. In addition to VAERS IDs being deleted without reason,[268] questions surround unusual delays in the publishing of reports, and above all: *Why the whole system is being all but ignored by key stakeholders—HHS, FDA, and CDC* (chapter 5)?

There is evidence that VAERS data were entered into the publicly available dataset much later than one would expect, dramatically lessening their utility as early warning safety signals. The duration between reporting of an AE and recording into the VAERS publicly available data, varies from a few days to many months. It is conceivable that death AEs have extended processing times for the issuance of death certificates, but there is no other valid reason for other AEs, severe or mild, to have delays with regard to data entry—especially not delays greater than four weeks.

After the rollout of the COVID-19 injections, a large backlog of data had accumulated and more trained staff were hired to expedite data entry.[269] To correct the backlog, data were retroactively added to the VAERS database far later than would be expected; the delay may be explained (though in no way justified) by manual curation of the initial large backlog of data. The additional staff appear to have cleared the backlog, but they are still not assessing the data with standard analyses—*a crucial failure to perform the basic due diligence required of our public health agencies.*

Again, VAERS was designed to reveal potential risk signals from data, but if these signals are not analyzed, they are not useful as warnings and pharmacovigilance becomes meaningless. Public health policy decisions might have been made differently if the true rates of reported SAEs and deaths had been available in a timely fashion. Similarly, if individuals knew of SAEs and deaths occurring early in the rollout, they might have exercised their right to informed consent and declined these injections, or waited for more safety data to come in. The delays in publishing AE reports constitute a grievous failure by FDA, CDC, and HHS in the performance of their main duties. The neglect of standard analysis and interpretation, in the face of an unprecedented number of SAEs, can only be considered a betrayal of public trust.

CONCLUSION

It cannot be stressed enough that effective antiviral responses against the SARS-CoV-2 pathogen, in the form of both cellular and humoral immune responses, have been reported in peer-reviewed studies—natural immunity is superior to injection with a foreign antigen (chapters 1, 5).[270] In addition, intramuscular injection is not an efficient way to induce mucosal immunity as required in the case of a pathogen that gains entry to the human body by respiration. Because of the low infection fatality rate, indicative of effective and robust natural (mucosal) immune responses, it is especially unclear why experimental modified mRNA products were fast-tracked through testing, production, and administration to the public, resulting in what might be the largest-scale health/medical disaster in history. It is obstinately clear from the literature, case/clinical studies and pharmacovigilance databases, that the COVID-19 injectable products are not safe or effective. The provably do not prevent infection or transmission, and in fact increase the likelihood of re-emergent COVID-19 (chapter 7). As part of the World Health Organization's own minimum requirements for a functioning pharmacovigilance system, substandard products need to be removed from circulation to ensure patient safety. VAERS data is sending a message loud and clear and has been since January 2021: the COVID-19 injectable products are substandard with regard to safety and efficacy, and should be removed from the market to reduce further public harms. In addition, any current product utilizing the modified mRNA LNP-based platform should be discontinued from use.

CHAPTER 7

IMMUNOLOGICAL HARMS OF THE MODRNA "VACCINES"

By Byram W. Bridle, PhD

As discussed in chapter 1, a real vaccine requires a single shot to protect a healthy person with a mature immune system from getting or spreading an infectious disease. It must also have an excellent short-, mid-, and long-term safety profile based on intense active monitoring in unbiased trials, with a parallel control group receiving only saline solution. A real vaccine confers immunity upon an individual for the remainder of their life through "immunological memory," enabling the immune system to respond rapidly and robustly anytime it sees the pathogen in the future. A real vaccine will *only benefit* and *never harm* the immune system.

THE BENEFITS OF COVID-19 SHOTS WERE EXTREMELY LIMITED

Unfortunately, a retrospective analysis of the COVID-19 modRNA shots demonstrates that their immunological benefits were, at best, few and limited. The shots were designed to target the original Wuhan strain of SARS-CoV-2 and were tested in healthy relatively young people who were at low risk of getting severe COVID-19. Even in that context, the shots were authorized for a global rollout based on their ability to mediate a small reduction in the absolute risk of getting COVID-19. For example, according to Pfizer-BioNTech's original clinical trial data, their COVID-19 shot was able to reduce the chance of getting COVID-19 by only 0.84 percent.[271] Further, the shots quickly became outdated, as a plethora of novel variants took over (chapters 1, 5). The potential for SARS-CoV-2 to cause harm seemed to peak with the Delta variant, but then the virus became less dangerous while simultaneously becoming more transmissible—a common course for a virus evolving to survive long term.[272]

So, while the COVID-19 shots induced short-lived immune responses, limited to a single, "obsolete" part of the virus, these were far from conferring immunity against SARS-CoV-2. Additionally, these immune responses focused on generating antibodies in the blood—not the place where SARS-CoV-2, a respiratory virus, usually infects people. As noted, the immune responses induced by the shots yielded only a small reduction in the absolute risk of symptomatic COVID-19 disease in people who were at relatively low risk of severe COVID-19 to begin with (chapter 5). However, with no impact on infection or transmission, these modest benefits should have been carefully weighed against their known and yet-to-be-determined harms. As the benefits were limited, injecting billions of healthy people with the COVID-19 shots *would only have been warranted if the risks were known to be extremely minimal.*

Sadly, the "warp speed" development of the shots left little time to adequately study potential harms, especially in high-risk populations that were largely excluded from clinical trials (chapters 1, 5). We now know that the COVID-19 shots can cause a wide range of harms, many detailed in this book. These include damage to the immune system itself—*the exact opposite of a vaccine's stated purpose.*

COVID-19 SHOTS FAILED TO RECAPITULATE NATURALLY ACQUIRED IMMUNITY

When judging if a vaccine works, we must always compare it to the gold standard of naturally acquired immunity, resulting from infection and recovery. Considering antiviral immunity, it is important to note that some scientists, like Dr. Anthony Fauci, mistakenly imply that naturally acquired immune responses are generally of poor quality against many respiratory viruses, including influenza viruses and SARS-CoV-2. One of their biggest criticisms is that any protection provided by a natural immune response against these viruses is short-lived.[273]

However, this fails to recognize that the reason people get the flu and COVID-19 again and again is not because of some shortcoming of naturally acquired immunity, but because the viruses that cause these diseases are prone to rapid mutation. *This is simply part of nature, making repeat exposure inevitable.* Each cold and flu season, people are exposed to what are often fundamentally different versions of these viruses. When it comes to viruses that naturally mutate, we can always get reinfected once they change enough to bypass our immunity to the original strain.[274] However, if we don't isolate ourselves from these viruses for excessive periods, and ensure our immune systems are functioning optimally through things like moderate exercise and proper nutrition, most of them will not be able to mutate enough to cause anything more than mild disease for most people.

So, how did the COVID-19 jabs fare in comparison to the gold standard of naturally acquired immunity? *Bluntly, naturally acquired immunity against SARS-CoV-2 was* superior in every way *to the COVID-19 shots.*[275] Naturally acquired immunity was broader and more balanced, meaning previously recovered people generated antibodies targeting multiple components of SARS-CoV-2, not just a single target like the modRNA shots, which were focused exclusively on the spike protein.[276] Naturally acquired immunity also enabled the immune systems of previously infected people to mount antibody responses targeting respiratory tissues, the frontline of infection, and much smaller antibody responses in the blood—obviously not the first place to fight a respiratory infection,[277] and one that carries the risk of autoimmune reactions if too many antibodies are produced, as in the case of the modRNA jabs.

It is not surprising that modRNA shots failed to recapitulate the effectiveness and durability of naturally acquired immunity—a gold standard that is admittedly hard to meet. What was shocking, however, was the blatant disregard of public health authorities for naturally acquired immunity against SARS-CoV-2.[278] There was even evidence, as common sense would suggest, that exposure to previous coronaviruses could provide at least partial protection against the related coronavirus known as SARS-CoV-2.[279] The preposterous notion that the immune system had suddenly lost its ability to protect humankind against a "novel" virus *must never again be allowed to dictate public health policies.*

THE PEOPLE MOST IN NEED OF COVID-19 VACCINES HAD COMPROMISED IMMUNE SYSTEMS

The basic premise of vaccination to protect against COVID-19 was false, because many of the people most in need of protection—including the elderly and people with multiple chronic illnesses or risk factors like obesity—could not respond properly to even ideal vaccines. These are typically the people most at risk from *any* infectious disease, because their immune systems are compromised.[280]

As we get older, our immune system ages, a process called "immunosenescence." The immune systems of frail, elderly people are also more prone to trigger excessive inflammation, the primary cause of severe COVID-19—in effect exacerbating the disease.[281] However, these same issues also prevent them from responding to vaccines nearly as well as younger healthy people. In the case of many chronic diseases such as cancers, a hallmark of compromised immune systems is their *inability to respond robustly to even real vaccines*.[282]

Some fortuitous biological differences protected children against SARS-CoV-2, such as low concentrations of the ACE2 receptors that SARS-CoV-2 needs to infect cells in their airways.[283] It is important to note, however, that the same ACE2 receptors are expressed at concentrations similar to adults in tissues throughout the child's body beyond the airways.[284] This means children are at much lower risk from natural infection with SARS-CoV-2 compared to adults—*but equally susceptible to harms caused by the spike protein when it is unnaturally introduced throughout the body via the COVID-19 shots.*

In summary, the people who most needed protection from SARS-CoV-2 were the same people who could not respond properly to COVID-19 shots, which failed to even confer immunity in young healthy people (chapter 1). Surrounding these high-risk individuals with people who had superior, naturally acquired immunity against SARS-CoV-2 would have been safer than surrounding them with "vaccinated" people who had, at best, suboptimal and short-lived immune responses.[285] Yet counterintuitively, people who got the COVID-19 shots were encouraged to visit and work with the high-risk demographic.[286] Meanwhile, easy-to-do testing for evidence of superior naturally acquired immunity was never implemented.[287]

EVIDENCE FOR IMMUNOLOGICAL HARMS

The COVID-19 modRNA shots were clearly doomed to failure for reasons that should have been obvious to any competent immunologist from the outset. Unfortunately, there is also abundant evidence that the shots also inflicted long-term immune damage.

The COVID-19 Shots Promoted Infection

A number of studies present evidence that COVID-19 is being disproportionately diagnosed among people who took the "vaccines," with more doses correlating with higher risk.[288] This peer-reviewed published science aligns with public health databases, although as we will see, in many cases public health authorities have sought to conceal this data from the public.

Figure 7.1, below, based on data later suppressed by the provincial government of Alberta, Canada, suggests that COVID-19 shots caused substantial acute harm to the immune system. The expectation is that breakthrough cases of COVID-19 should be relatively random post-vaccination, coinciding with waves of infections. However, there was an unusual clustering of cases and hospitalizations due to COVID-19 shortly after receiving a first dose. This is suggestive of immunological suppression, leading to enhanced risk of acquiring COVID-19.

For those tempted to suggest that people receiving shot number one were just particularly unlucky in the following two weeks, please refer to Figure 7.2, which shows similar clustering in proximity to the second dose, followed by the far more random occurrences of breakthrough cases that one would expect. As noted, *these data were removed from public view by provincial public health authorities as soon as their implications became clear.*

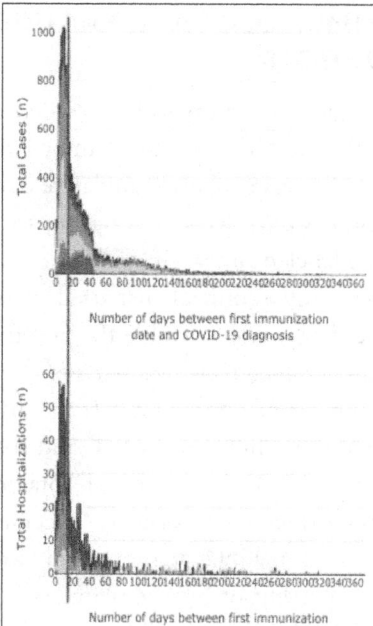

Figure 9.1: Cases of COVID-19 and associated hospitalizations unexpectedly clustered within proximity to inoculation. Of people who got COVID-19 following the first dose of a COVID-19 'vaccine', the majority developed the disease within 14 days (upper graph). The same applied to hospitalizations (lower graph). The vertical red line drawn through the graphs is at fourteen days post-inoculation. Only people beyond this time were defined as 'vaccinated'. So, a large proportion of people impacted by this effect of vaccination were defined as being 'unvaccinated'. These data were obtained from Alberta Public Health on January 14, 2022 (https://www.alberta.ca/stats/covid-19-alberta-statistics.htm).

These data are no longer publicly available.

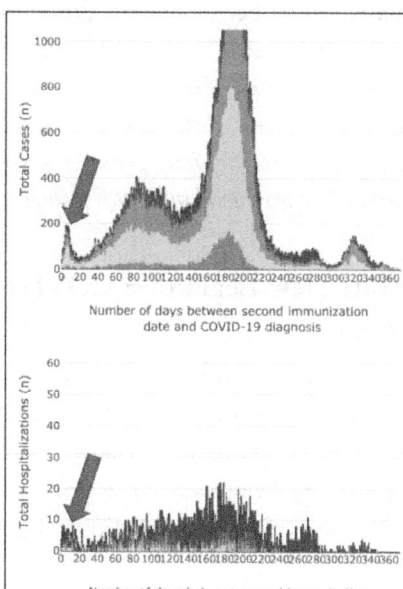

Figure 9.2: Cases of COVID-19 and associated hospitalizations unexpectedly clustered within proximity to inoculation. Of people who got COVID-19 following the second dose of a COVID-19 'vaccine', there was an unusual clustering of cases (top graph; shown by red arrow) and hospitalizations (lower graph; shown by red arrow) attributed to COVID-19 in proximity to receipt of the vaccine. This was followed by cases that followed a pattern typical of waves of an infectious disease. These data were obtained from Alberta Public Health on January 14, 2022 (https://www.alberta.ca/stats/covid-19-alberta-statistics.htm).

These data are no longer publicly available.

ATTEMPTS TO HIDE THE IMMUNOLOGICAL FAILURES AND HARMS OF COVID-19 SHOTS

In fact, there have been many egregious attempts to hide evidence of the immunological harms caused by the COVID-19 shots. Among the best-known strategies to mislead the public was to show cumulative data about cases of COVID-19 by "vaccination" status, with no attempts to identify the naturally immune among those labeled "unvaccinated."

New Zealand was among the many countries that tried to play this trick, but, given enough time, the data could not hide the fact that cases had been occurring *disproportionately among those who received COVID-19 shots*.[289] Breaking down the total number of cases of COVID-19 by "vaccination" status, including groups that were "fully vaccinated" and "boosted," the "unvaccinated" accounted for only 4.08 percent of total cases of COVID-19. In contrast, those who had received a primary "vaccine" series, with or without boosting, accounted for 95.92 percent of all cases. This is disconcerting, because only 89.4 percent of New Zealanders had completed a primary course of the COVID-19 shots as of this analysis.[290] In other words, the data clearly show that cases of COVID-19 have occurred disproportionately among the "fully vaxxed"—and this, despite the massive bias built against the "unvaccinated" described above. So, although the data would suggest that the 89 percent who are "vaccinated" account for 96 percent of the cases, the reality is much worse, due to intentional bias. This is a horrifying outcome for a novel medical intervention. *Vaccines should never increase the risk of acquiring the disease they have been designed to target, and people should* never *be mandated or pressured into taking such a product.*

Canadian Data Corroborate New Zealand's: COVID-19 Shots Increase Risk of Disease

Data from the government of Ontario, Canada, breaks down cases of COVID-19 occurring over time based on "vaccination" status, beginning with the wave of infections caused by the Omicron variant of SARS-CoV-2. When the Omicron wave hit, provincial health authorities could no longer conceal that cases of COVID-19 were being disproportionately diagnosed among the "vaccinated."

Troubling data from the province of Quebec, Canada, also demonstrate that cases of COVID-19, beginning with the Omicron wave, have been diagnosed disproportionately among people who took COVID-19 shots. Specifically, these data demonstrate that COVID-19 has been diagnosed 82 percent and 294 percent more often among those who received two versus three doses, respectively, as compared to the "unvaccinated."

The data even appear to dispel the lingering argument that "vaccinated" people are better protected against severe outcomes of disease than the "unvaccinated." According to these results, a single dose of a COVID-19 shot was, by far, the most protective—yet nobody, not even the companies that made the shots, would advocate for a single dose. Even if these data were taken at face value, it suggests that people who took three doses are still being hospitalized due to COVID-19 at a greater rate than the "unvaccinated." No matter which way one interprets these findings, one conclusion is crystal clear: the scientific data demand that the COVID-19 shots be stopped.

It is of course extremely concerning that most public health data showing cases of COVID-19 disproportionately occurring among the "vaccinated" were removed from public view, once it became apparent that this was not a transient phenomenon—falsifying the prevailing narrative.

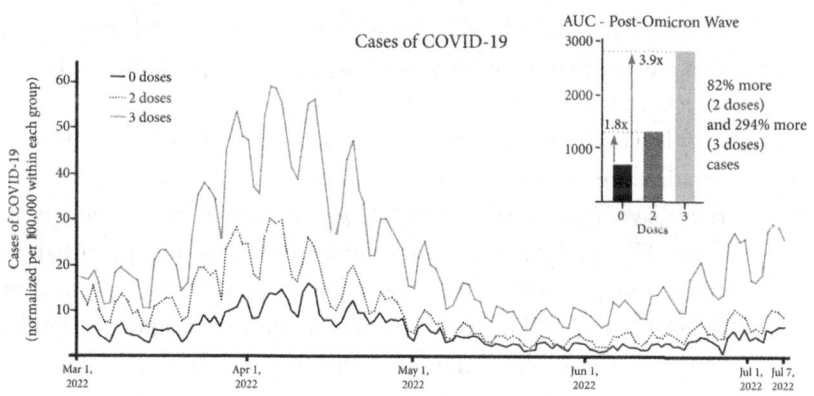

Figure 3: Cases of COVID-19 Occurring Disproportionately Among the "Vaccinated."
The larger of the two graphs shows cases of COVID-19 based on "vaccination" status. The smaller graph in the upper right-hand corner depicts the area under each curve (AUC), which is a way to evaluate the accumulation of cases over time. Data for these graphs came from the National Institute of Public Health of Quebec (INSPQ), Health Montreal, Quebec Ministry of Health and Social Services.
Original source: https://www.ledevoir.com/documents/special/2020-07-22-evolution-covid19-quebec/index.html

These data were not provided beyond July 7, 2022.

Accruing evidence that the shots made people more likely to get COVID-19 leaves no doubt that mandating them was not only unnecessary but wholly counterproductive. Naturally, it also raises the question:

What mechanisms could explain how COVID-19 shots are making people more susceptible to infection?

POTENTIAL MECHANISMS OF HARM

- *Loss of white blood cells.* White blood cells, also called "lymphocytes," are the primary weapons used by the immune system to fight off viral infections. From the earliest clinical trials, it was known that COVID-19 shots could cause a condition called "lymphopenia," or a decrease in the number of white blood cells circulating in the blood.[291] A reduction in circulating white blood cells would be expected to increase susceptibility to getting infected with viruses, including SARS-CoV-2, and could explain the phenomenon of acute susceptibility to COVID-19 after people got their first modRNA shot—as shown in Figure 1. The data shown in Figure 2 suggest this phenomenon might contribute to susceptibility to infection with SARS-CoV-2, after the second dose as well.

- *Induction of tolerance to SARS-CoV-2.* Primary scientific evidence shows that repeated dosing with modRNA COVID-19 shots causes SARS-CoV-2 spike-specific antibodies to switch from types that have antiviral mechanisms of action to a type known as IgG4, which lack effective antiviral mechanisms.[292] This suggests that people who received COVID-19 shots, unlike those with naturally acquired immunity, could progressively lose what little protection they have against SARS-CoV-2, *particularly as they receive more doses*. Worse, IgG4-type antibodies even have the potential to cause some people to become tolerant to the spike protein of SARS-CoV-2.[293] This could result in some "vaccinated" people, especially those who had more than two doses, *becoming even more susceptible to COVID-19 than if they had never received the shots in the first place*.

- *Vaccine-enhanced disease.* Historically, coronavirus vaccines have been plagued by a problem known as "vaccine-enhanced disease," in which a vaccine *actually makes the disease worse*.[294] This can also result from other inappropriate immune responses, such as the exacerbation of inflammation in the lungs of vaccinated monkeys infected with SARS-CoV-1, cause of the original SARS outbreak in 2003.[295] In view of this history, the risk of vaccine-enhanced disease should have been definitively ruled out prior to the public rollout of the COVID-19 shots. However, safety testing takes time. Remarkably, as the shots were being rolled out, briefing documents submitted to FDA stated: "…risk of vaccine-enhanced disease over time, potentially associated with waning immunity, remains unknown and needs to be evaluated further in ongoing clinical trials and in observational studies that could be conducted following authorization and/or licensure."[296] In plain language, this means that instead of properly evaluating the potential for the shots to increase the severity or risk of acquiring COVID-19, public health authorities decided the risk could be assessed within the global population—*essentially enrolling humanity in a vast experiment.*

- *Immunological imprinting.* An immunological phenomenon known as "immunological imprinting" (also sometimes referred to as the principle of "original antigenic sin") essentially states that a person's immune system will become permanently trained to respond to the first version of a foreign pathogen it encounters, including various classes of viruses and bacteria. This means that later, on encountering a similar but not identical pathogen, our immune system activates immune memory cells and produces antibodies targeted to the historic threat, which are likely less effective against the newly evolved pathogen. Immunological imprinting has been demonstrated in endemic viruses including influenza, RSV, HIV, cytomegalovirus (CMV), dengue, and other coronaviruses.[297]

In the case of the COVID-19 modRNA "vaccines," immunological imprinting occurs when the immune system learns to target different parts of the spike protein (chapter 4). Antibodies binding to some parts of the spike protein can neutralize the virus, but antibodies keyed to other parts of the spike provide little or no protection. *However, the immune system retains immunological memory of these ineffective targets anyway.*

As SARS-CoV-2 mutates to evade nonlethal immunological pressure from the COVID-19 shots, the new mutations naturally tend to occur in parts of the spike protein that allow a person to neutralize the virus. Therefore, there is no need for the virus to change parts of the spike protein where antibodies are ineffective for neutralizing the virus.

When new "vaccines," like the bivalent COVID-19 "boosters" or fall 2023 monovalent "booster," are used, they will cause immunological imprinting to take effect. Specifically, the new spike protein (derived from the Omicron variant) differs from the spike in the Wuhan variant in regions that cause the virus to be neutralized—but still shares the non-neutralizing parts.

Since the immune systems of people who received the original modRNA injections retain memory of non-neutralizing parts of the spike protein, they automatically produce extremely high concentrations of essentially useless antibodies against these irrelevant targets. *This strong but ineffective response to inactive parts of the spike protein comes at the expense of antibodies that could actually be neutralizing and protective.* In other words, people who received modRNA injections coding for the original Wuhan strain of SARS-CoV-2 cannot respond nearly as well to new variants with mutated spike proteins, and those receiving "boosters" are likewise sacrificing an important part of their immune response.

In contrast, those with naturally acquired immunity maintain much better protection, because their immune systems have mounted full-spectrum responses to many other components of the virus, such as the proteins of the central nucleocapsid structure, which don't change as much, but still allow neutralization. This would be an example of the COVID-19 shots causing the immune system to change in a way that places people at risk of not being able to mount proper immune responses against SARS-CoV-2 and related future pathogenic coronaviruses.

COVID-19 "VACCINES" ARE MORE DANGEROUS TO PEOPLE WITH PREEXISTING IMMUNITY

The superiority of naturally acquired immunity against SARS-CoV-2 was never acknowledged throughout the COVID-19 pandemic. This is particularly egregious because evidence suggests that harmful side effects of the COVID-19 shots were *more common and more severe in people with preexisting immunity against SARS-CoV-2*, possibly due to autoimmune response.[298] At the very least, people should have been tested to determine if they had preexisting immunity against SARS-CoV-2 before offering them a COVID-19 shot—an easy test to perform, with a number of vendors, which has been largely neglected, despite obvious utility.[299] Such testing would also have provided accurate data about the immunity status of the population, which, in turn, would have enabled more informed predictive modeling and policy decisions.

A RISK-BENEFIT ANALYSIS

At the population level, no public health agency seems to have considered the possibility that a mass rollout of COVID-19 shots would not only fail to confer immunity but could in fact contribute to the emergence of immune-evasive variants of SARS-CoV-2. The COVID-19 shots were pushed most vigorously upon high-risk demographics such as the elderly, sick, and immunosuppressed. These people received the highest number of shots—*despite not being represented in the original clinical trial population and not being able to respond immunologically to vaccines*. A proper risk-benefit analysis for these people would have accounted for the expected very poor efficacy of the COVID-19 shots, along with the cumulative risks of getting multiple doses—a recognized danger (chapters 1, 5, 6, 13).

The shortcomings and harms of the modRNA "vaccines," still only partially understood, call into question future use of modRNA technology to control infectious disease. One thing is certain: there needs to be a massive amount of research conducted to properly understand modRNA-based agents. In the meantime, for the safety and health of the global population, there needs to be a complete moratorium on this technology.

CHAPTER 8

CARDIAC AND CARDIOVASCULAR DAMAGE FROM THE MODRNA "VACCINES"

By Dr. Peter A. McCullough, MD, MPH

Some of the most serious potential dangers of the modRNA "vaccines" are injuries to the heart and circulatory system, including myocarditis (inflammation of the heart muscle) and thrombosis (blood clots). These injuries raise the risk of heart failure and strokes. In addition to sudden death, both conditions can also result in long-term damage, leading to disability and premature death later on.

Public health authorities have admitted that the modRNA "vaccines" cause myocarditis and blood clots but significantly understate the incidence rate, falsely claiming these dangerous side effects are "very rare."[300] While US public health authorities have neglected to determine how common these conditions really are, international research indicates that myocarditis and blood clots pose an unwarranted hazard, especially to healthy young people.

MYOCARDITIS AND PERICARDITIS

Myocarditis refers to inflammation of the myocardium, the heart's muscle tissue. It is most likely to affect adolescent boys and young men after the second dose of modRNA pro-vaccine but has been observed in all ages and both sexes post-"vaccination." Myocarditis and pericarditis—a related condition affecting the pericardium (the tissue lining the outside of the heart)—result when the spike protein generated by the modRNA pro-vaccine triggers an inflammatory response in those tissues.

More research is required to understand how the "vaccines" cause inflammation of heart tissue, but there are a number of plausible overlapping explanations, centering on the fact that the spike protein generated by the modRNA pro-vaccine is itself pathogenic (disease-causing). Because the modRNA shots don't remain in the upper arm, at the site of injection, but circulate throughout the body, "vaccination" exposes a wide variety of organs and tissues to the harmful spike protein, including three important kinds of heart cells: (1) endothelial cells, lining the inside of the heart; (2) myocytes, the muscle cells that make the heart pump; and (3) pericytes, which play key roles in cardiac function and repair, including protecting blood vessels.

- A study by Salk Institute researchers in March 2021 showed that the spike protein can damage endothelial tissue by lowering levels of ACE2, an enzyme that helps control the activity of mitochondria, the "powerhouses" of animal cells, fragmenting the mitochondria and causing inflammation.[301]

- A study published in December 2021 showed that the spike protein disrupted the activity of pericytes, resulting in inflammation of the heart tissue and damage to blood vessels.[302]

- Research first presented in July 2022 showed that the spike protein is also toxic to myocytes, or heart muscle cells.[303] A study published in September 2023 found "vaccine" modRNA in myocardial cells up to thirty days after injection, highlighting the lasting threat to these critical heart cells.[304]

- Linking these findings together, in January 2023 a study showed that myocarditis is strongly linked to the level of "free" (i.e., not neutralized by antibodies) spike protein in blood plasma, indicating the spike protein itself is pathogenic.[305]

Myocarditis could be caused by spike protein damage alone or in concert with other processes suggested by scientists, including autoimmune reactions.[306] Whatever the precise mechanisms, all the different explanations are grounded in the fact that the modRNA injections don't stay in the vaccination site, as originally claimed, but spread throughout the body, triggering harmful reactions wherever they go (chapter 4).

POST-VACCINATION MYOCARDITIS IS MORE COMMON THAN OFFICIAL CLAIMS

The CDC has stated that myocarditis resulting from modRNA "vaccination" is "rare," "usually mild," and "resolves quickly," with an estimated incidence of one symptomatic case per 2,800 males aged twelve to seventeen within three weeks of the second dose.[307] However, these estimates are based on flawed and incomplete data, and fail to address the issue of "hidden" or "subclinical" myocarditis, often occurring without symptoms, which can still result in serious heart damage.

Studies conducted overseas suggest significantly higher rates of post-"vaccination" myocarditis in high-risk groups:

- A Hong Kong study estimated the incidence of myocarditis and pericarditis at around 1 in 2,700 adolescent males after the second Pfizer shot.[308]
- A study of 4,928 Taiwanese high school students found 17.1 percent experienced cardiac symptoms after receiving the second dose of the Pfizer "vaccine," including one case of myocarditis and four others with "significant arrhythmia."[309]
- Mansanguan et al. used a prospective cohort study in children ages thirteen to eighteen on the second administration of Pfizer and found the rate of adjudicated myocarditis and pericarditis was 2.3 percent. Out of 301 Thai high school students screened, 29 percent experienced cardiac symptoms, including one student diagnosed with myopericarditis, as well as four with suspected subclinical myocarditis and two with suspected pericarditis.[310]
- LePessec et al. used a prospective cohort design measuring cardiac troponin, an inflammatory marker, on the third administration of mRNA in health-care workers and found that 2.8 percent of subjects experienced elevated troponin.[311]
- A South Korean study published in June 2023 documented 480 cases of post-"vaccination" myocarditis, including twenty-one deaths, suggesting mortality rates far exceeding negligible estimates from US public health officials.[312]

All these figures must be judged against the very low mortality rate from COVID-19 infection among healthy children and teenagers, most of whom have already been infected with the virus at least once, according to the CDC, and therefore enjoy natural immunity far superior to "vaccination" (chapters 1, 5, 7).[313]

Claims that myocarditis associated with COVID-19 infection is more common and more severe than myocarditis resulting from "vaccination" are not supported by scientific evidence. An Israeli study compared 196,992 individuals who experienced acute COVID-19 infection with a control group of 590,976 individuals, representing the baseline rate in the population. The study showed that 0.0102 percent of individuals with COVID-19 infection were diagnosed with myocarditis or pericarditis, comparable to the control group rate of 0.013 percent, leading the authors to conclude: "Post COVID-19 infection was not associated with either myocarditis... or pericarditis.... We did not observe an increased incidence of either pericarditis or myocarditis in adult patients recovering from COVID-19 infection."[314]

It should be noted that myocarditis associated with COVID-19 infection is more prevalent among older adults than younger adults, and is significantly correlated with comorbidities associated with age. US research from December 2022 showed 77.6 percent of myocarditis cases with COVID-19 infection in hospitalized patients occurred in individuals ages fifty-plus, compared to just 6.1 percent occurring in individuals ages eighteen to twenty-nine (who were also more likely to have significant comorbidities like type 2 diabetes, heart disease, and obesity).[315] Put simply, myocarditis with COVID-19 infection is a disease of the old and sick, while myocarditis with modRNA "vaccination" is a disease of the young and healthy.

The very low rate of symptomatic myocarditis and pericarditis associated with COVID-19 infection in the Israeli study (0.0102 percent = 1/9,804) must be weighed against the findings discussed above, suggesting symptomatic myocarditis rates of 1/301 to 1/2,700 in healthy adolescent boys and young men post-"vaccination." On that note, an independent analysis of VAERS data warned: "In boys with prior infection and no comorbidities, even one dose carried more risk than benefit according to international estimates."[316] In light of CDC's own finding that most children have already experienced prior infection, *even one dose must be considered too risky for healthy young people across the board.*[317]

Studies purporting to show postinfection incidence of myocarditis higher than the incidence of post-"vaccination" myocarditis are limited by a common methodological flaw in defining the study population. Typically, these studies focus on cases of myocarditis following a positive COVID-19 test.[318] However, the composition of these study groups naturally tends to be skewed by selection bias toward individuals seeking out PCR tests, who are more likely to be experiencing symptomatic COVID-19 infection in the first place, *and therefore more likely to experience severe disease, including myocarditis*.[319] Study groups for postinfection myocarditis naturally tend to exclude most asymptomatic and subclinical cases, which, however, outnumber cases confirmed by PCR tests *by a multiple of three or more*, depending on the location and period of the pandemic.

The exclusion of large numbers of asymptomatic or mildly symptomatic cases, who by definition experience lower rates of infection-related myocarditis, must significantly change the observed results, and thus any comparison of the incidence of viral myocarditis with the incidence of myocarditis post-"vaccination."[320] For example, in February 2022 seroprevalence testing showed that 57.7 percent of the US population had experienced COVID-19 infection, or around 200 million people, compared to a total of fewer than 75 million test-confirmed cases up to that time.[321] Therefore any analysis of the incidence of postinfection myocarditis, or any other condition, using test-confirmed cases would be off by a factor proportional to the prevalence of undiagnosed COVID-19 infections—the actual population-level numbers of infected and recovered as reflected in seroprevalence figures.

At the same time, underreporting of "vaccine" adverse effects, as discussed in chapters 5 and 6, likely applies to post-"vaccination" myocarditis, including evidence of substantially higher rates of asymptomatic myocarditis accompanying "vaccination" than is officially acknowledged.

A pre-pandemic study of myocarditis following vaccination for another disease, smallpox, concluded that "passive surveillance significantly underestimates the true incidence of myocarditis/pericarditis" after vaccination, with a rate over two hundred times the population background rate. The authors emphasized that long-term effects are largely unknown.[322] The Thai study by Mansanguan et al., referenced above, found that 58 percent of post-modRNA "vaccination" myocarditis cases were asymptomatic, while the Swiss study by LePessec et al. found elevated troponin in otherwise healthy subjects.[323] A study of 566 patients at a preventive cardiology clinic using PULS—an assessment tool measuring cardiac stress chemicals—showed dramatically elevated levels of key biomarkers signaling cardiac damage after modRNA "vaccination," increasing the cohort's assessed average five-year risk of acute coronary syndrome from 11 percent to 25 percent, despite absence of symptoms.[324]

LONG-TERM RISKS

Official claims that most cases of myocarditis following modRNA "vaccination" are "mild" and get better on their own ignore the possibility of lingering heart damage well after symptoms resolve.[325]

Studies of long-term outcomes in myocarditis patients conducted before the pandemic consistently show increased risk of heart failure and hospitalization, sometimes years after the initial incident. A Danish study tracked 1,557 patients diagnosed with myocarditis from 1996–2016, and concluded, "Myocarditis in younger patients without prior cardiac disease was associated with a long-term excess risk of [heart failure] hospitalization, and death," with an incidence of heart failure hospitalization over four times the control group and a death rate double the control group.[326]

While only a few small studies of long-term outcomes following COVID "vaccine"-induced myocarditis have been published, they suggest cause for concern. Researchers at Vanderbilt University followed 151 patients who experienced myocarditis after "vaccination" with cardiac MRIs at least ninety days later, and found roughly half (47 percent) showed "late gadolinium enhancement," a sign of myocardial fibrosis or scar tissue on the heart.[327] Among the larger study cohort of "recovered" individuals, 26 percent were still taking medication for their condition at least ninety days later, and 20 percent of survey respondents said they still had trouble with everyday activities. Three smaller studies reported similar findings, with the majority of patients showing signs of cardiac injury up to six months later.[328] The authors registered concern about the possibility of lasting damage, noting the lack of knowledge about the long-term prognosis of post-"vaccination" myocarditis.

This concern is well-founded. Myocardial scar tissue can disrupt electrical signaling in the heart, leading to heart failure, particularly when exposed to stress response hormones, called catecholamines, which are released in large amounts during exercise. Up to 20 percent of acute myocarditis cases may go on to develop dilated cardiomyopathy, a condition in which the walls of the heart's chambers stretch and become thinner, again raising the risk of heart failure.[329] Individuals who suffer post-"vaccination" myocarditis are also at risk of chronic myocarditis, or long-lasting inflammation of the heart tissue, which can continue without resolution for months or even years, leaving lingering debility.

mRNA "VACCINE" ➔ MYOCARDITIS ➔ OUTCOMES

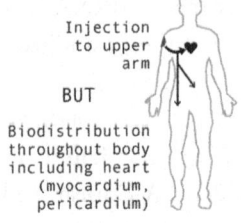

Injection to upper arm
BUT
Biodistribution throughout body including heart (myocardium, pericardium)

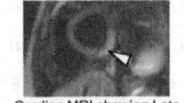

Cardiac MRI showing Late Gadolinium Enhancement (LGE)

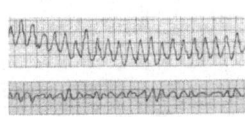

ARRHYTHMIAS
• Ventricular Tachycardia
• Ventricular Fibrillation

RISK FACTORS
♂ Peak risk men ages 18-24
Genetic predisposition: SCN5A mutation
• "Hot lots" of well-manufactured, high-purity mRNA adenoviral DNA
• Cumulative spike protein exposure
• Pericyte uptake of mRNA and production of spike protein

DIAGNOSIS
• Presenting, ~90% hospitalized
• ECG changes
• Troponin, BNP, ST2, Galectin 3
• Arrhythmias
• Ventricular dysfunction
• Positive MRI for LGE (see above)
• Biopsy shows spike-protein+ inflammation

COLLAPSE

SYMPTOMS
57% SUBCLINICAL (few/no symptoms)
• 43% symptomatic: chest pain, effort intolerance, palpitations, near/syncope ("passing out") fever, malaise, myalgia

DETECTION
 IF DETECTED: NO EXERCISE
• Meds, defibrill. in high-risk patients; repeat testing for resolution
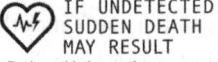 IF UNDETECTED: SUDDEN DEATH MAY RESULT
• During athletic exertion
• While asleep in early morning hours

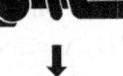
"SUDDEN ADULT DEATH SYNDROME"

© 2023 Dr. Peter McCullough

Guidance papers in cardiology for years before COVID-19 stressed the importance of abstention from sports in the setting of myocarditis. It is well known that the surge of adrenaline with exercise can trigger lethal arrhythmias and sudden death. This is of great concern because the vast majority of patients who have received the "vaccine," including many healthy young athletes, have not been screened for myocarditis.

BLOOD CLOTS, HEART ATTACK, AND STROKE

Thrombosis (blood clots) caused by the modRNA "vaccines" can trigger heart attacks and strokes in "vaccinated" individuals, leading to disability or death, as well as a variety of other injuries to the circulatory system. As with myocarditis and other "vaccine"-related injuries, public health authorities have understated how often thrombosis occurs after "vaccination," while neglecting to undertake the large-scale screening studies needed to determine its actual frequency.

More investigation is required to understand how the modRNA pro-vaccines cause blood clots, but once again many of the most plausible theories are based on the fact the spike protein itself is harmful (chapter 4):

- The spike protein binds angiotensin-converting enzyme 2 (ACE2) directly to platelets and endothelial cells, setting off a "coagulation cascade" and forming blood clots.[330]
- The spike protein binds and disables heparan sulfate, a chemical that usually regulates heparin, a clotting factor, making clotting more likely.[331]
- The spike protein interacts with fibrinogen, a protein that plays a key role in coagulation, to form blood clots that are especially resistant to the body's natural anti-clotting chemicals.[332]
- The spike protein causes hemagglutination, or clumping of red blood cells, via electrostatic attraction between glycans (long carbohydrate molecules) on the tip of the spike and complementary glycoconjugates (carbohydrates bonded to lipids or proteins) on the red blood cells.[333]
- Interaction between the spike protein and toll-like receptor 2 (TLR2) causes thrombosis by encouraging the formation of "neutrophil extracellular traps"—tangles of fiber created by white blood cells to catch foreign pathogens.[334]
- Interaction between the spike protein and toll-like receptor 4 (TLR4) causes platelet-related thrombosis.[335]
- Spike proteins have been found in blood clots from patients who suffered heart attacks or strokes during COVID infection, again suggesting the spike protein is a pathogen on its own.[336]

While US public health officials maintain that cardiovascular risks of the modRNA pro-vaccines are rare, once again data from foreign countries tell a different story:

- A study of 265,339 hospital visits by "vaccinated" individuals in Norway, Finland, and Denmark found that the Moderna modRNA "vaccine" increased the risk of coronary artery disease by 13 percent, coagulation disorders by 26 percent, and cerebrovascular disease by 21 percent, while Pfizer increased the risk of coagulation disorders by 12 percent and cerebrovascular disease by 9 percent. Both modRNA "vaccines" also showed increased rates of thrombocytopenia, or low blood platelets, and central venous thrombosis, when a blood clot forms in the brain.[337]

- A study of 1.8 million Pfizer recipients in the UK found that the first shot increased the risk of venous thromboembolism, or blood clots in veins, by roughly 12 percent.[338]

Foreign studies have focused specifically on vascular injuries in the brain:

- An English study of over 12 million Pfizer recipients found a 38 percent increase in hemorrhagic strokes fifteen to twenty-one days after "vaccination," in which a ruptured blood vessel causes bleeding in the brain, along with increased risk of other neurological disorders.[339]

- A study of over 5.5 million Pfizer "vaccine" recipients in Hong Kong found a 169 percent increase in hemorrhagic strokes in the thirteen-day period following the second shot.[340]

- A study of 9.5 million English Pfizer "vaccine" recipients found a 258 percent increase in cerebral venous sinus thrombosis, in which a blood clot forms in the venous sinuses, potentially causing hemorrhage.[341]

Long-term negative outcomes are a real concern. One of the most comprehensive studies to date examined the incidence of blood clots leading to retinal arterial and vascular occlusion (when a clot blocks blood vessels serving the eye) in 739,066 "vaccinated" subjects, over a two-year period following "vaccination," comparing them with a matched cohort of unvaccinated subjects. The study found "vaccinated" individuals were 119 percent more likely to suffer from retinal vascular occlusion—which can result from blood clots arising anywhere in the body—adding that they "had significantly increased risk of retinal vascular occlusion *2 years following vaccination*"[342] (emphasis added).

Based on these data, where retinal vascular disease strongly predicts fatal and nonfatal atherosclerotic events, we can anticipate a sharp rise in myocardial infarction (heart attack), stroke, and peripheral vascular disease, warranting intervention and amputation. Additionally, it is very likely that the "vaccinated" are to some extent hypercoagulable, or prone to blood clots. That means the risk of blood clots (venous thromboembolism) with the usual provoking incident (surgery, prolonged immobilization, estrogen use) is even greater among the "vaccinated," for years into the future.

Once again, all these findings must be weighed against the very low risk of COVID-19 infection to healthy young people, including cardiovascular complications such as blood clots, with one study concluding, "Thrombodic or thromboembolic events are rare in pediatric patients with COVID-19 infection and MIS-C."[343] Like other serious complications, when blood clots have occurred in children with COVID-19 infection, they are associated with preexisting major comorbidities like cancer, morbid obesity, or other risk factors that make the patients more likely to develop severe disease in general.[344]

Studies claiming to show higher incidence of blood clots with COVID-19 infection than post-"vaccination" suffer from the same testing bias described above: they exclude large numbers of asymptomatic individuals who are less likely to experience these complications. Like myocarditis, the risks of blood clots from the modRNA "vaccines" must be judged in view of widespread natural immunity resulting from prior COVID-19 infection among young people, conferring protection far superior to "vaccination."[345]

CHAPTER 9

NEUROLOGICAL INJURIES FROM THE MODRNA "VACCINES"

By Matt Bain, MD

Neurological injuries are a long-established potential side effect of all vaccines but have generally been rare and transient, resolving on their own fairly quickly.[346] In recent decades new vaccines have been withdrawn from the market after even modest numbers of neurological injuries, the most notable of which was the withdrawal of the 1976 H1N1 swine flu vaccine following an increased incidence of Guillain-Barré syndrome in patients in New Jersey, after vaccination.[347] By contrast, the COVID-19 modRNA "vaccines" have been linked to large numbers of neurological injuries, yet mystifyingly remain on the market—an unprecedented failure of oversight by public health authorities.

This chapter offers only a preliminary overview of this emerging data. Injuries related to SARS-CoV-2 modRNA injections will require years of research before we can fully understand all the potential mechanisms inflicting nervous system damage. As things stand, simply trying to determine how many people have suffered neurological injuries from the modRNA shots is challenging, due to the lack of adequate safety monitoring by public health agencies. However, the available evidence indicates neurologic injuries are both *far more common and more severe than official claims.*

I first publicly articulated my opposition to the modRNA injections in public testimony to Indiana legislators in February 2022.[348] One year later, I reluctantly resigned as assistant professor of neurology at a large academic medical center where I'd spent my whole career in general neurology practice, managing patients in both outpatient and inpatient settings, due to the same concerns over modRNA "vaccine" safety.

I have never considered myself "anti-vax." In fact, in fall 2020, my initial enthusiasm for the concept of COVID vaccination prompted me to volunteer for the AstraZeneca trial of its DNA-based adenovector "vaccine," only to have the study stalled by surprising neurological injuries. Just a few months later, this was followed by my personal experience diagnosing the same kind of neurologic adverse effects seen with the AstraZeneca adenovector product, many of them serious, in patients who had recently received the modRNA shots.

As the pandemic unfolded, the censorship and quashing of discussion of adverse effects from the modRNA "vaccines," and the disregard for the sanctity of the physician-patient relationship—particularly compulsory compliance by practitioners with "vaccine mandates," in conflict with their own understanding of science—violated every principle of my practice as a physician. Sadly, bureaucratic edicts appear to have supplanted evidence-driven decision-making, and many brave professionals have been forced to choose between integrity and employment. Inspired by their example, we must at least try to begin to understand the wave of injuries we are now facing.

BACKGROUND: IMMUNOLOGY AND NEUROLOGY

The effort to establish a possible causal relationship between the SARS-CoV-2 injections and neurologic injury starts with having a sufficient index of suspicion to ask a patient whether, and when, she or he received an injection. When considering whether modRNA injection could be the cause of a patient's symptoms, the clinician must first exclude all other reasonably plausible causes. Other important questions include: Has the condition been reported with other vaccines? And what is the annual incidence of this diagnosis, meaning the rate at which the condition appears in a population under normal (pre-pandemic) circumstances over the course of a year? These two questions are critical, as there are many neurological illnesses whose proximate causes remain uncertain; for example, the exact cause for multiple sclerosis (MS) is not fully understood today, even though there are several hypotheses, including an association with Epstein-Barr virus.

As nearly all these conditions involve impairment or dysregulation of the immune system, it is helpful to have some familiarity with normal immune function to appreciate the mechanisms involved (chapters 1, 5, 7). The immune system is composed of the *innate immune system*, the first line of defense, and the *adaptive immune system*, which can deliver a more targeted, seek-and-destroy response.

- The white blood cells of the *innate immune system* consist of cell types (e.g., macrophages, natural killer T lymphocytes, and microglia) that are nonspecific in their ability to attack foreign material (e.g., viruses, toxins and non-self proteins), generally leading to inflammatory responses.

- The *adaptive immune system* is more refined in its ability to specifically target certain pathogens and foreign material, typically with responses mediated by the antibodies formed to different parts of the virus. The adaptive immune system (informed by CD4+ helper T lymphocytes and their interaction with antigen presenting cells [APCs]), also has "memory" of previous exposures, which can last for years.

The cells of the adaptive immune system must be "trained" in tissue outside the bone marrow (thymus gland, spleen, and lymph nodes) to recognize "self" cells (meaning the body's own cells) through their interactions with a collection of genes called major histocompatibility complex I (MHC I) that are expressed on all "self" cells. Major histocompatibility complex II (MHC II) is expressed on the surface of antigen-presenting cells (dendritic cells, macrophages, microglia) that bring foreign pathogens to the attention of the immune system and are critical to the formation of B lymphocytes (immune cells which form antibodies), cytotoxic T lymphocytes, and autoimmune responses. Microglia are the primary APCs for the central nervous system and play an important role in inflammation and neurodegeneration.

FIRSTHAND CLINICAL OBSERVATIONS OF NEUROLOGICAL INJURIES

I have treated the following cases of neurological injury from January 2021 to present. Each diagnosis has been represented in the Vaccine Adverse Event Reporting System (VAERS) and, in many cases, the medical literature. While they serve as only a partial illustration of the many neurologic adverse events that have been reported following administration of SARS-

CoV-2 modRNA injections, they suggest potential common mechanisms for other neurological injuries following the injections.

1. *Acute transverse myelitis (ATM).* This is acute inflammation of the spinal cord resulting in symptoms including weakness, sensory loss, loss of bowel/bladder control, loss of regulation of blood pressure/heart rate (dysautonomia), and pathologically brisk muscle stretch reflexes (MSRs). ATM was the first diagnosis I encountered in previously healthy patients following modRNA injections. Since the beginning of 2021, I have treated seven patients with acute transverse myelitis following the injections—both men and women, ranging in age from late twenties to sixties. Before the modRNA shots, in an average year I would typically treat no more than one new case of acute transverse myelitis.

    o *Incidence:* Before the pandemic, the annual incidence of transverse myelitis was estimated at between one and five cases per million, with MS a common cause. Transverse myelitis has been reported following routine vaccination for many years, but the incidence following the modRNA shots appears to be *several orders of magnitude greater than all other shots combined.* In 2017 a review article catalogued the number of cases of ATM following all vaccines administered in the United States from 1985 to 2017, tallying 119 cases over the thirty-three-year interval.[349] As of July 2023, 663 cases following SARS-CoV-2 modRNA injections have been recorded in the US. For comparison, the annual incidence recorded among *all* vaccines in the review was 3.7, versus an annual incidence with the SARS-CoV-2 modRNA injections of 265.2. The incidence of ATM alone should have stopped distribution of the modRNA injections.

    o *Mechanisms:* While the cause of transverse myelitis is not fully known, it is believed to be primarily autoimmune (referring to any condition in which the immune system attacks the organism's own body).[350] Pathologically, it is characterized by perivascular infiltration of inflammatory cells and axonal (the portion of the nerve containing nerve fibers) injury in addition to demyelination (destruction of the insulating myelin sheath, composed of lipids and proteins, which encases nerve cell extensions).[351] It can occur following a host of viral infections, as well as in the context of MS, systemic lupus erythematosus (SLE), paraneoplastic conditions related to underlying cancers, and vascular inflammation.

- A. As attested by the litany of MS therapies targeting T lymphocyte activity (interferons and drugs targeting both CD4+ and CD8+ T lymphocytes) and B lymphocytes, these sophisticated immune cells play a critical role in the disease process that ends up causing demyelination and axonal injury, making it impossible for them to conduct electrical signals normally.[352]

- B. The spike protein's ability to cross the blood-brain barrier and cause direct inflammation is likely a cause. Microglial cells carrying the spike protein into the central nervous system provide another likely mechanism for inflammation.[353] Molecular mimicry, bystander activation, and destruction of the myelin due to direct binding of spike protein are also plausible explanations.

- C. Its association with SLE suggests a possible vasculitic mechanism, which has been suggested in other studies.

○ *Prognosis.* The first patient I treated for transverse myelitis ultimately had resolution of her symptoms after eleven months, which is a typical time period for recovery from this diagnosis. However, other patients have been less fortunate in their recoveries, with several suffering lasting neurological injuries.

2. *Acute disseminated encephalomyelitis (ADEM).* A disease process of the central nervous system (the brain and spinal cord) that causes acute inflammation, also resulting in demyelination, or the loss of nerve cells' insulating myelin sheath, ADEM is often difficult to distinguish clinically and radiographically from new-onset multiple sclerosis. Cerebrospinal fluid findings are nearly identical between the two in the acute setting.[354] Most cases are

characterized by one or several small contrast-enhancing lesions in the white matter of the brain and/or spinal cord on MRI. Of the four patients I have treated, two had very large (tumefactive) lesions at the time of presentation, occurring within a month of an modRNA injection. None of the patients had any history of neurologic complaints prior to receiving an modRNA injection but quickly became severely neurologically impaired.[355]

- *Incidence.* Before the pandemic, the estimated annual incidence of ADEM varied widely from five to ten or more cases per million. Like ATM, it often follows a viral illness but has also been seen following vaccination, for example, the measles-mumps-rubella vaccine and a higher incidence following the modRNA injections. As of this writing, sixty-eight cases of ADEM have been reported to VAERS following SARS-CoV-2 injections, resulting in an annual incidence of 27.2. As always, it should be remembered *this likely represents underreporting of adverse events.*[356]

- *Mechanisms.* The spike protein's inflammatory properties and ability to induce adaptive immunity can result in acute, delayed, and chronic inflammation, of which demyelination is but one manifestation (chapter 4). Certain patients may have a genetic predisposition to developing acute demyelination, which the injections unmask (e.g., neuromyelitis optica or anti-MOG syndrome).[357]

    A. Because of alterations introduced during their manufacture, the modRNA injections have been shown to largely evade the innate immune response in favor of augmenting an adaptive immune response (chapter 1) and may do so sufficiently to result in autoimmune destruction of the insulation (myelin) of the central nervous system by means of excess antibody production (chapter 7).

    B. Microglial cells, a specialized subset of white blood cells necessary for normal immune function in the nervous system, can transport spike protein into the central nervous system for months, if not years, thereby acting as a catalyst for chronic inflammation. The S1 subunit of the spike protein binds directly to the ACE-2 receptor in the brain, activating microglia, resulting in the production of tissue-damaging reactive oxygen species.[358]

C. The lipid nanoparticles containing the modRNA coding for the pathogenic spike protein give it unique access to *tissues usually isolated and protected from other organ systems*. A Japanese disclosure of biodistribution studies assessing the Pfizer modRNA injection (chapter 4) found that the lipid nanoparticles containing spike protein modRNA distributed rapidly (within forty-eight hours), with high affinity to tissues including the brain, easily traversing the blood-brain barrier. Additional studies have demonstrated that the spike protein itself also crosses the blood-brain barrier. Therefore, *the spike protein has easy access to the central nervous system by at least three known mechanisms*: via lipid nanoparticle, direct access by the spike protein, and introduction through microglia.

D. The spike protein has been shown to downregulate interferon regulatory factor 9 (IRF9), which leads to decreased production by the liver of sulfatide, a fundamental component of myelin, the primary insulation of nerves. This can lead to chronic demyelination.[359]

E. Other possible mechanisms include *molecular mimicry*, in which non-self-antigens cross-react with self-antigens; *bystander activation*, in which an overzealous immune response releases additional self-antigens that then stimulate nearby self-reactive T lymphocytes; and *epitope spreading*, similar to bystander activation, except that the released self-antigens stimulate the development of new self-reactive T lymphocytes.[360]

- *Prognosis.* Often described as a monophasic illness, recurrence of symptoms within three months suggests that a patient may develop chronic demyelination.[361] Alternatively, patients with undiagnosed MS may present with ADEM as their first episode. At minimum, patients with ADEM will require monitoring for ongoing demyelination.

3. *Stroke.* Ischemic stroke is the result of sudden loss of blood flow to the brain. Approximately 87 percent of strokes occur when a blood clot travels from one location in the vascular system to the brain (ischemic strokes). (The other type—hemorrhagic strokes—occur when excessive bleeding occurs suddenly within or on the surface of the brain, typically due to a ruptured blood vessel.) Both types of strokes have been reported in high numbers following the rollout of the modRNA injections (chapters 5–7). I have treated several patients with stroke, both in the setting of active COVID infection and following SARS-CoV-2 modRNA injections. Cases in patients who had received an injection, however, did not occur in the setting of overwhelming acute inflammation, as was always the case in patients who had an active COVID infection. Concerningly, those with stroke following administration of SARS-CoV-2 modRNA preparations whom I have treated had no other discernable risk factors.

   - *Incidence.* A total of 8,954 ischemic strokes and 472 hemorrhagic strokes following SARS-CoV-2 injections have been reported to VAERS as of this writing. The annual incidence of stroke in the US is approximately 800,000 (CDC). Acknowledging almost certain underreporting, the strokes attributed to the modRNA injections alone reported only to VAERS comprise over 11 percent of the annual incidence of stroke in the US.

   - *Mechanisms.* In an ischemic stroke, a blood clot forms in the heart or a blood vessel and then travels to the brain. Blood clots often form in response to vascular inflammation, such as that seen in ruptured arterial plaques (atherosclerosis). The clot then breaks loose and travels further downstream within the blood vessel, resulting in permanent loss of the brain tissue supplied by that blood vessel, unless the clot is quickly dissolved or removed. As noted in chapter 8, the mechanisms of stroke following the modRNA injections likely include multiple causes.

    A. The spike protein downregulates ACE-2 in the vascular endothelium, resulting in decreased mitochondrial function, as published by the Salk Institute, and can cause vascular inflammation and hypertension, both common contributors to stroke.[362] These mechanisms are suggested in strokes occurring in two of my patients with nontraumatic, acute bilateral carotid dissections (tearing of the inside lining of the blood vessel leading to acute clot formation). While unilateral carotid dissection is not uncommon, bilateral dissections are particularly rare.

    B. The spike protein can also cause blood platelets to stick together (aggregate) abnormally, leading to clot formation. These clots, in turn, break loose and plug (embolize) arteries beyond where the clot initially formed, resulting in stroke.[363]

    C. Spike protein's interaction with fibrinogen, a pro-clotting factor, makes the clots more difficult for the body to dissolve.[364]

    D. Cardiac conduction abnormalities (arrhythmias) and functional changes in heart muscle contractions are common causes for clot formation and subsequent stroke. Given the well-documented propensity for the modRNA injections to cause direct inflammation of the heart muscle, both impaired mobility of the heart wall (hypokinesis) and arrhythmia have been observed following their administration (chapters 6, 8).

- *Prognosis.* Even with "clot-busting medicines" (thrombolytics) and mechanical clot removal, stroke continues to be one of the leading causes of death and disability the world over. Unfortunately, most who have them will never fully return to their previous level of function.[365] Again, the overwhelming evidence of increased incidence of stroke following the modRNA injections should have halted their distribution.

4. *Small-fiber neuropathy.* This is a disease of the peripheral nervous system (nerve extensions outside the brain and spinal cord) as opposed to the central nervous system. Small, unmyelinated or lightly myelinated nerve fibers are injured, resulting in symptoms ranging from sensory loss to painful, burning, or itchy sensations of the skin (paresthesias), and abnormal sensations triggered by non-painful stimuli (dysesthesias) in a patchy pattern throughout the limbs and torso. Many patients have likely had mild symptoms of neuropathy from the modRNA injections but have not sought evaluation, thinking that their symptoms were due to skin irritation. Skin punch biopsies have confirmed small-fiber neuropathy in many cases, including my own patients.[366]

    o *Incidence.* The incidence of all-cause small-fiber neuropathy is estimated at 13 per million.[367] The number of cases of neuropathy/small-fiber neuropathy reported to VAERS at the time of writing (summer 2023) is 3,351, correlating with an incidence of 1,340 among those who have received modRNA injections over the past thirty months, not accounting for underreporting.

    o *Mechanism.* The mechanisms for sporadic small-fiber neuropathy are varied, occurring as a consequence of metabolic diseases (e.g., diabetes), autoimmune processes, pharmacologic toxicity, chemical toxicity (e.g., alcohol), and vasculitis (inflammation of the blood vessels). It has been observed following other vaccines, including the human papilloma virus vaccine. Direct toxicity from the spike protein is likely the primary contributor, but the role of the lipid nanoparticle cannot be overlooked. The vasculitic mechanism previously described is a possible contributor, as are autoimmune mechanisms targeting myelin.

    o *Prognosis.* Depending on the mechanism, the symptoms of small-fiber neuropathy can be short-lived, lasting only a few weeks, to long-term, lasting years. In any case, patients are left with symptoms that can disrupt sleep and impair their ability to carry out work-related activities, as with some of my patients. The role of intravenous immunoglobulin should be considered in refractory cases.

5. *Acute inflammatory demyelinating polyneuropathy (AIDP/Guillain-Barré syndrome)* is commonly seen after viral infections and has been associated with certain bacterial infections, but is also widely known to follow flu vaccination.[368] Guillain-Barré syndrome (GBS) is a neurologic emergency, as a patient's symptoms can progress rapidly from weakness in the legs to respiratory paralysis, within twenty-four hours in some cases. These patients are often intubated in the ICU for weeks at a time. While many recover with proper medical support, a large percentage are left with some degree of permanent weakness.

   o *Incidence.* AIDP historically occurs with an incidence of 1 case per million flu vaccines annually. The incidence of AIDP following the SARS-CoV-2 injections has consistently been four to five times the incidence associated with the annual flu vaccine. As of this writing, 920 cases have been reported to VAERS.[369]

   o *Mechanism.* The mechanism of injury is almost certainly autoimmune. As has been demonstrated with *Campylobacter jejuni* infection and GBS, molecular mimicry is likely involved, leading to destruction of the lipid-rich myelin sheath insulating the nerves.[370] Antigen-presenting cells trigger activation of T lymphocytes, and their differentiation into T-helper 1 (Th1) and T-helper 2 (Th2) subtypes, both exerting different effects based on the cytokines they release. Th1 cells cause direct nerve inflammation through macrophage activation, whereas Th2 cells facilitate indirect nerve inflammation by activating B lymphocytes, which produce antibodies.[371] It has also been suggested that the spike protein can bind directly to sulfatide (a primary component of myelin) and cause both direct and secondary inflammation.[372] Because adequate blood flow is necessary for proper nerve function—for example, neuropathy in diabetes is largely due to blood vessel failure—a vasculitic cause should also be considered in view of the spike protein's ability to cause vascular inflammation. An overzealous inflammatory response mediated, in part, by T lymphocytes, is also likely a factor.

- o *Prognosis.* Many of these patients require months of physical therapy and medications to ease pain resulting from prolonged immobility. Skin ulcers can result from lying in bed for prolonged periods.

6. *Bell's palsy.* Noted early in the modRNA injection rollout,[373] Bell's palsy involves varying degrees of paralysis of one side of the face from inflammation of the VIIth cranial nerve (there are twelve cranial nerves that originate from each side of the brainstem to the upper cervical spinal cord). This paralysis can last days to weeks.

   - o *Incidence.* The number of cases of Bell's palsy recorded in VAERS following the modRNA shots as of this writing is 4,251. Conservative estimates suggest the incidence of Bell's palsy among the modRNA injections is three times that in the general population, with the onset of symptoms ranging from one day to roughly four months after injection.[374]

   - o *Mechanisms.* Traditionally, the cause of Bell's palsy is "unknown." However, viral reactivation is believed to be the likeliest mechanism.[375] This is illustrated in the occurrence of Ramsay Hunt syndrome, which is facial paralysis associated with painful lesions of the ear and occasional hearing loss on the same side due to reactivation of the chickenpox virus (varicella zoster).[376] Impaired functioning of CD8+ T lymphocytes (memory T cells) is the likeliest mechanism.[377] However, direct nerve injury from the spike protein must also be considered; as previously discussed, it may cause direct nerve injury by inducing inflammation as it binds directly to one of the main components of the myelin sheath—sulfatide. Molecular mimicry and bystander activation are also plausible mechanisms.[378]

   - o *Prognosis.* While many cases can improve significantly, patients are often left with disfiguring weakness of one side of the face and involuntary movement (spasms and fasciculations) of the affected side, which can be lifelong.

7. *Myasthenia gravis (MG).* A disease of fluctuating weakness that frequently involves the eye, facial, and swallowing (bulbar) muscles, myasthenia gravis can also be systemic, affecting the respiratory muscles. Patients often require mechanical ventilatory support when they are in a myasthenic crisis. I have treated two patients with MG with symptom onset one month after a SARS-CoV-2 modRNA injection. Both patients presented with double vision and swallowing difficulty. Both had antibodies to the acetylcholine receptor, which is the commonest mechanism for the weakness associated with this diagnosis.

    o *Incidence.* As of this writing, 351 cases following the modRNA injections have been reported to VAERS, and several cases have been reported in the medical literature. The annual incidence of myasthenia gravis in the US is estimated at twenty per million at the upper limit. A review of the number of cases of MG following all vaccines administered in the US from 1990–2017, as reported to VAERS, found seventy-one new cases over the twenty-eight-year interval, with an incidence of 2.1, as opposed to an incidence of 140 with the modRNA injections alone (at the time of writing, summer 2023).[379]

    o *Mechanisms.* MG is a quintessential autoimmune process and can become life-threatening when systemic symptoms have developed. In the traditional model, the body makes an autoantibody that attaches to the acetylcholine receptor (AChR) on the muscle membrane opposite the nerve ending (axon terminus), which releases the neurotransmitter acetylcholine, rendering the muscle incapable of contracting, resulting in weakness.[380] T lymphocytes are critical to the development of MG as they stimulate B lymphocytes to produce antibodies to the AChR. Other antibodies such as those formed against muscle specific kinase (MUSK), lipoprotein-related peptide 4 (LRP4), and titin can also cause myasthenic symptoms through different mechanisms.[381] Overstimulation of T lymphocytes or their dysregulation is implicated as a cause of MG following modRNA injections, as T lymphocytes critically must learn to distinguish between self and non-self-proteins in lymphoid tissue as part of their normal maturation, as noted.

- ○ *Prognosis.* Treatment of myasthenia gravis invariably involves immunotherapy ranging from steroids and steroid-sparing immunotherapy to intravenous immunoglobulin (IVIg), plasmapheresis, and recently approved monoclonal antibodies. Those who require advanced therapy often experience long-term adverse effects of the treatments themselves. For many patients this is a debilitating lifelong illness. Again, the number of cases associated with the modRNA injections should have been sufficient to suspend their distribution.

8. *Central nervous system (CNS) lymphoma.* This is overgrowth of a single white blood cell line (diffuse large B cell in 95 percent of cases), which selectively involves the brain, spinal cord, and the tissue encasing them (meninges). Most cases are fatal.[382] I have treated one patient, and a suspected second, with CNS lymphoma likely related to SARS-CoV-2 injections. Eleven cases have been reported to VAERS as of this writing. Diagnosis can be challenging, as it often mimics other processes, such as infection (meningitis/encephalitis), metastatic disease, and MS.[383] Brain biopsy is frequently necessary to achieve the diagnosis. Impaired T lymphocyte activity resulting in abnormal cytokine production is implicated as the cause, leading to overstimulation of B lymphocytes.[384] Impaired immunosurveillance (the normal process by which unhealthy cells are identified and destroyed by the immune system) is also likely (chapters 1, 4, 7).

9. *Idiopathic intracranial hypertension (IIH)/pseudotumor cerebri.* Often resulting in headaches, impaired vision, and eventually blindness if untreated, IIH is due to decreased absorption of cerebrospinal fluid in the brain, which causes increased pressure around the optic nerves, leading to compression and dysfunction.[385] There are numerous causes for the condition including cerebral venous sinus thrombosis (CVST, or blood clots in the veins of the head; see chapter 8). One risk factor is elevated body mass index (BMI). Lumbar puncture (spinal tap) is required for definitive diagnosis. In some cases, ventriculoperitoneal shunting is required for treat-

ment if medications fail. It is difficult to determine if the lipid nanoparticle or the spike protein is the more likely cause. The risk of vaccine-induced immune thrombotic thrombocytopenia (VITT) leading to microclot formation in the brain is highly concerning.[386] Notably, the patients I have treated for IIH following the modRNA injections have *not* been overweight, one of the main risk factors in usual practice.

10. *Migraine.* Migraine is a primary headache disorder characterized by vascular irritability, resulting in severe unilateral to global throbbing head pain, associated with autonomic symptoms (e.g., light sensitivity, sound sensitivity, nausea, vomiting, vertigo, or diarrhea). This is without doubt one of the most common diagnoses in neurologic practice, with conservative prevalence estimates at around 12 percent of the US population; that said, *I have treated countless patients with worsening migraine symptoms within days to weeks of modRNA injections.* The literature reflects an incidence for headache of nearly 50 percent following the second of the injections in the initial series.[387] While even now the exact mechanisms of migraine are not fully understood, there are innumerable triggers for them; given the vascular nature of migraines, endothelial irritation (endotheliitis) is likely. Migraines are believed to originate in the brainstem, with the Vth nerve (trigeminal nerve) nucleus playing an important role. The vagus nerve may play a role as an antigen-presenting mechanism, transmitting the inflammatory spike protein to the brainstem.[388]

11. *Malignancy.* Clinicians have noted a surge in reactivation of malignancies previously in remission (in some cases for many years) following modRNA injections, resulting in central nervous system malignancies and cancers presenting with metastatic disease to the central nervous system—again likely due to the spike protein—implicated in COVID-19-related cancers.[389] One such patient had been in remission from breast cancer for over ten years and presented with multiple cranial neuropathies (infiltration of the cranial nerves by cancer cells, resulting in weakness of face and throat muscles) within several weeks of having received an modRNA injection. Studies have demonstrated that the S2 sub-

unit of the spike protein strongly interacts with the tumor suppressor proteins p53 and BRCA 1/2, potentially resulting in faulty DNA repair.[390] Reduced activity of a protein critical to the repair of ribosomal DNA—RNA polymerase I (Pol I)—and the release of specific microRNAs from exosomes—following the production of modRNA injection-induced spike protein—are additional mechanisms potentially leading to impaired DNA repair.[391] Faulty DNA repair, coupled with weakened immunosurveillance resulting from the modRNA injections, is a potentially devastating combination.[392] Additionally, the modRNA in the injections has been modified during its manufacture to keep it from being destroyed by the innate immune system, and it has been demonstrated to be reverse-transcribed into DNA within six hours of administration.[393] Long interspersed nuclear elements, comprising approximately 17 percent of our genome, can become active in some cases (notably with LINE-1, an endogenous reverse transcriptase), providing a mechanism by which spike modRNA can be reverse transcribed and integrated into the genome. This has, in fact, been shown to occur in human liver cells following administration of modRNA injections.[394] The very presence of LINE-1 is an indicator of cancer and poor prognosis in several diseases.[395] The potential implications of indeterminate expression of spike protein through these mechanisms may not be realized for many years.

12. *Prion diseases and amyloid plaques.* Prions are self-replicating misfolded proteins, which contain no genetic information but cause other proteins in the brain to misfold, leading to incurable neurodegenerative conditions. The most notable of these is the human equivalent of "mad cow" disease—Creutzfeldt Jakob disease (CJD), and its variant form (vCJD), both uniformly fatal after presenting with rapid onset memory loss (dementia).[396] While speculative, clinical evidence suggests a possible connection between the injections and these conditions; one patient with rapidly progressive dementia within four months of an modRNA injection tested positive with a markedly high level of the protein associated with CJD, using the current diagnostic test of choice (RT-QuIC).

- *Incidence.* The increased incidence of Parkinson's disease reported in VAERS suggests this phenomenon should be considered. The tendency for the spike protein to facilitate aggregation of pathologic proteins, coupled with the injections' suppression of BRCA1, is a potentially ominous combination for the development of multiple neurodegenerative conditions. If even a fraction of the 19 cases of CJD and the 215 cases of ALS recorded in VAERS thus far are related to the modRNA injections, they must be investigated.
- *Mechanisms.* The spike protein itself may trigger misfolding of proteins to form amyloid plaques, leading to multiple neurodegenerative conditions.
    A. An article from 2021 noted that the S1 receptor binding domain (RBD) of the spike protein binds to heparin and heparin-binding proteins.[397] Heparin binding accelerates aggregation of pathologic amyloid proteins in the brain, including A-β (Alzheimer's disease), α-synuclein (Parkinson's disease, multiple systems atrophy), tau (cortical basal degeneration, progressive supranuclear palsy, Alzheimer's disease), prion (CJD) and TDP-43 RRM (tandemly tethered RNA recognition motif domains, ALS, frontotemporal dementia, Alzheimer's disease).[398]

    B. It has also been demonstrated that the S1 RBD of SARS-CoV-2 is unique among all other beta-coronaviruses, in that it contains a prion-like domain (PrD), giving it greater affinity for the ACE-2 receptor.[399]

    C. The modRNA injections are glycoprotein-rich, which leads to enhanced formation of potential G-quadruplexes (pG4), which may facilitate misfolding of the PrD of the S1 RBD, akin to the way prion proteins (which contain multiple G-quadruplex forming motifs) are believed to bind to their own mRNA, which codes for them, causing misfolding.[400]

- *Prognosis.* One of the challenges with prion and prion-like neurodegenerative diseases is that they often take years to present with symptoms once the process of abnormal protein accumulation has started. If a patient continues to produce large amounts of spike protein following a SARS-CoV-2 modRNA injection, it is possible the process of abnormal protein accumulation, such as that seen in prion and amyloid illnesses, could be accelerated, given the propensity to increase aggregation of these proteins.

13. *Other Disorders.* In addition to the diseases mentioned above, my practice has included several other conditions frequently catalogued as adverse events following modRNA injections.
    - *Orthostasis/postural orthostatic tachycardia syndrome* (POTS), or lightheadedness made worse with standing, is likely due to spike protein binding endothelial ACE-2 receptors or activated macrophages binding to the endothelium.[401] Another likely mechanism for orthostasis is direct involvement of the vagus nerve (the Xth cranial nerve, which originates in the lower brainstem and travels widely throughout the body, providing autonomic/parasympathetic innervation). The 15,829 cases reported to VAERS at the time of this writing imply multiple contributing mechanisms.
    - *Tinnitus* is incessant ringing in the ears felt to be secondary to direct injury to the cochlea in the inner ear. The inner ear cells of the cochlea have abundant ACE-2 receptors. The spike protein can potentially damage these delicate inner ear cells by directly binding to the ACE-2 receptor, or through direct toxicity. The lipid nanoparticle may also cause direct toxicity. The 10,243 cases reported to VAERS by summer 2023 attest to its significance.[402]
    - *New onset seizures* have also been observed. The mechanism for new-onset seizures is unclear, but excitotoxicity, in which certain neurotransmitters released excessively or in abnormal ways can have toxic side effects, provides a plausible explanation.[403] VAERS catalogues 6,926 cases as of summer 2023.

- *Cognitive decline* following administration of modRNA injections, including "brain fog," has been widely reported.[404] The vascular effects of the injections, direct toxicity of the spike protein, the tendency to aggregate A-β and tau proteins, and suppression of BRCA1 are all potential mechanisms. The 150 cases of Alzheimer's disease and 2,913 cases of dementia reported to VAERS as of summer 2023 are a signal that must be followed closely.

- *Shingles* resulting from reactivation of the dormant chickenpox virus (varicella zoster) in peripheral nerves causes a painful skin rash, though sometimes the rash is not present ("sine herpeticum"). A notable increase in shingles following the modRNA injections has been observed.[405] One of my patients developed zoster brachial plexitis, resulting in pain and weakness of the left arm with a patchy red rash that started between four and six weeks after having received an modRNA injection. MRI showed contrast enhancement of all trunks of the brachial plexus, and spinal fluid showed active inflammation with PCR positive for varicella zoster virus. The few cases of this kind of plexitis reported in the literature have nearly all been in immunocompromised patients, highlighting an important mechanism of injury. Viral reactivation resulting from impaired T lymphocyte function (CD8+ memory T cells, in particular) is the likeliest cause.[406] Impaired type I interferon signaling, a critical process in coordinating appropriate innate and adaptive immune responses, is also implicated.[407] The staggering 11,329 cases of zoster/shingles reported in VAERS following the modRNA injections, as of this writing, implies multiple mechanisms at work, including those suggested in Bell's palsy.

CONCLUSION

Underreporting of vaccine injuries is a well-known shortcoming of pharmacovigilance systems like VAERS, as discussed in more depth in chapter 6.[408] In my own professional experience, I cannot recall a single patient chart documenting whether, or when, a patient received an modRNA injection. *Needless to say, no one can find a correlation between an injection and a diagnosis, if the relevant information is never gathered.* Worse yet, doctors rightly fear being labeled "science deniers," obstructionists to the vaccination campaign, or "anti-vaxxers"—quite possibly at the cost of their careers. Professional ostracism and public criticism await anyone who speaks out against the prevailing narrative.

This grim injustice does not change our ethical obligations as healthcare providers. As clinicians, investigators, and scientists we must ask questions, do our own research, and form independent opinions. Our oath and our commitment as providers must always be to our patients. At a minimum, we owe them objectivity and transparency.

We should also refuse the counsel of fear. Above all, I wish to emphasize there is cause for hope, with efforts underway to identify compounds that show promise in breaking down spike protein and reducing inflammation, thereby helping to minimize any potential adverse effects. The primary mainstays used to treat neurologic autoimmune illness—IVIg (intravenous immunoglobulin) and plasmapheresis (a modified form of hemodialysis)—will inevitably find broad utility in many of these conditions. The roles for emerging therapies, such as monoclonal antibodies targeting Aβ (lecanemab and donanemab), may need to be considered for new indications.[409]

We must also look outside the bounds of traditional medicine to consider therapeutics that not only break down the spike protein, but facilitate a healthy general immune response.

- Nattokinase, a product of fermented soy, has been shown to help break down circulating spike protein.[410]
- Omega-3 fatty acids are critical for healthy blood vessels.[411]
- Adequate levels of vitamins D and K are necessary to coordinate a proper immune response.[412]
- B-vitamins and alpha lipoic acid have been shown to facilitate nerve repair.[413]

Moreover, a number of botanicals forgotten by Western medicine offer a range of benefits:

- Artemisia enhances Th2 response and decreases nitric oxide–induced damage.[414]
- Andrographis, an anti-inflammatory, reduces platelet aggregation and promotes regulatory T cell development.[415]

- Japanese knotweed has been shown to cross the blood-brain barrier and reduce inflammation.[416]
- Cat's claw has been shown to inhibit and reduce both Aβ and tau proteins.[417]
- Lion's mane mushroom may facilitate remyelination of damaged nerves.[418]
- Turmeric plays an important role in reducing inflammation in a number of different conditions.[419]

By utilizing the most promising therapeutics across disciplines, rather than limiting ourselves to allopathic (often called "modern Western medicine") approaches alone, we can begin to restore and maintain neurologic function in the face of injuries resulting from the modRNA injections, whose magnitude has no historical precedent. Whatever challenges we face in the years to come, as Proverbs 13:12 reminds us, "Hope deferred makes the heart sick, but a longing fulfilled is a tree of life." May we encourage one another to maintain hope even in the darkest circumstances.

CHAPTER 10

CANCER RISKS OF THE MODRNA COVID-19 "VACCINES"

By Jane Orient, MD

Humanity has been plagued by cancer for centuries, and despite the progress of medical science, this disease remains lethal and very difficult to treat. Consequently, people fear being diagnosed with malignancy more than with any other serious illness.[420] In the pre-COVID world, the dread of cancer transcended ideological views and political affiliations, as reflected in numerous initiatives from Republican and Democratic administrations, typically with bipartisan congressional support.[421] Yet, with the introduction of the novel modRNA COVID-19 "vaccines," administrators and experts have inexplicably changed their stance toward cancer prevention "180 degrees"—from imposingly strict to breathtakingly lax.

Historically, in the battle against cancer, governmental agencies, academia, and professional medical societies have prudently advised the two best strategies for preventing cancer are: (1) elimination of existing carcinogens and (2) prevention of the introduction of new carcinogens into the environment. Therefore, public health authorities have emphasized the detection of even the slightest carcinogenic properties of chemical compounds found in any product to which humans are frequently exposed, especially food and drugs. New therapeutic agents, including vaccines, were subject to meticulous premarketing testing and post-marketing surveillance aimed at screening potential carcinogenic properties.

However, a shocking exception from those prudent and well-established safety measures was made for the novel modRNA COVID-19 "vaccines"—and the excuses offered by policymakers responsible for this cavalier strategy of "shortcuts" are unconvincing at best.

INADEQUACY OF PREMARKETING SAFETY STUDIES OF MODRNA "VACCINES"

The two most relevant types of premarketing studies for cancer prevention are *carcinogenicity* and *genotoxicity* studies.

- Carcinogenicity studies test the probable risks of new drugs to cause malignancies. Such tests are usually conducted in rodents, because they have physiological and genetic characteristics similar to humans. Typically, carcinogenicity studies involve exposing rodents to different doses of the new drug for a long period, *usually eighteen to twenty-four months*, and then examining their tissues for any signs of cancer.

- Genotoxicity studies examine the potential of new drugs to induce genetic damage in humans. Such genetic damage can lead to mutations that are associated with cancer. Genotoxicity studies are performed "in vitro" and "in vivo" using different types of cells and organisms. In vitro studies use isolated cells or tissues from humans or animals to test the direct effects of the new drug on DNA or chromosomes. In vivo studies use laboratory animals, such as rodents, to test the systemic effects of the new drug on different organs and tissues. The most commonly used tests for genotoxicity are the bacterial reverse mutation test (Ames test), the mammalian cell gene mutation test, the in vitro chromosome aberration test, the in vivo micronucleus test, and the in vivo comet assay.[422]

Carcinogenicity and genotoxicity studies are regulated by a set of guidelines issued by governmental agencies such as the Food and Drug Administration (FDA), European Medicines Agency (EMA), and other national and international organizations.[423] Carcinogenicity and genotoxicity studies are among the most time-consuming, costly, and effort-intensive types of nonclinical safety studies for new drugs. However, due to their immense importance in preventing approval of potentially cancer-causing drugs, governmental agencies in charge of new drug approval have historically been strict in requiring performance of those studies. As noted, however, a puzzling exception to this rule was granted for the novel COVID-19 "vaccines."

As evidenced by the package inserts and official reports of American, European, and Australian drug-approving agencies for both approved modRNA "vaccines," Comirnaty (Pfizer) and Spikevax (Moderna), *no carcinogenicity studies* were performed.[424] Bewilderingly, all those governmental agencies, typically so strict about potential carcinogenicity, agreed that not submitting the carcinogenicity studies for those novel "vaccines" was "scientifically acceptable" and "consistent with guidelines." They explained further that such studies are unnecessary because the components of the new "vaccine" formulations are lipids and natural nucleosides that are "not expected" to have carcinogenic potential.

Genotoxicity studies were not done for Comirnaty, based upon the stated rationale that its components (LNPs and modRNA) are not expected to elicit genotoxic effects.[425] However, oddly enough, several genotoxicity studies *were* done for the Spikevax (Moderna) modRNA vaccine.[426] Specifically, those studies examined genotoxic potential of the final Spikevax formulation, and a novel excipient SM-102, which is one of the four lipids contained in the "vaccine's" lipid nanoparticle (LNP) system. The following guidelines-compliant tests were used: a bacterial reverse mutation test; in vitro mammalian cell micronucleus test in human peripheral blood lymphocytes; and in vivo mammalian bone marrow erythrocyte micronucleus assay in the rat. According to the "vaccine" manufacturer, its results indicated that a relevant genotoxic risk was not expected for this product.[427] No explanation was provided for why such studies were performed and why their performance was consistent with guidelines, *when it was determined previously that such studies were not necessary*, and nonperformance was consistent with guidelines for a very similar modRNA "vaccine"—Comirnaty.

The absence of carcinogenicity studies, inconsistent performance of genotoxicity studies, and the dubious explanations presented are very concerning. They represent irrational, unaccountable deviations from established, prudent practices for cancer prevention. The categorical safety principle that has been violated here can be summarized as follows: cancer is rightfully the most dreaded disease, any new drug (including vaccine) may increase its risk by yet unknown mechanisms, and the proven best way to detect such risk is by performance of experimental carcinogenicity and genotoxicity studies.

This imperative is both simple and powerful. It should not be overridden by the optimistic expectations of "no harm," but it also requires no "enhancements" in the form of speculations about potential mechanisms that could increase such a risk. While investigators in other fields of medicine have already adduced *clear causal mechanisms for some categories of acute "vaccine" injury* (documented in other chapters), cancer's notorious complexity, variety, and long disease etiology mean we are only starting to understand the modRNA shots' true *long-term cancer risks*. Therefore, any discussion of carcinogenicity must necessarily remain circumspect in presenting hypothetical mechanisms of harm. The history of medicine is full of theories that seemed to be plausible, only to be proven wrong upon empirical examination, and the risk is manifold here in view of the bewildering complexity of carcinogenicity and oncogenomics. Above all, these facts caution both against *inflating* the cancer risks of the modRNA "vaccines" and against *understating* them, as regulators may well have.

The decision about approval of any novel medical modality should not be based upon the wishful expectations of optimists nor on gloomy speculations of pessimists. Plainly, it should be based on analyzing the empirical data derived from well-designed experimental studies—*and in the case of the COVID-19 modRNA "vaccines," those were not performed.*

This unprecedented, extremely risky gamble received the blessing of governmental entities established specifically to prevent such a hazardous situation. One would expect that the academic establishment would react with harsh criticism of the grave recklessness of those decisions. Sadly, only very few scholars voiced their concern about the dearth and inconsistency of the essential premarketing studies.[428] The vast majority of mainstream academia remained silent on this issue.

INSUFFICIENCY OF POST-MARKETING PHARMACOVIGILANCE

As demonstrated above, the premarketing safety studies of modRNA COVID-19 "vaccines" were woefully inadequate. To be generous to the public health authorities, one could argue this phase was rushed due to the global emergency caused by the COVID-19 pandemic. However, one would expect that the insufficiencies of premarketing studies "forced by the acute crisis" would then be compensated for by robust post-marketing pharmacovigilance. Shockingly, this has not occurred.

One of the most essential parts of post-marketing pharmacovigilance is tracking "safety signals."[429] Detection of a new or known side effect that may be caused by a drug or vaccine, typically based on multiple reports, requires further investigation and ultimately regulatory actions if confirmed to be valid.[430] Safety signals can be detected from a variety of sources, such as spontaneous reporting systems (e.g., VAERS), clinical trials, observational studies, and even social media.[431]

Safety signals are crucial for identifying and preventing potential harms from vaccines. However, a safety signal by itself *is not direct evidence* of a vaccine side effect. Rather, it is a cautionary hypothesis that, analyzed in the context of other data and existing scientific knowledge, may provide justification for further investigation. Not all safety signals indicate a true causal association between a vaccine and an adverse event. Some safety signals may be due to chance, bias, confounding, or other factors.[432] The key issue here is that safety signals *cannot be arbitrarily dismissed* without careful investigation. Similarly, one should not pick and choose only those signals that fit one's agenda.

Public health authorities have displayed a counterintuitive lack of interest in searching for safety signals of potential carcinogenicity of the modRNA "vaccines," in any available sources, including the VAERS and V-safe databases they themselves manage. As discussed in chapter 6, VAERS, established in 1990, is a post-marketing passive surveillance program, comanaged by CDC and FDA, that collects information submitted by the public about adverse events occurring after administration of vaccines.[433] V-safe (discussed in chapter 5), is a smartphone-based COVID-19 "vaccine" active-side-effects surveillance program established by CDC specifically for those "vaccines" during their authorization under emergency use authorization (EUA), discontinued in May 2023.[434]

It is puzzling that the same agencies that created these databases have shown minimal interest in using them to examine the inconvenient question of potential carcinogenicity of the new "vaccines." The limitations of VAERS are well known, *but the reports still present safety signals which deserve investigation.*

Meanwhile other sources of information have also sent up red flags, as social media and alternative news outlets became saturated with numerous personal testimonies about cancer developing or accelerating in patients after COVID-19 "vaccination."[435] Such reports are known as "anecdotal data," deemed irrelevant in the current dominant paradigm of evidence-based medicine, in accordance with its dogma that "the plural of anecdote is not evidence."[436] However, *such reports also still constitute safety signals*, in accordance with the widely accepted definition.

With safety signals arising from multiple sources, one would assume, based upon their past responses, that health authorities would spring into action in accordance with their own guidelines. Instead, they responded with an aggressive public relations campaign to discredit and silence anyone who dared bring up VAERS data, supported by draconian Big Tech censorship (foreword, chapters 5, 6).[437]

CONCEPT OF "NEGATIVE EVIDENCE" APPLIED TO THE QUESTION OF CARCINOGENICITY OF COVID-19 VACCINES

The foregoing facts demonstrate that—contravening logic, expectations, and precedent—public health regulatory agencies failed miserably to ensure the adequacy of premarketing safety studies of modRNA "vaccines" regarding their possible carcinogenicity. Furthermore, those agencies were unable or unwilling to conduct the necessary high-quality post-marketing pharmacovigilance. They initially ignored, and later tried to suppress, the clear presence of safety signals related to potential carcinogenicity (chapter 5). They performed no follow-up investigations of those safety signals, which should be routinely done under such circumstances. They issued no advisories to the public and implemented no administrative measures, despite the obvious need to do so.

Such *counterintuitive lack* of logically expected research efforts and regulatory actions by the institutions charged with protecting the public safety can be described as the presence of *"negative evidence."* The term "negative evidence" is used to denote the *surprising absence of data or actions that logically should be present in a specific setting, in light of statute, common sense, and past practice.*[438] Discovery of negative evidence provides valuable clues that the essential information *is being deliberately obscured to prevent the uncovering of sinister acts or agendas*. Awareness of negative evidence, and its implications, should serve as a wakeup call for the public and spur elected officials to use their electoral mandates to protect their constituents.

SEEKING POTENTIAL CARCINOGENIC MECHANISMS OF THE MODRNA "VACCINES"

In the information age, due to robust internet connectivity, the free flow of information has become hard to control, even by the most tyrannical governmental and Big Tech censorship. In such settings the tacitly observed correlation between COVID-19 "vaccines" and development of cancers could no longer be hidden. The public became aware of those terrifying correlations and started to demand answers and explanations.

Yet, the traditional sources of authority, expertise, and information—such as governmental agencies, academia, and mainstream press—refuse to acknowledge any correlation between modRNA "vaccines" and cancer. The medical establishment maintains firmly that there is not only *no reliable scientific evidence* but in fact *no reasonable theoretical basis* to suggest that the modRNA COVID-19 "vaccines" might cause cancer.[439]

The presence of such enormous discrepancy between public observations and the opinion of the previously respected authorities is bound to cause distress and confusion, resulting in more public demands for preferably *simple, plausible, universal, and incontestable explanations* of the mechanism by which the novel modRNA "vaccines" could cause cancer. While those demands are understandable, they are very unlikely to be met soon, due to numerous factors.

Public expectations reflect the understandable wish that any new pathological phenomenon can be explained through simple reasoning—without the need for cumbersome experiments and research data collection. In such a process, the author of the "explanation" just picks the pieces of the "proper information" from the pool of existing knowledge and connects them together. Typically, however, reality is exactly opposite to such a scheme. The current "pool of knowledge" does not contain all possible information about the world. A novel agent, such as an modRNA "vaccine," may act by a well-known mechanism, but it can also induce its effect by as yet unknown means. Moreover, from a simple logistical standpoint, the matter of carcinogenetic properties of COVID-19 vaccines is too complex to be tackled by individuals working separately, without substantial financial and technical resources.

Nonetheless, many "vaccine"-skeptical physicians and scientists have proposed various hypotheses that could explain the tacitly observed correlation between COVID-19 "vaccines" and cancer. The interested reader is encouraged to review the papers containing those hypotheses.[440] However, without confirmation from experimental studies, even the most elegant hypothesis will remain a mere conjecture.[441] Sadly, members of the medical establishment with the requisite expertise have united around the idea that the modRNA "vaccines" are entirely safe and refuse to engage in respectful debate with those who question the official narrative. Instead, such dissidents and their hypotheses, presented in good faith, are mercilessly mocked by mainstream academicians—as epitomized by the infamous paper published in the prestigious *British Medical Journal*: "Everything Causes Cancer? Beliefs and Attitudes towards Cancer Prevention among Anti-Vaxxers, Flat Earthers, and Reptilian Conspiracists: Online Cross Sectional Survey."[442]

This is an extremely disheartening reality. The unfortunate and unavoidable fact is that fully coming to the grips with the cancer risks of the modRNA "vaccines" would require all the resources and power of traditional academia and public health agencies. In the current world, characterized by the politicization of science, public health officials and their clients in academia are unlikely to grant their ideological opponents access to those resources.[443]

In these difficult circumstances, instead of proposing to formulate one neat and plausible hypothesis, a more sensible approach is to concentrate on seeking a better general command of the underlying principles of oncogenomics and pharmacoepidemiology, as discussed below.

THE ROLE OF ONCOGENOMICS

Oncogenomics, which concerns cancer-associated genes and their expression, is key to understanding the mechanisms by which carcinogens can cause the malignant transformation of benign tissue into a cancer. Familiarity with principles of oncogenomics is critical to understanding how the modRNA "vaccines" may be causing cancers.

Due to its multilayered complexity, oncogenomics must be approached with humility even by clinical oncologists and general geneticists. Pathologies that we call "cancer" are extremely complex. Their in-depth study requires numerous years of specialized training and direct research experience, along with sophisticated research systems found only in the leading scientific centers.

Nonetheless, anyone with a basic scientific background can familiarize himself with many essential concepts of oncogenomics with the proper effort. Those who would like to study this subject in greater depth can peruse a number of useful texts that are listed at the reference here.[444] As always, technical jargon is one of the main obstacles for new students. The following is a quick overview of some oncogenomic concepts.

1. *Cancer.* The term "cancer" has been defined in the not-so-remote past as the group of distinct diseases that shared the six essential hallmarks described by Robert Weinberg and Douglas Hanahan: neoplastic autonomy, insensitivity to anti-growth signals, evasion of apoptosis, immortality of cells, sustained angiogenesis, and local invasion and distal metastases.[445]

2. *Oncogenes and tumor suppressor genes.* These are the two main types of cancer genes. Oncogenes are genes that promote cell growth and reproduction, which can induce cancer when activated inappropriately. Tumor suppressor genes inhibit those processes, keeping cell division in check. A defect of tumor suppressor genes resulting from loss-of-function mutation causes their inactivity, inducing in turn the uncontrolled growth of cells leading to cancers.[446]

3. *Mutation.* The process of alteration occurring in a gene is mutation. Typically, such alteration affects the function of the gene, but not always. For instance, a "silent" mutation causes a change in the DNA sequence, but despite that alteration, the DNA still translates into the same protein sequence. In another example, several other codons call for signals to stop the process of protein synthesis, and the protein is ejected from the ribosome "early." In this case, the mutation would be a "nonsense" mutation, because the protein would be incomplete. In a "conservative missense" mutation, the replacement amino acid is similar in function and shape to the amino acid being replaced, and the change in protein function may be minor. In a "non-conservative missense mutation," a completely different kind of amino acid is added to the chain, perhaps a nonpolar versus a polar one. This will likely change the shape, structure, and function of the protein.

The terms "mutation" and "mutant" can cause confusion since they may be used in different contexts to denote different processes in human and non-human subjects. In human genetics, a mutant is a genetic variant of low population frequency. When used in the context of inheritance, mutation implies a recent sequence change (either germline or somatic), in contrast to inheritance from a carrier parent. When describing genetic processes in nonhuman organisms, the name mutant refers to a population that harbors a specific, atypical variant, such as antibiotic resistance. The types of mutation relevant to this editorial include:

- Gain-of-function mutation (GOF). Also known as an "activating mutation," this type of mutation enhances the gene product in such a way that its effect becomes stronger. This quantitative gain is called "an enhanced activation." GOF can also modify the gene to change its function qualitatively—that is, to produce an entirely different function than the original one. Such new functions may be abnormal and detrimental to the organism, or can be beneficial. GOF research was associated with the recent controversy over the origin of the SARS-CoV-2 virus.[447]

- Loss-of-function mutation (LOF). Also called "an inactivating mutation," an LOF mutation results in the gene product having less or no function. In other words, LOF causes partial or full inactivation of the gene. A well-known example of disease caused by an LOF is cystic fibrosis.[448]

- Other noteworthy type of mutations (some already mentioned above) include: "nonsense mutation," which creates a premature stop codon; "missense mutation," which creates amino acid change; a "synonymous" mutation, which does not change protein sequence; and a "frameshift" mutation, which shifts the reading frame of the DNA, in turn altering the triplet codons for protein translation, creating an entirely new protein sequence downstream of the mutation.

4. *Malignant transformation.* This process converts normal (benign) tissue into neoplastic (malignant) tissue. This occurs through the formation of novel oncogenes, the inappropriate over-expression of normal oncogenes, or by the under-expression or disabling of tumor suppressor genes.[449]

5. *Carcinogens.* There are two types of environmental factors that are capable of inducing carcinogenesis: non-genotoxic (NGTX) or activation-dependent, and genotoxic (GTX) or activation-independent. Viruses can also be carcinogenic.[450]

    o NGTX carcinogens have no direct interaction with DNA; they most likely induce malignancies by disrupting cellular structures and by modifying the rate of cell proliferation, or by altering the processes that enhance the odds of genetic errors.

    o GTX carcinogens are typically electrophiles (molecules that attract electrons) that are capable of interfering directly with DNA via formation of covalent bonds. This process leads to formation of DNA-carcinogen complexes, also known as "DNA adducts." These complexes cause various types of DNA damage, including cleavage of the DNA strands, removal of DNA bases (hydration), formation of cross-links between the two helices, and chemical bonds between adjacent bases. Those structural changes cause modifications of the coded DNA genetic information. Such mutations are typically fixed by DNA repair mechanisms; however, if DNA replication occurs prior to the action of a repair mechanism, mutations are bound to become permanent, resulting in malignant transformation.

    o Viruses and their components have been long recognized as carcinogens. In fact, viral infections are estimated to play a causal role in at least 11 percent of all new cancer diagnoses worldwide.[451]

6. *Nucleic acids.* In addition to messenger RNA (mRNA), ribosomal RNA (rRNA), and transfer RNA (tRNA) involved in protein synthesis, there are also regulatory RNAs, which play a role in gene expression.

    Before discovery of regulatory RNA, it was assumed that only proteins could act as regulators of gene expression. Those proteins were known as repressors and activators. They had specific short binding sites within enhancer regions near the genes to be regulated.[452] However, later studies have shown that RNAs are also involved in the process of gene regulation in a variety of organisms. Bacteria and archaea have regulatory RNA systems.[453] In eukaryotes there are several kinds of RNA-dependent processes regulating the expression of genes at various points.

RNA interference (RNAi) is a ubiquitous intracellular process mediated by small RNA species, through which specific RNAs are targeted for editing, degradation, or clearance. RNAi plays important roles in the regulation of gene expression, developmental processes, cellular defense, and epigenetic effects. RNAi technology (also called antisense technology) has been used in the laboratory to test the function of a gene by preventing its expression. Its use has been attempted clinically as a means of posttranscriptional gene silencing to reduce expression of viral or cancer genes, or to lower cholesterol. The specific therapies are sometimes referred to as antisense oligonucleotides (ASOs; AS-ODNs).

There are ongoing early attempts at developing therapeutic applications using RNAs in the fields of hematology, oncology, and neurodegenerative disease. These may utilize long non-coding RNAs to shut down blocks of chromatin epigenetically; enhancer RNAs to induce increased gene expression;[454] PIWI-interacting RNAs (piRNAs) that interact with PIWI (P-element-induced wimpy testis), a class of proteins that may regulate stem cells and appear to be aberrantly expressed in some cancers;[455] and microRNAs (miRNAs), specific short RNA molecules that can base-pair with mRNAs.

7. *Reverse transcription* is a process in which a complementary DNA (cDNA) is generated from an RNA template. This generation is mediated by the enzyme reverse transcriptase (RT). RTs are used by various viruses such as HIV and hepatitis B to replicate their genomes. Most importantly, the oncogenic RNA viruses, such as Rous sarcoma inducing virus, rely on this process as well.[456]

ROLE OF CANCER PHARMACOEPIDEMIOLOGY IN STUDYING VACCINE-CANCER ASSOCIATIONS

While familiarity with theoretical oncogenomics is very important, overreliance on theoretical methods has limitations for solving the practical clinical problem. The best theory, even validated by laboratory experiments, will remain mere conjecture if not confirmed by a large amount of real-world data.

What sets cancer pharmacoepidemiology apart from classic pharmacoepidemiology is the significant challenge of establishing causality *when the carcinogenic effects of a "vaccine" may only manifest with a substantial delay of up to several years after "vaccine" administration.* The long period of cancer development and the relatively low incidence of individual cancers impede the ability of traditional pharmacovigilance systems to identify drug-cancer associations. Data systems based upon spontaneous reporting of adverse effects, such as VAERS, are the most affected by this long delay. Most patients simply do not make connections between "vaccination" and appearance of cancer, due to the long interval between those two events. Consequently, analyses based on large-scale medical data sets are essential to provide solid data on potential effects of "vaccines" on cancer incidence.[457]

However, formal oncopharmacological studies are the gold standard that would complement perfectly the oncogenomic theory to produce the ultimate and irrevocable proof of the COVID-19 "vaccine" carcinogenicity.[458] US public health officials are of course aware of the power and impact that well-designed pharmacoepidemiologic studies of drug-vaccine associations can have[459] and are using their enormous leverage—in the form of control over cancer pharmacovigilance reporting and lab research—to suppress any attempts at independent inquiry about the safety of COVID-19 "vaccines." However, it is creating *negative evidence* in the process.

CONCLUSION

The introduction of potentially highly carcinogenic COVID-19 "vaccines," in the setting of a worldwide pandemic emergency, has revealed that public health authorities are much more interested in promoting the "vaccine" produced by their major donors than in protecting the public from the disease. The more acute side effects of this "vaccine"—such as myocarditis, blood clots, neurological injuries, and sudden death—started to appear right away. Currently, we are bracing for the next wave of delayed, but equally horrific, side effects of this "vaccine" in the form of newly induced and accelerated cancers. The public must demand that the responsible agencies start doing the duties they have so shockingly neglected. In the meantime, dissenting researchers must keep challenging officialdom about the negative evidence in the field of cancer pharmacovigilance.

CHAPTER 11

COVID-19 "VACCINE" EFFECTS ON WOMEN OF REPRODUCTIVE AGE AND PREGNANCY

By James A. Thorp, MD

This chapter reviews the well-documented adverse effects of the COVID-19 experimental gene therapies—inappropriately referred to as "vaccines"—on women's fertility, fetal viability and pregnancy, live births, and maternal health. The modRNA shots are still endorsed by public health agencies for use in pregnant women, despite clear signs of the dangers to reproductive health in lab data from Moderna, post-marketing safety data gathered by Pfizer, and demographic data showing dramatic shifts in fertility.[460] This chapter also exposes deliberate deceptions in the campaign to persuade the public that the modRNA shots were safe, effective, and necessary in pregnancy.

The potential for modRNA "vaccines" to negatively affect reproduction was first established in laboratory trials by Moderna examining fetal development in pregnant rats, the results of which were only released after a FOIA request (chapters 2, 5).[461] Subsequently, clear evidence of reproductive harms has emerged in pharmacovigilance systems like the US Vaccine Adverse Event Reporting System (VAERS) and European Medicines Agency's EudraVigilance database, as well as Pfizer's own post-market safety monitoring data, released by court order after an FOIA request.[462]

As a practicing physician with forty-four years of obstetrical experience—including active clinical practice over the last four years, during which I reviewed ultrasound images from 27,000 pregnant women—I was in a unique position to directly observe the physiological impact of first COVID-19 and then the modRNA shots on the health of pregnant women and their fetuses. This chapter will present a discussion of my own clinical observations, followed by a brief discussion of how the modRNA shots may be hurting women's fertility. After summarizing evidence of negative global impacts on fertility from population-level metrics, it concludes with an account of the government takeover of professional medical societies, turning them into nothing more than marketing channels for CDC.

WAS COVID-19 A MAJOR THREAT TO GENERAL AND REPRODUCTIVE HEALTH?

Any evaluation of potential reproductive harms from the modRNA shots must begin by assessing the actual threat posed by COVID-19 infection to pregnant women, as a first step toward a rational cost-benefit analysis for any experimental intervention. In stark contrast to alarming messages from public health authorities, studies conducted throughout the pandemic have shown *pregnant women are at no greater risk of severe COVID-19 than their nonpregnant peers.*

A May 2021 study of around 11,000 pregnant and nonpregnant women, all hospitalized for COVID-19 viral pneumonia, found the mortality rate among hospitalized pregnant women was *significantly lower than their nonpregnant hospitalized peers* (0.8 percent versus 3.5 percent). This also held true among the subset admitted to ICU, where 3.5 percent of pregnant patients died, compared to 14.9 percent of nonpregnant patients. Among those who received mechanical ventilation, in-hospital death occurred in 8.6 percent of pregnant patients, compared to 31.4 percent of nonpregnant patients.[463]

Later, the same authors conducted a larger study of 23,574 female inpatients, aged fifteen to forty-five, diagnosed with COVID-19, who were discharged from 749 US hospitals between April 2020 and May 2021. The second study's results closely echoed the first, finding, "In-hospital mortality occurred in 1.1 percent of pregnant patients and 3.5 percent of nonpregnant patients hospitalized with COVID-19 and viral pneumonia." Further, the authors reported that pregnant women were no more likely to be intubated than nonpregnant ones, while "among patients who were admitted to an ICU, mortality was lower for pregnant compared with non-pregnant patients."[464]

Since COVID-19 posed no special threat to healthy pregnant women, even speculative harms to women's reproductive health from the modRNA shots should have been considered unacceptable out of hand.

Next, any discussion of possible harms to pregnancy from the modRNA shots should consider the overall evidence of the modRNA shots' general pathogenic potential (ability to cause harm) in human beings. On that note, within weeks of introduction, Pfizer's own post-market safety monitoring (per its 5.3.6 Cumulative Analysis submission to FDA, detailed in DailyClout's *Pfizer Papers*) showed the COVID-19 gene therapy to be the *most lethal medical intervention ever rolled out to the public in medical history.* To our knowledge, no other drug, medicine, vaccine, or medical intervention has ever been associated with 1,223 deaths in the first ten weeks after rollout to the public (December 14, 2020, through February 28, 2021). By historic standards, based on this number alone, all modRNA genetic therapies masquerading as "vaccines" should have been removed from public consumption in December 2020 (chapters 5, 6).[465]

EVIDENCE OF REPRODUCTIVE HARMS IN VAERS

The Vaccine Adverse Event Reporting System (VAERS) maintained by FDA and CDC documents a clear danger signal for fertility at the time of writing (May 24, 2023). One of the most visible signs of trouble is the much higher volume of reports for "infertility," "female infertility," "male infertility," and "abnormal fertility tests" published in VAERS for the COVID-19 shots over a 2.3-year period, *compared to the volume of reports for influenza vaccines and all other vaccines over 33 years of use.* The rate of such reports eclipses the rates for all other vaccines by a massive margin. A proportional reporting ratio (PRR), comparing the rate of adverse event reports for the COVID-19 shots to other vaccines, was calculated exactly as recommended by CDC/FDA. According to CDC/FDA's own guidelines, a signal of twofold or greater breaches their safety signal; VAERS data reveals an increase *far exceeding this baseline, but no official action has followed.*

In Figure 1, below, there are 171 cases of infertility for the COVID-19 shots in just 2.3 years, compared to just one case in 33 years for influenza vaccines, yielding a PRR of 171. Likewise, there were only 121 cases for all other vaccines for 33 years, yielding a PRR of 20.3.

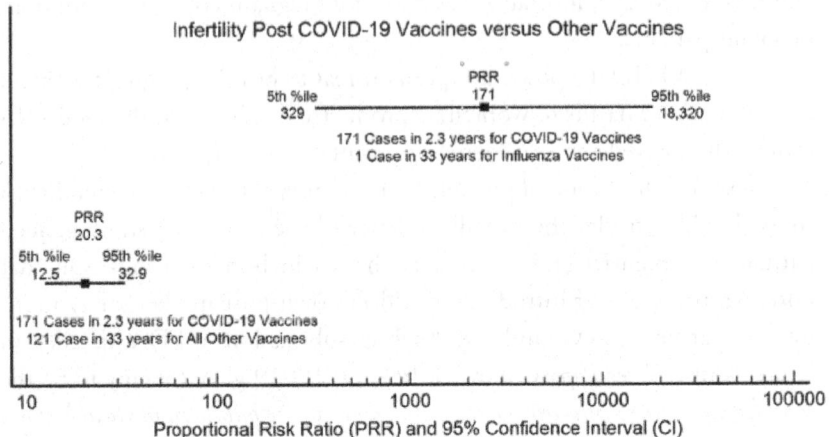

Our own investigational study compared the number of adverse events reported in VAERS following COVID-19 "vaccination" in pregnant women to adverse events reported following all influenza vaccines since 1998.[466] The results of this VAERS investigational retrospective study are catastrophic: FDA and CDC use a twofold increase as triggering a safety signal, yet we found a *fifty-seven-fold increase in miscarriage, and a thirty-eight-fold increase in fetal death (stillbirth)* following COVID-19 "vaccination," when compared to influenza vaccines. Eighteen distinct adverse events types, including abnormal menses and seventeen other major pregnancy complications, all exceeded CDC and FDA safety signals.

PFIZER POST-MARKET MONITORING

The high frequency of adverse events affecting women's fertility associated with the modRNA shots is confirmed by Pfizer's own post-market safety monitoring, which was released in two phases by court order in 2021 and 2022, after FOIA requests, then analyzed by expert volunteers organized by author Naomi Wolf's DailyClout. Their invaluable analysis, collected in a volume published January 2023,[467] and a follow-up volume due out October 2024, emphasizes that reported harms to female fertility outnumber harms to male fertility by several orders of magnitude, meaning women bear the brunt of the impact of the experimental shots in the reproductive category.

In the first phase, ending February 28, 2021, covering the period of drug product development and the first three months of distribution under the emergency use authorization (EUA), Pfizer's internal database recorded 673 incidents relating to pregnancy and lactation.[468] Many incidents reported in the Pfizer first phase of post-market safety monitoring analyzed by the WarRoom/DailyClout researchers were minor, including injection site pain and dizziness, but a number were serious. These included 53 cases of spontaneous abortion, 39 of which occurred in pregnant women with no risk factors; a case of fetal tachycardia one week after the mother was "vaccinated"; two cases of spontaneous membrane rupture in the second or third trimester, leading to premature delivery; and two cases of a fetus accidentally receiving the "vaccine" via the placenta, in both cases followed by extremely premature delivery and death due to respiratory distress.

It should be noted that a CDC study from mid-2021—claiming to find no safety issues in a cohort of around 10,000 "vaccinated" pregnant women—focused narrowly on preterm birth and low birthweight in women "vaccinated" in their second or third trimester, leaving other crucial issues unaddressed—such as miscarriages, maternal mortality, and all events in first-trimester modRNA shot recipients.[469]

The Pfizer post-market data analyzed by the WarRoom/DailyClout volunteer experts covering the first phase, through February 28, 2021, paints a very different picture from the reassuring CDC study. Page 12 of the Pfizer 5.3.6 document details adverse obstetrical events that Pfizer attempted to hide for seventy-five years. The document is poorly written, perhaps to obfuscate the data, but the danger signals of miscarriage and stillbirth are definitive. In a cohort of 270 pregnant mothers, there were danger signals documenting an 81 percent rate of miscarriage (spontaneous abortion) in the first trimester, a fivefold increase in stillbirths (fetal death at or after twenty weeks), an eightfold increase in neonatal mortality rate, and a 14.7 percent complication rate in breastfed infants.

Extending the time frame to March 15, 2022, Pfizer's second phase of post-market safety monitoring elaborated the same pattern, with increasing numbers of adverse events affecting pregnancies as more pregnant women received the shots. By that time, Pfizer documents analyzed by DailyClout revealed 1,809 cases of spontaneous abortions in "vaccinated" pregnant women. By March 2022 over 200,000 women had received a COVID-19 "vaccine" during pregnancy, suggesting an alarming incidence of lost pregnancies.[470]

The DailyClout analysis of Pfizer data uncovered large numbers of other reproductive harms and dysregulations, especially regarding menstrual cycles. The list included 27,685 cases of heavy menstrual bleeding; 15,083 cases of irregular menstruation; 13,989 cases of delayed menstruation; 13,904 cases of pain during menstruation; 12,424 cases of bleeding between periods; and 11,363 cases of absent menstruation.[471]

MENSTRUAL HARMS EXTRAORDINARILY PREVALENT

Echoing the DailyClout analysis of Pfizer's post-market safety monitoring, *menstrual irregularities are far and away the most common harm to women's reproductive systems recorded in safety databases around the world.* As of August 2022, the European Medicines Agency recorded 126,155 reports of menstrual disorders following modRNA injection, including 37,255 reports of heavy bleeding, 18,013 reports of missed periods, and 12,754 reports of bleeding between periods.[472] The trend has been widely discussed by social media users and even acknowledged in a handful of mainstream media reports. However, Big Tech censorship, medical sexism and gaslighting, and the persistence of harmful cultural taboos mean many women likely remain unaware that their menstrual disorders are part of a wider trend.

The mere fact that talk of menstrual irregularities has cropped up in mainstream news media, despite the global censorship regime (chapter 5), shows the very wide prevalence of these side effects.[473] Even pro-modRNA-"vaccine" commentators have criticized the medical establishment for ignoring menstrual changes.[474] Others have detailed the social and cultural factors that lead clinicians to minimize or dismiss women's experiences.[475]

In their rare public acknowledgments of menstrual disorders caused by the modRNA shots, public health authorities and mainstream media have consistently downplayed the severity of menstrual impacts, falsely assuring women and their loved ones that the side effects are always mild and short-lived.[476] *In fact, they can be severe, even life-threatening; they may also point to long-term damage to women's reproductive health.*

Social media has been a key channel of communication and support for women experiencing menstrual disorders after the modRNA shot, and data from online communities offer some insight into the actual prevalence of reproductive injuries from the injections, as a substitute for the screening studies neglected by public health authorities. At a time when reliable, unbiased research is scarce, and public health authorities are actively censoring scientific journals, online surveys can provide useful signals—

especially in cases where an extremely rare condition suddenly crops up in large numbers.

Tiffany Parotto and colleagues published their initial manuscript from MyCycleStory.com documenting extraordinarily high rates of menstrual abnormalities beginning in 2021.[477] After the distribution of the COVID-19 gene products, they observed a marked increase of women sharing irregular menstrual experiences on social media platforms, prompting interest in formal surveys. One survey launched in April 2021 had more than 150,000 respondents.[478] To expound on those findings and gather a wider array of general and menstruation-related symptom data, Parotto and colleagues created a new user-centered survey at MyCycleStory.com.

In the MyCycleStory.com survey, 292 women (4.83 percent of the sample) reported having experienced symptoms consistent with a rare, severe form of abnormal vaginal bleeding—the vaginal passage of a decidual cast. A decidual cast is composed of the endometrial layer in juxtaposition to the uterine cavity, called the decidua. While these were self-reported, according to Google metadata, search terms for "decidual cast shedding" substantially increased during the months of April, May, and June of 2021. Just to put these figures in perspective, the survey identified 292 cases of patients experiencing this event in only 7.5 months in 2021, compared to fewer than 40 cases published in the medical literature spanning 109 years.

The second manuscript from the MyCycleStory.com team, currently in the process of submission for publication, deals with menstrual disorders possibly resulting from "shedding"—the transfer of components of the experimental shot or the resulting spike proteins from one person to another via personal contact.[479] The entity being transferred could include a variety of candidates including, but not limited to, spike protein, lipid nanoparticles, or the pseudouridine-containing modRNA in the vaccine. Research has demonstrated exocrine excretion of modRNA, meaning shedding is very much a possibility, including via sweat and sexual contact.[480] Pfizer "vaccinated" clinical trial participants were advised to avoid any exposure to pregnant woman by way of inhalation, skin contact, or sexual exposure.[481] *It is concerning that the same precautions were not given as warning and protection after the rollout to the public.*

INFLAMMATION A LIKELY MECHANISM OF HARM

More investigation of reproductive harms from the modRNA shots is required. However, as indicated above, many of the injuries cluster in broad categories, suggesting possible common mechanisms of harm. Most importantly, the modRNA shots display powerful inflammatory properties, due in large part to the highly toxic spike protein they produce using cellular machinery. The lipid nanoparticle (LNP) and modified RNA (modRNA) components also have confirmed inflammatory properties (chapters 1, 5).

Inflammation can endanger the health of women and fetuses in all stages of pregnancy. Pre-pandemic research showed that inflammatory responses in pregnant mothers and unborn fetuses lead to increased risk of preterm birth, obstetric complications like ruptured membranes, and neurological handicaps and cerebral palsy, among other long-term risks, as "reprogramming of the fetal immune response may predispose to diseases in adulthood."[482] Additionally, "inflammation can lead to a fetal systemic inflammatory response syndrome, which may involve multiple organ systems, including the fetal brain."[483]

FIRSTHAND CLINICAL OBSERVATIONS

My observations include a dramatic increase in menstrual abnormalities that did not appear until after the rollout of the COVID-19 "vaccines" in 2021. I have observed a dramatic rise in couples seeking advice for infertility, *which does not appear to be isolated to women*, as the modRNA shots have been linked to male factors beyond the scope of this chapter, such as oligospermia, abnormal sperm motility and morphology, loss of libido, and erectile dysfunction.[484] This is not unexpected, as the lipid nanoparticles have been shown by biodistribution studies to concentrate in the ovaries and testes of lab rats (chapters 4, 5). The cationic lipids, modified mRNA, and lysosomal DNA may also be concentrated in these organ systems crucial to human reproduction.

My observations also include a substantial increase in malformations affecting every organ system of embryos and fetuses, including congenital cystic hygroma, hydrocephalus, neural tube defect, cardiac defect, congenital diaphragmatic hernia, and others.[485] Like many of my colleagues, I have observed a sharp increase in placental abnormalities, specifically including calcifications or calcium deposits, particularly in the abdomen and particularly the liver; lacunae, or blank spots that may indicate developmental defects; and infarcts, or areas of dead tissue—all noted only after the rollout of the COVID-19 "vaccines." We hypothesize that many of these are the results of inflammation triggered by the modRNA shots, also associated with an unprecedented increase in lymphadenopathy. Calcifications occur in many human tissues that are generally the final common pathway of an inflammatory process including apoptosis, necrosis, and cell death.[486] We believe the calcification process may be driven by energy-dependent mechanisms, with loss of intracellular and extracellular ion gradients.[487]

Figure 2 summarizes our observations in the ultrasound images of post-"vaccinated" placental images. There are three important findings in common—calcifications (c), infarcts (i), and lacunae (L)—associated with the COVID-19 "vaccines." The infarcts may be associated with thrombosis/embolus (blood clots) and will morphologically evolve in appearance depending upon the proximity to the event.

Figure 2

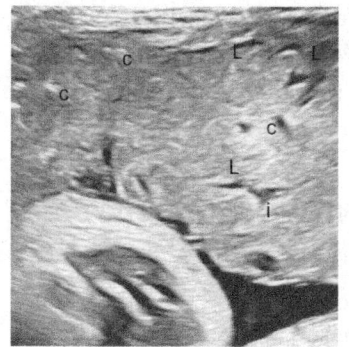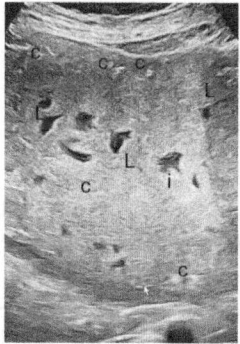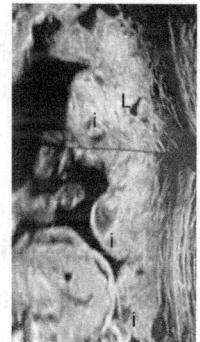

Three separate placental ultrasounds documenting the pathological effects of COVID-19 vaccines. Three important observations are noted including the presence of calcifications [c], lacunae [L], and infarcts [i].

Also observed in my clinical practice is a concerning increase in both spontaneous premature delivery as well as "indicated" (deliberately induced) preterm birth because of severe complications that are increased by the modRNA shots, including severe placental dysfunction, fetal growth restriction, bleeding, placental abruption, severe early onset preeclampsia, and others. My observations have further documented a substantial rise in placental bleeding complications of pregnancy, placental abruptions, severe postpartum hemorrhages, postpartum hysterectomy, and autoimmune complications in pregnancy. I have observed a substantial increase in risk of immune and autoimmune complications in the newborns and infants of mothers who were "vaccinated."

Similarly, I have observed increases in fetal death (also known as stillbirth), defined as the death of the preborn fetus at or after twenty weeks of gestation. The rates of fetal death are clearly increased, as shown by Pfizer's 5.3.6 post-marketing data analyzed by the WarRoom/DailyClout analysis teams, with a fivefold increase based upon a baseline stillbirth rate of 5.8 per 1,000 births.[488] I have noted substantial rises in the number of patients admitted to the neonatal intensive care unit (NICU), as well as in neonatal and infant death rates. These observations are echoed by whistleblower reports from the US and Canada, and align with population-level fertility trends, discussed below.[489]

This overview has covered just a small portion of the harms to women and pregnancy observed by this author in medical practice. Unfortunately, a full presentation of all personal clinical observations of harm resulting from the modRNA shots is beyond the scope of this chapter. "Vaccine" injuries and complications not discussed here may still be valid complaints, deserving investigation and compensation for women and children who have been harmed.

EVIDENCE FROM BIRTH RATES AND OTHER VITAL OUTCOMES

While global birth rates have gradually declined since 2000, they plummeted following the rollout of the COVID-19 gene therapy, with diverse global rates ranging from a 5 percent to 20 percent decrease (a 10 percent drop in birth rates is catastrophic). This alarming trend is buttressed by widespread increases in preterm births, stillbirths, and maternal mortality—reversing decades of progress in a few years.

Backers of the modRNA shots have argued that negative trends in obstetric outcomes are due to COVID-19 itself, presented as the leading cause of maternal mortality in some countries. COVID-19 posed a threat to the overall and reproductive health of a small number of pregnant women, especially those with major comorbidities like diabetes, obesity, heart disease, or autoimmune conditions. But as noted above, it poses no greater overall risk to pregnant women than their nonpregnant peers. Meanwhile, correlations between the rollout of modRNA shots and the timing of demographic declines are strongly suggestive of a causal relationship.

It should be emphasized, again, that *any fall in population-level fertility trends cannot be attributed solely to changes in women's fertility*. As noted, a growing body of andrology (male fertility) research—not presented here—reveals negative impacts of the modRNA shots on the *male reproductive system*, including decreases in motile sperm count and semen concentration, lasting months.[490]

1. *Birth rate declines.* Significant declines in birth rates were observed in high-"vaccination" countries and areas including the US and European Union in 2021–2022. Some of these drops can be attributed to couples deciding to defer conception, or other circumstances imposed by the pandemic. However, most of the declines occurred *after* lockdowns and other major disruptive measures were withdrawn. Further, *quarterly and monthly data from European countries reveal a strong temporal correlation between mass modRNA "vaccination" and changes in birth rates*,[491] as well as various negative pregnancy-related outcomes.

   ○ *United States.* In 2020, the first year of the COVID-19 pandemic, US live births fell 4 percent to 3,605,201. Following a partial recovery in 2021, the expected rally fizzled, and birth rates continue to trend well below their pre-pandemic total.[492] In 2021, total US live births were 2.2 percent below their 2019 total, at 3,664,292. In 2022, to the surprise of experts the total number dropped again to 3,661,220, 2.3 percent below the 2019 total. In July 2022, the abrupt change in the US birth rate over the previous year prompted the US Congressional Budget Office (CBO) to revise its long-term population forecasts, explaining:

   "Changes to projected rates of fertility, mortality, and net immigration mean that the population will be older, smaller, and grow more slowly, on average, than CBO projected last year. CBO now expects the population to be 1.7 percent smaller (equaling 6.5 million fewer people) in

2051 than it projected last year.... Downward revisions to the size of the population age 24 or younger—stemming from reductions to the agency's projection of fertility rates—account for 66 percent of the overall reduction in the annual population estimates for the years from 2022 to 2051.... As a result, CBO now anticipates an average of 170,000 fewer births per year from 2022 to 2031 than it did last year. That difference grows over the projection period as fewer babies born in the first decade grow into adults of childbearing age in later decades. CBO expects there to be 230,000 fewer births annually, on average, from 2043 to 2051 than it projected last year."[493]

o *European Union.* Every country in Europe saw birth rates decline in 2022—two years into the pandemic and following the introduction of the modRNA injections. An analysis by Initiative Corona showed an EU-wide decline of 7 percent in births in 2022, corresponding to about 110,000 "missing" births, with national declines ranging from 1.3 percent in France to 18.8 percent in Romania.[494] Among the three largest EU members:

   i. *Germany.* Total German live births plunged 10.3 percent in 2022, to under 700,000, surprising demographers.[495] As in the US, it is noteworthy that this decline occurred when other possible explanations like lockdowns and resulting economic disruptions were no longer factors. Analysis of monthly figures for live births reveals a strong temporal correlation with the onset of mass modRNA injection. After steady year-over-year increases in monthly live births during 2021, numbers dropped sharply in January 2022, ten months after the beginning of the German mass injection campaign.[496] Births per month continued to trend down in the first quarter of 2023.[497] The authors of a study documenting steep drops in Germany and Sweden remarked: "There is no association of the fertility trends with changes in unemployment, infection rates, or COVID-19 deaths. However, there is a strong association between the onset of vaccination programmes and the fertility decline nine months after this onset. The fertility decline in the first months of 2022 in Germany and Sweden is remarkable. Common explanations of fertility change during the pandemic do not apply in its aftermath."[498]

ii. *United Kingdom.* The UK also saw an unexplained decline in 2022. Once again, an analysis of monthly figures shows a strong temporal correlation between the sudden reversal in birth rates, beginning ten months after the onset of the mass modRNA injection campaign in the UK in April 2021.[499] After year-over-year increases through February 2022, monthly live births in England and Wales show an accelerating decline from March 2022 onward, with year-over-year drops of 2.4 percent in March, 3.8 percent in April, 0 percent in May, 4.5 percent in June, 6 percent in July, and 4 percent in August—the most recent month for which data was available at writing.[500]

iii. *France.* Total births fell 2.6 percent to 723,000 in 2022.[501] Examination of monthly birth numbers shows a pronounced decline beginning in August 2022, twelve months after the government introduced a coercive "health pass" requiring COVID-19 shots to take part in public life.[502] Further monthly declines have followed in 2023, raising alarms about a "fertility crisis."[503]

o *Other countries.* Birth rates also fell sharply in other developed countries in 2022—including Japan, South Korea, and Singapore—although established trends of long-term declines in birth rates, predating the pandemic, make it difficult to assess the overlapping impacts of underlying social factors and the experimental modRNA shots.[504]

2. *Preterm births, stillbirths, and maternal mortality.* Critics have pointed to other possible explanations besides injuries from the experimental injections for declining birthrates, such as couples deciding to defer conception and women's increasing participation in the workforce. However, significant increases in other negative obstetric (pregnancy-related) outcomes—namely preterm births, stillbirths, and maternal mortality—cast further doubt on these benign explanations. Again, it is noteworthy these negative trends were not apparent in 2020, the first year of the pandemic, *but only emerged in 2021–2022*, making it less likely they are due primarily to COVID-19 infection.

   A) *Preterm births.* Premature births increased in countries around the world from 2021–2022, possibly reflecting pregnancy complications resulting from the modRNA shots. No major increases in premature births were recorded during COVID-19 lockdowns in 2020, in a global study of twenty-six countries, with many seeing decreases in preterm birth rates in the first year of the pandemic.[505] In 2021, however, the trend reversed sharply, with large increases in preterm births.

   o *United States.* After years of declining preterm births, including a small drop in 2020, in 2021 the US preterm birth rate increased 0.4 percent to 10.48 percent, "the highest reported figure since at least 2007."[506] This included a 4.5 percent increase in preterm births among "singleton" (single-child) pregnancies, generally at lower risk for prematurity.[507]

   o *South Korea.* Preterm birth rates were already increasing in South Korea before the pandemic, reflecting various factors including increasing maternal age. However, the rate of increase accelerated markedly in 2021. From 2011–2019, the preterm birth rate increased from 5.9 percent to 8 percent, for an average annual increase of 0.26 percent.[508] After decreasing to 7.7 percent in 2020, the share of preterm births jumped to 9.2 percent in 2021, an annual growth rate almost sixfold the 2011–2019 average.[509]

- ○ *Israel.* An Israeli study found that pregnant women who were "vaccinated" in the second trimester were more likely to have a preterm birth than unvaccinated women (8.1 percent of "vaccinated" women compared to 6.2 percent of unvaccinated).[510]

B) *Stillbirths.* It remains challenging to find consistent, accurate global and national data on stillbirths.[511] However, many developed countries with established reporting systems saw increases in stillbirth rates correlated with the mass modRNA injection campaigns, suggesting a direct impact on developing fetuses. Once again, most countries saw stillbirth rates *decrease* in 2020, only to have them rebound strongly in 2021, the second year of the pandemic. This points again to the possibility that the modRNA shots, not COVID-19, were to blame.[512]

While cases of stillbirths associated with COVID-19 infection in pregnant women have been reported, all evidence suggests they are "very rare" and generally associated with maternal comorbid conditions like obesity and diabetes, which make pregnant women more vulnerable to severe COVID-19 disease.[513] A CDC study purporting to show that pregnant women diagnosed with COVID-19 have a stillbirth rate (1.26 percent), double pregnant women without COVID-19 (0.64 percent), failed to account for an unknown number of previous or current, undetected COVID-19 infections in healthy pregnant women—mild or asymptomatic cases, never diagnosed, followed by successful deliveries.[514] The CDC study authors acknowledged these limitations, noting that "identification of COVID-19 status, underlying medical conditions, gestational age, and stillbirths might be misclassified." As a result, the study likely overstates the real prevalence of stillbirths among healthy pregnant women who test positive for COVID-19 with few or no symptoms. Meanwhile, national data show stillbirths correlated closely with the onset of mass "vaccination" campaigns, *not* with waves of COVID-19 infections.

- *Germany.* According to German researchers, a sudden rise in stillbirths was observed beginning the same time as the mass "vaccination" campaign—the second quarter of 2021—and the rate remained elevated through the first three quarters of 2022. The researchers explicitly point to a cause other than COVID-19 infections:

  "Regarding the number of stillbirths, a stable course is observed until the end of the first quarter of 2021. In the second quarter of 2021, a sudden increase in stillbirths is observed, despite the stable course of live births until the end of 2021. Compared to the quarterly number of stillbirths per 1,000 total births in the years 2019 and 2020, the number of stillbirths increased by 9.4 percent in the second quarter of 2021, and by 19.4 percent in the fourth quarter of 2021. In 2022, the stillbirth rate stays unusually high, reaching a maximum in the third quarter.... The findings of this study raise the question of what happened in spring 2021 that led to a sudden and sustained increase in mortality, although no such effects on mortality had been observed during the early COVID pandemic so far."[515]

- *United Kingdom.* The stillbirth rate in England and Wales fell from 3.9 per 1,000 births in 2019 to 3.8 in 2020. However, the following year more than erased this progress, as the stillbirth rate jumped 7.9 percent to 4.1 per 1,000 births in 2021—the first increase in seven years and comparable with the 2018 figure, according to the UK Office of National Statistics.[516]

- *Switzerland.* Stillbirths followed a similar pattern in Switzerland, with the rate falling 7.5 percent from 4.0

stillbirths per 1,000 births in 2019 to 3.7 in 2020, followed by a 19 percent jump to 4.4 stillbirths per 1,000 births in 2021.[517]

- *Netherlands.* From 2020–2021 the overall birth rate in the Netherlands increased 0.2 percent, to 10.162 births per 1,000 people, while over the same time frame the number of stillbirths jumped 6 percent, to a total 887 for the year in 2021.[518]

C) *Maternal mortality.* Given the generally high prevalence of injuries and death among modRNA shot recipients documented in this book, it comes as no surprise they may also be associated with increased maternal mortality, via a range of disease processes including preeclampsia, thromboembolism (blood clots), and heart failure. As with other reproductive harms, it is telling that *maternal mortality didn't increase sharply until 2021*, suggesting another cause besides complications from COVID-19 infection.

- *United States.* After increasing at an average rate of 3.2 maternal deaths per 100,000 live births from 2018 to 2020, in 2021 the US maternal mortality rate (measured as the death of a pregnant woman during pregnancy, childbirth, or within forty-two days of delivery) soared by 9.1 to 32.9 maternal deaths per 100,000 live births. This represents a *roughly threefold increase* in the growth rate over the previous period.[519] The total number of US maternal deaths increased 40 percent in 2021 compared to 2020, dwarfing the 1.4 percent increase in the total number of live births in the same timeframe. According to an analysis by the US Government Accountability Office, COVID-19 infection was responsible for around a quarter of maternal deaths in 2020–2021, but this cannot account for the full 51 percent increase over pre-pandemic levels, from an annual average of 18.8 maternal deaths per 100,000 live births in 2018–2019 to an annual average of 28.4 in 2020–2021.[520] In terms of raw numbers, total maternal deaths in the US *more than doubled* from 1,412 in 2018–2019 to 3,271 in 2020–2021. Subtracting around 800 maternal deaths due to COVID-19 from the 2020–2021 figure, this still leaves *over 1,000 excess, unexplained maternal deaths* in that period compared to the pre-pandemic baseline.

- *United Kingdom and Ireland.* Total maternal deaths in the UK and Ireland increased from 185 over the triennial 2017–2019 period, to 229 in 2018–2020, and 239 in 2019–2021. Excluding 33 maternal deaths due to COVID-19 from the rolling three-year comparisons, maternal deaths in 2019–2021 remained 11 percent higher than the most recent pre-pandemic total (206 in 2019–2021 versus 185 in 2017–2019).[521]

WHO IS RESPONSIBLE FOR EXPOSING PREGNANT WOMEN TO AN EXPERIMENTAL GENETIC THERAPY?

The modRNA shots are dangerous and unnecessary for healthy young people across the board. However, authorization of the experimental injections for use in pregnant women in the absence of long-term safety data, and in the face of laboratory results pointing to reproductive harms, represents a particularly egregious ethical transgression. Continuing to push the shots on pregnant women in the face of mounting evidence of reproductive harms from post-market safety monitoring *can only be viewed as a deliberate assault on women's fertility, and thereby humanity's future.*

The reckless marketing of this untested gene therapy has relied on corrupt medical journals, heavily dependent on advertising revenue from the pharmaceutical industry, purveying bad science and misinformation to persuade doctors that the modRNA shots are safe, effective, and necessary for healthy pregnant women. Independent observers have documented serious scientific lapses and errors in academic publications, suggesting a deliberate, coordinated campaign to deceive pregnant women and their doctors.[522]

Unfortunately, the corruption of scientific publishing is nothing new. In 2009, Dr. Marcia Angell, a well-known, respected physician and longtime editor of the *New England Journal of Medicine (NEJM)*, stated the following:

> It is simply no longer possible to believe much of the clinical research that is published, or to rely on the judgment of trusted physicians or authoritative medical guidelines. I take no pleasure in the conclusion, which I reached slowly and reluctantly over my two decades as an editor of *The New England Journal of Medicine*.[523]

Public health authorities and professional medical societies have colluded to amplify the scientific misinformation published in trusted journals, and threaten any health-care providers who express doubt with professional retribution. The list of organizations distributing misinformation to women and their doctors includes the American College of Obstetricians and Gynecologists (ACOG).

A timetable of events—from December 14, 2020, to the completion of the Pfizer 5.3.6 rollout on February 28, 2021—makes it obvious that the rollout of this dangerous gene-based therapy in pregnancy was planned well before December 2020. The most concerning part of this timeline is the fact that key officials from HHS, CDC, and ACOG were well aware of the Pfizer 5.3.6 data as investigated by WarRoom/DailyClout experts, which showed that the modRNA shots were the most lethal medical products ever brought to the public market—with 1,223 deaths over ten weeks—before recommending them for pregnant women anyway.[524]

In fact, in February–March 2021 HHS/CDC/FDA chose to roll out a $13 billion program through the "COVID-19 Community Corps" (CCC)—a powerful new, government-funded, public outreach and advocacy organization—to unleash a highly deceptive marketing campaign.[525] Their task was to convince the world that this experimental gene product was safe, effective, and necessary in pregnant women, among other groups.

Operating through the COVID-19 Community Corps, HHS awarded billions of federal dollars to recruit what it referred to as "trusted community leaders" who could push the "vaccines" using people's most private relationships. These "trusted messengers" would be unique in their ability to permeate all facets of private life. HHS sought to identify credible and influential community leaders, enlist them to join its COVID-19 Community Corps, and then exploit these "trusted sources" to convince others to get "vaccinated."[526]

The key was finding people with not just *local* but uniquely *interpersonal* influence. As Harvard public health professor Jay Winsten—who has advised previous administrations—explained to *CBS News* in a December 2020 article about the HHS' monumental effort, "You want to go for the low hanging fruit, those that are easiest to pick and harvest." Noting that the focus should be on finding locally influential people to push the "vaccines," Winsten added, "People trust their own doctors, their own nurses, their own pastors, their own social networks. That's very, very different from a distant figure."[527]

Along with over 275 other organizations, 25 of which were health and medical organizations, the American College of Obstetricians and Gynecologists (ACOG) was a founding member of the COVID-19 Community Corps, ultimately receiving millions in federal grant money.[528] Shortly thereafter, on July 30, 2021, ACOG began endorsing COVID-19 "vaccination" in pregnancy, even though the clinical trials failed to include pregnant women and even attempted to exclude them.

Perhaps no other medical organization had as much potential to persuade Americans to get "vaccinated" as ACOG. A pregnant patient's relationship with her ob-gyn is one of the most intimate physician-patient relationships in medicine. Government capture of ACOG allowed it to capitalize on this sacred doctor-patient relationship, using ob-gyn doctors as pro-"vaccine" "trusted messengers." Additionally, convincing pregnant women to take novel modRNA shots would yield an exponential harvest of "low hanging fruit." Women reportedly make 90 percent of health-care decisions for their households; convincing pregnant women to take the COVID-19 shots was almost a guarantee that they would become pro-"vaccine" "trusted messengers" within their own families as well.

Moreover, the optics were exceptionally good for persuading other "vaccine"-hesitant Americans to roll up their sleeve for the experimental shots. If the COVID-19 "vaccines" were considered safe enough to administer to pregnant patients (and thereby trans-placentally to their unborn babies), presumably they would be safe enough for everyone. If HHS and CDC could capture ACOG and convince its ob-gyn members to push the shots on their patients, this would be a bonanza for reaching the "vaccine" hesitant—what HHS Deputy Assistant Secretary Mark Weber referred to as the "moveable middle."[529]

HHS' grand marketing strategy was highly successful. The methods utilized by HHS to push the COVID-19 "vaccines," including the creation of COVID-19 Community Corps, were so vastly different from any other HHS effort that an academic article was published in *Journal of Health Communication* in April 2022 detailing the process and commending its success targeting interpersonal relationships.[530]

Today the HHS campaign to push the COVID-19 "vaccines" is far from over. Having entered its third phase in 2022, it has evolved into a highly targeted approach using both paid and "earned" media strategies. As explained in the article, the HHS campaign:

> …focuses more on precision marketing to identify subgroups with vaccine hesitancy, working directly with communities and using trusted messengers in those communities to deliver messages without the Federal government being directly involved (even though the information may come from a Federal source).

ACOG: A CASE STUDY OF GOVERNMENT CAPTURE OF MEDICAL NON-PROFIT ORGANIZATIONS

On February 1, 2021, ACOG was awarded the first of what would eventually be three HHS and CDC "cooperative agreement" grants made during the pandemic. Under these grants, ACOG would receive over $11 million in federal money over coming years.[531] But there was a catch: as confirmed by documents obtained in a Freedom of Information Act (FOIA) request, by accepting the federal grant money, ACOG relinquished independent control over its COVID-19 recommendations for patients to CDC. Receipt of grant money by ACOG was contingent on ACOG's full compliance with CDC guidance on COVID-19 infection and control,[532] even when CDC rules were contradicted by science.

Although heavily redacted, the FOIA documents revealed startling information about the extent of control CDC wielded (and still wields) over ACOG. For example, the FOIA documents show that CDC grants totaling $3,300,000 were awarded to ACOG on September 2, 2021, for two separate programs, entitled "Engaging Women's Health Care Providers for Effective COVID-19 Vaccine Conversations" and "Improving Ob-Gyns' Ability to Support Covid-19 Vaccination, Mental Health, Social Support."[533] As part of receiving funds under these awards, ACOG is required to "comply with existing and or future directives and guidance from the [HHS]

Secretary regarding control of the spread of COVID-19."[534] The award is also expressly contingent on ACOG's agreement "to comply with existing and future guidance from the HHS Secretary regarding the control and spread of COVID-19."[535] In addition, ACOG must also "flow down" these terms to any person or entity who receives a "subaward."[536] Moreover, CDC is expressly authorized to terminate any award due to material failure to comply with "the terms and conditions of the federal award."[537]

The FOIA documents show CDC working *through* ACOG, in essence exploiting ACOG's authority and sway, to influence not only doctors and patients but also a host of public health entities and "partner organizations" that take their guidance from ACOG.[538]

CDC RECOMMENDS COVID-19 "VACCINES" FOR PREGNANT WOMEN

On April 23, 2021, during a high-profile White House COVID-19 press briefing, CDC director Dr. Rochelle Walensky announced CDC's new recommendation that all pregnant women receive the COVID-19 "vaccine."[539] Apparently basing this recommendation on a misleading CDC study published just days before, Walensky publicly declared that the vaccines appeared to be safe for pregnant women.[540] *However, the study showed precisely the opposite.*

The researchers followed outcomes in 3,958 vaccinated pregnant women between mid-December 2020 and the end of February 2021. During this ten-week window, 827 women completed their pregnancy, of which 712 (86.1 percent) were live births and 115 (13.9 percent) pregnancy losses. Of the pregnancy losses, 104 were spontaneous abortions (miscarriages), the vast majority of which (92.3 percent) occurred before thirteen weeks of gestation. Upon review of the data, however, 700 women (84.6 percent) weren't "vaccinated" until the third trimester, long after most miscarriages (spontaneous abortions) occur. Nonetheless, authors included these 700 third-trimester "vaccinations" in the denominator of the first trimester miscarriages when they calculated the spontaneous abortion rate. Based on their statistical sleight of hand, authors pegged the spontaneous abortion rate at 12.6 percent (104/827) when, in fact, it was truthfully 82 percent (104/127) in the relevant (first) trimester. It should be noted that the miscarriage rate was remarkably close to the Pfizer 5.3.6 study's finding of a ten-week post-market miscarriage rate (81 percent) first brought to light by the WarRoom/DailyClout analysis.[541]

For comparison, a 2013 study estimated the chance of miscarriage at 21.3 percent during the fifth week of pregnancy, falling to 5 percent in the sixth week and then 2 percent to 4 percent during the second half of the first trimester.[542] The astonishingly high miscarriage rate revealed in the CDC study is comparable to the efficacy of the popular "abortion pill" RU486, which carries an FDA black box warning to alert consumers to major drug risks.[543] And yet the CDC study concluded there were no obvious safety concerns.

ACOG FOLLOWS CDC'S LEAD

On July 30, 2021, ACOG, along with the Society for Maternal Fetal Medicine (SMFM), recklessly endorsed the modRNA shots in pregnancy, even though the clinical trials failed to include pregnant women.[544] Now bound under terms and conditions of the cooperative agreements grants, ACOG dutifully fulfilled its mission as a "trusted messenger" by pushing the COVID shots on pregnant women with virtually no scientific justification.

It should be noted that ACOG's July 30, 2021, announcement strongly recommending COVID-19 "vaccination" in pregnancy was a sharp about-face from the organization's previous stance on the issue. Website archives show that—for the months of the pandemic preceding July 30, 2021 (December 2020 through July 21, 2021)—ACOG's official recommendation was to allow pregnant women the freedom to choose, stating throughout the first half 2021: "In the interest of patient autonomy, ACOG recommends that pregnant individuals be free to make their own decision regarding COVID-19 vaccination."[545] Yet ACOG's recommendation abruptly changed on July 30, 2021. In place of patient autonomy, independent clinical judgment, and informed consent about the known and unknown risks of the COVID-19 "vaccines," ACOG's recommendations would now follow CDC's guidance, announced by CDC director Walensky on April 23, 2021—that novel, experimental gene therapy "vaccines" with zero long-term safety data were somehow shown to be safe in pregnancy.

Once again, the suggestion that pregnant women must be innately immunocompromised—parroted in the email to clinicians from the American Board of Obstetrics and Gynecology, recommending modRNA "vaccination" for pregnant women—*is flatly false*. As noted above, pregnant women do not appear to be at greater risk from COVID-19.[546]

ATTEMPTS TO SILENCE DISSENT

To their lasting shame, professional medical societies have cooperated with state medical boards to unleash a campaign of harassment, coercion, censorship, and media bullying of individuals who publish research or espouse views contradicting the propagandistic claim the modRNA shots are "one hundred percent safe and effective." Targeted individuals have been falsely accused of personal and/or scientific misconduct, threatened with potential litigation, and punished with loss of their licensures, board certification, and livelihoods.

In September 2021, professional bodies that govern medical certification—including the American Board of Obstetrics and Gynecology, American Board of Internal Medicine, Federation of State Medical Boards, American Board of Medical Specialties, and American College of Nursing—banded together to issue threats against physicians and nurses who publicly questioned the safety, efficacy, or necessity of the COVID-19 "vaccines," including in pregnant women.[547]

The totalitarian turn by medical professional groups, coordinated by government agencies and pharmaceutical lobbyists, and abetted by academic publishers and the mainstream media, is perhaps the most disturbing and dangerous development of the COVID-19 pandemic. The high degree of cooperation between all these elements, beginning early in the pandemic, points to the existence of a coordinating authority not accountable to the American people.

CONCLUSION

In this chapter we present overwhelming evidence that the experimental modRNA product, falsely marketed as a "vaccine," was rolled out to the global population of pregnant women despite being the most lethal medical product ever, according to Pfizer's 5.3.6 documents.[548] HHS-CDC-ACOG, instead of being transparent and removing the lethal product from the market, tried to hide the damning Pfizer data for up to seventy-five years, while falsely promoting the modRNA "vaccines'" safety, efficacy, and necessity in pregnancy. This campaign of falsehood, with its terrible price of human misery, must be ended immediately.

CHAPTER 12

RISKS TO CHILDREN

By Kelly Victory, MD

Without question, the global response to the COVID pandemic has been characterized by nonscientific, misguided, and counterproductive public health measures, as well as confusing and contradictory messaging. *Children especially suffered mercilessly throughout the duration of the crisis, not from the virus itself, but from draconian lockdowns, unnecessary school closures, futile and cruel mask mandates, and the resultant social isolation and loss of educational opportunities.* The risk of COVID disease to children was grossly overstated, while the crucial role of natural immunity was vehemently and incorrectly denied (chapters 1, 5, 7). Subsequently, experimental modRNA injections were aggressively rolled out with inadequate testing and a paucity of data on both safety and efficacy (chapters 2–5). Many schools and municipalities rushed to mandate the experimental shots, and *some even attempted to circumvent long-established requirements for parental consent.* Arbitrary and capricious public health measures were foisted upon children and their families, while confusing, nonscientific, and frequently contradictory messaging became the norm.

Now, parents and others tasked with protecting the welfare of children are faced with the daunting task of navigating a health-care system that behaved irrationally in response to a global public health crisis, as well as trying to distill sound guidance from health-care practitioners and state and federal authorities who grossly overreacted and so can no longer be trusted as sources of coherent, science-based guidance regarding the potential risks and benefits of childhood vaccination. Unfortunately, this will only undermine confidence in more familiar vaccines, including those with established efficacy and favorable risk-benefit profiles—profoundly negative but entirely predictable "blowback" from the irresponsible rollout of the modRNA shots to children, already reflected in declining uptake for all childhood vaccines.[549]

Since the mid-1990s, challenges to the safety of immunizations have gained prominence in both public and scientific debate. As federal oversight and regulation of biological products, including vaccines, has increased, so too has the public's awareness of the process. In 1999, the Immunization Safety Review Committee was established by the Institute of Medicine (IOM) to evaluate the evidence on possible causal associations between immunizations and certain adverse outcomes, and to assess the broad significance of any potential immunization safety issues and how they might ultimately impact vaccination recommendations. Tragically, this fundamental commitment to the cautious and measured assessment of both vaccine risks and benefits for children was *completely abandoned during COVID-19*. This chapter questions the rationale for "vaccinating" children who face minimal risk—if any—from the virus when there is a clear risk from the "vaccine" itself.

TYPICAL VACCINE DEVELOPMENT

For many of the questions regarding the potential impacts of the experimental modRNA shots technology on children, unfortunately the simple and honest answer is, "We don't know—and we probably won't for a long time." This is due to the unprecedented speed with which the injections were developed and ultimately authorized for children, which logically means *there is no long-term safety data of any kind*.

According to Johns Hopkins University School of Medicine, "A typical vaccine development timeline takes five to ten years, and sometimes longer, to assess whether the vaccine is safe and effective in clinical trials, complete the regulatory approval processes, and manufacture sufficient quantity of vaccine doses for widespread distribution."[550]

This typical prolonged timeline allows for extensive animal testing, elimination of toxic components, and preliminary evaluation of vaccine efficacy during the "preclinical stage." These preclinical trials are followed by multiple "clinical trials" to further assess safety, dosing, and immune response in human subjects, engaging larger and more diverse groups of healthy volunteers as testing progresses. By Phase III clinical trials, tens of thousands of volunteers may be enrolled, including both treatment and placebo groups, allowing for evaluation of short- and long-term safety as well as vaccine efficacy. These trials are critical, as certain rare side effects may only become evident in larger groups.

After a successful Phase III trial, the vaccine developer would typically submit an application to FDA for a biologics license. Before approval of the license, FDA inspects the manufacturing facilities; engages in testing of vaccine lots for purity, potency, and safety; and oversees labeling of the product.

The usually long and complex process of vaccine development involves well-established stepwise, standardized procedures and regulations, with no guarantee that a product will *ever* be successfully brought to market. Many candidate vaccines that appear to be safe, and induce protective immune responses in preliminary animal trials, subsequently fail in human studies. Likewise, initially promising immune responses are frequently found later to be inadequate to induce meaningful immunity, or to be only transitory. Furthermore, clinical trials that deliver robust and enduring immune responses may subsequently reveal pathogenic changes in various organ systems years after the initial inoculation. It is worth noting that, despite decades of research and trial efforts, safe and effective vaccines have *never* been created for numerous viruses—including herpes, norovirus, Coxsackievirus, and a multitude of previous coronaviruses.

Following full FDA approval, a variety of post-marketing vaccine-monitoring systems, such as the Vaccine Adverse Event Reporting System (VAERS), track adverse events potentially related to the new product. Pharmacovigilance systems have been used successfully in multiple previous investigations to identify vaccines associated with increased incidence of adverse events, and vaccines have been withdrawn from use for a much lower incidence of serious harm than that associated with the modRNA vaccines (chapters 5, 6, 9). In 1976, the swine flu vaccine was pulled for purportedly causing Guillain-Barré syndrome in only 1 in 100,000 adults and following reports of 25 potentially associated deaths out of a total of 43 million doses (1 death per 1.7 million doses). Likewise, in 1998–1999, the rotavirus vaccine was withdrawn from the market following 15 reported cases of intussusception, a type of bowel obstruction where the intestine folds in on itself. Although officials stated that "no firm link had been drawn between the vaccine and the children's illnesses," they concluded that *the most reasonable response* was to withdraw the product from the market and recall all remaining doses, as interim data "continued to suggest" an association of around 1 in 10,000 between the bowel issues and the shots.[551]

Although raw data from VAERS is not sufficient to conclusively determine whether a vaccine has caused a particular adverse event, CDC and FDA are *obligated* to carefully review and fully investigate these submissions to determine if there is verifiable causation (chapters 5, 6). To date this has not occurred, despite hundreds of thousands of adverse events, and tens of thousands of deaths, reported to VAERS since the beginning of the COVID "vaccine" roll-out. As of this writing in fall 2023, the COVID "vaccinations" are still on the market despite a serious adverse event rate between 1 in 800 and 1 in 1,000.

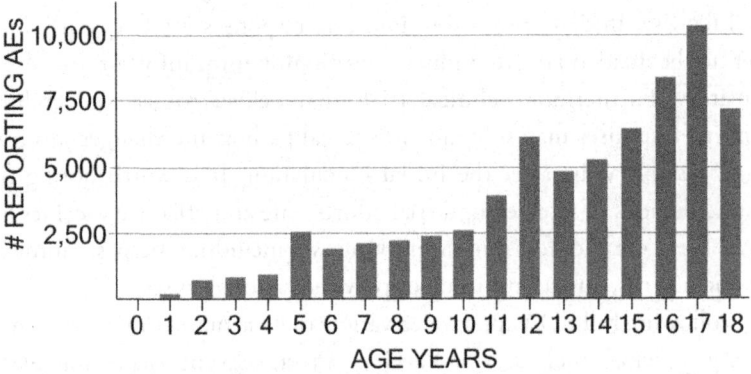

Source: VAERS foreign and domestic data. Analysis by: Dr. Jessica Rose

One of the foundational constructs in medicine is that we *never* use a drug or therapeutic, even if fully approved, in groups of people on whom that intervention was never tested. Children, along with pregnant women, the elderly, those with underlying autoimmune diseases, and the COVID-recovered, were specifically *excluded* from prerelease testing.

It is undeniable that the COVID modRNA injections went through only a fraction of the typical vaccine development process (chapters 2, 3, 5). Preclinical animal testing was minimal, and the very limited clinical trials conducted were rudimentary and of short duration—and in the case of children included very small numbers of subjects. In Pfizer's trial for children ages six months to five years, only 1,678 total children received the "vaccine," and the observation period prior to data submission was only six months—the shortest ever for a childhood vaccine.[552] This study was *both too small and too short in duration* to adequately assess the incidence of adverse effects such as myocarditis, neurological injuries, and blood clots. As of October 1, 2023, the currently available modRNA "vaccines" for children six months to sixteen years old are still only available by emergency use authorization (EUA)—that is, they have not achieved standard biologics license application (BLA) approval. They remain entirely experimental.

Even with the noblest of intentions, there is no substitute for time in medicine. Long-term safety data do not exist because the injections are simply too new to have collected this information. Despite these gross testing limitations, the experimental injections were rolled out widely and indiscriminately to the masses. Now, with ever-mounting evidence of grievous harms resulting from the "vaccines," we are left to grapple with the inexplicable: Why are they still on the market?

RISK-BENEFIT ANALYSIS

There is nothing in medicine that doesn't rightly begin with a thoughtful and well-reasoned risk-benefit analysis. This analysis requires the comparison of the true risk of a situation, treatment or therapy, relative to its potential benefits. Not uncommonly, *both the "risk" and the "benefit" components of the equation are different for various groups.* Younger patients may have greater or lesser risk from a particular condition and may also stand to gain more or less benefit from a particular intervention than older subjects. The risk-benefit calculation may be quite different between males and females, different ethnic groups, people with existing medical conditions, and so on. For a medical intervention that involves more than infinitesimal risk of harm to a particular subject, a clinician *must ensure that the amount of benefit clearly outweighs the amount of risk.*

The risk-benefit analysis directs health-care professionals to apply the "precautionary principle": the broad philosophical and legal concept that, if an innovation has the *potential* to cause harm, particularly when extensive scientific knowledge regarding the risks and benefits are lacking, then *caution* should take precedence. Rather than rushing to apply a new technology, the precautionary principle emphasizes hesitancy, circumspection, and critical review.

Furthermore, to protect patients from unnecessary anxiety and manipulation, there is a moral and ethical responsibility that information regarding medical risks and benefits be communicated in terms of *absolute* benefit and *absolute* risk, rather than *relative* benefit and *relative* risk. For example, to state that a potential intervention or therapy is "95 percent effective" in eliminating the risk of something that *only had a one-in-a-million chance of occurring in the first place* is, at best, grossly misleading (chapter 5).

The risk-benefit calculation is the critical foundation of all medical intervention and requires an honest and accurate analysis of both components of the equation. Very early in the campaign to roll out the experimental modRNA COVID injections, little had been proven about the actual risks from the shots, as no long-term studies had been conducted, and the short-term studies that were conducted purposefully excluded huge categories of people—including pregnant women, the elderly, those with underlying autoimmune diseases, those who had already had and recovered from COVID, and children.

Further complicating the lack of data necessary to adequately assess "vaccine" risk, the potential benefits of the injections were egregiously overstated. If a treatment or therapy is known to be "100 percent safe"—in other words, without any potential for present or future risk—then the efficacy or "benefit" of that intervention need not necessarily be proven. If, on the other hand, the potential for risks is more than zero, or unknown, then efficacy becomes critical relative to accurately calculating any potential benefit (chapter 3). While the public was repeatedly told that the "vaccines" were "greater than 95 percent" effective in preventing COVID infection, it quickly became clear that this protective element had been vastly inflated. Moderna's trial during the Omicron wave in 2021–2022 showed a bleak 44 percent effectiveness against symptomatic infection in six-month-olds to two-year-olds, and only 37 percent effectiveness in two- to five-year-olds. With reported "vaccine" effectiveness having dropped below 40 percent within a matter of months of the "vaccine" rollout, both "vaccine" manufacturers and public health officials began priming the public to expect not only one but likely multiple and repeated routine "booster" doses.

Although FDA and CDC have incessantly repeated their mantra that the modRNA COVID injections "met rigorous scientific and regulatory standards for both safety and effectiveness," they have relied—in error—on the development of injection-induced antibody elevations in making this claim. Key public health decision-makers are surely aware that the production of antibodies is a false surrogate of immunity and is not de facto evidence that a vaccine is effective (chapter 1). In fact, not only are antibody levels not indicative of protection from COVID infection, but the data are overwhelmingly conclusive that multiply "vaccinated" individuals actually have a higher risk of COVID infection than unvaccinated individuals, regardless of the presence of injection-induced antibodies (chapter 7).

To continue to promote an ineffective treatment with unquantified risks is to ignore the fundamental principles of risk-benefit analysis, *and thereby to jettison the moral, ethical, logical, and rational foundation of the practice of medicine.*

UNDERSTANDING CHILDREN'S TRUE RISK FROM COVID INFECTION

From the very beginnings of the pandemic, it was clear that children were at extraordinarily low risk of severe disease from COVID. Week-over-week analysis of national and state-by-state data revealed that children without serious underlying medical conditions were at *statistically zero risk of hospitalization or death.* Many more children were hospitalized with respiratory syncytial virus (RSV), pneumonia, and influenza.[553]

While concerns regarding the risk of COVID to the elderly and those with well-known comorbidities were initially well founded, *this was never true for healthy children.* Analysis of clinical data of 2,135 children ages two to thirteen who tested positive for COVID in China, between January 16, 2020, and February 8, 2020, showed that more than 90 percent of the children were either completely asymptomatic or had less severe symptoms than infected adults.[554]

Similar results were reported from Italy, Germany, the United Kingdom, and Scandinavia, with universally low rates of severe symptomatic disease and no fatalities in young children, including during the outbreak of the more virulent Wuhan and Delta strains.[555] The infection fatality rate (IFR) from COVID was found to be extraordinarily low for children, only 0.002 percent at age ten (roughly 1 in 50,000)—*including those with preexisting medical conditions*—compared to the significantly higher but still relatively modest IFR of 1.4 percent at age sixty-five.[556]

A large study of 48,000 children under the age of eighteen conducted by researchers at Johns Hopkins University found a COVID mortality rate of zero; furthermore, there were no hospitalizations among children without a severe preexisting medical condition such as leukemia. In fact, children were once again shown to be at a much greater risk of hospitalization and death from seasonal influenza and RSV than from COVID.[557] By July 2022, worldwide data showed that the COVID survivability rate for patients under the age of twenty, with infections confirmed by PCR tests, was 99.997 percent.

The extremely low mortality figure for children is based on fatalities among children with *confirmed* COVID infections, excluding the manifold larger cohort of children who experienced asymptomatic or very mild infection and were never tested. If this larger group of undetected cases were included in the study population, *the mortality rate would certainly be even lower*.

Despite the minimal risk to children's health from COVID, many have justified instituting draconian restrictions on their activities, as well as the blanket recommendations for COVID "vaccination," on the basis that children were likely to spread the virus to adults. Examination of data from US schools, however, reveals infection rates among children and school staff *far lower* than in the broader community.[558] Furthermore, there was no increase in COVID cases following the reopening of schools for in-person education, further dispelling this flawed rationale.[559]

In a study of North Carolina school districts with a composite student population of approximately 90,000, a total of 773 COVID infections were traced to interactions that occurred *outside* of school, while only 32 infections occurred as a result of exposures *in* school. Just as importantly, no incidences of child-to-adult transmission were identified at all.[560] These findings are consistent with those seen elsewhere around the world. Teachers in Swedish preschools caring for children ages one to six years, and in schools with children seven to sixteen years of age that remained open during the pandemic and did not require face masks, were not found to have an increased risk of contracting or being hospitalized for COVID relative to other occupations.[561]

NATURAL IMMUNITY

It has long been recognized that natural immunity to infection is far superior to "vaccine"-induced immunity (chapters 1, 5, 7). In early 2022, by a conservative estimate over 75 percent of children had already had COVID-19 and recovered through their own natural immune response. Therefore, these children should have been considered to have this natural protection for at least some period—*certainly long enough to allow for more extensive testing and evaluation of the experimental modRNA injections.*

Despite a continued, vehement argument from officials at CDC, NIH, and elsewhere that natural immunity quickly waned and was insufficient protection against recurrent disease, study after study has documented the strength and endurance of natural immunity to this virus. Gazit et al., for example, concluded that natural immunity confers longer-lasting and stronger protection against infection, symptomatic disease, and hospitalization than two doses of the "vaccines."[562] Likewise, a large study conducted by the Cleveland Clinic, published in July 2022, including data on more than 52,000 individuals, revealed that individuals with previous COVID infection did not receive additional benefit from COVID vaccination.[563]

After nearly three years of denying the robust and enduring nature of natural immunity to COVID, *The Lancet* finally published a definitive study concluding that the immunity acquired from natural infection confers protection that is on par with, if not better than, that from two doses of the experimental mRNA injections.[564] The study found that infection-acquired immunity cut the risk of hospitalization and death from a COVID reinfection by at least 88 percent for at least ten months.

"VACCINE"-INDUCED ADVERSE EVENTS IN CHILDREN AND ADOLESCENTS

Without question the COVID modRNA injections were subjected to a grossly curtailed testing period, as shown here (chapters 2, 3, 5). Whereas vaccines typically undergo a minimum of six to eight years of rigorous testing, these shots were rolled out to the public in a matter of months. As noted, testing on children was all but nonexistent, as they were specifically excluded from the preliminary clinical studies; a very small number of children were ultimately studied, only briefly, before the decision was made to extend the emergency use authorization to these younger age groups.

Not long after mass COVID "vaccinations" began in January 2021, worldwide reports of serious adverse reactions following injection began to surface. Of particular concern were adverse events seen in children, given their significantly lower risk from COVID infection itself, suggesting an unfavorable risk-benefit analysis.[565] Official calculations by UK public health authorities indicate that, depending on the severity of future strains, it would require giving COVID-19 "vaccines" to between 340,000 and 1.9 million children ages five to eleven *to prevent a single pediatric ICU hospitalization in that age group*—an absurdly skewed cost-benefit equation.[566]

Well before the injections were approved for use in young children, the incidence and risk of myocarditis was well-documented in teens and young adults. A study on patients conducted between December 14, 2020, and August 31, 2021, reported rates of myocarditis within seven days following "vaccination," significantly exceeding the expected rates for both males and females across multiple age ranges. The rates of myocarditis cases were highest after the second "vaccination" dose in adolescent males aged twelve to fifteen years (70.7 per million Pfizer doses), in adolescent males aged sixteen to seventeen years (105.9 per million Pfizer doses), and in young men aged eighteen to twenty-four years (52.4 and 56.3 per million doses of the Pfizer "vaccine" and the Moderna "vaccine," respectively).[567]

Researchers Gill et al., published in the *Archives of Pathology*, demonstrated that death during sleep occurs in teenagers with COVID-19 modRNA "vaccine"-induced myocarditis. Importantly, this study further demonstrated that these post-"vaccine" cases of cardiac insult have myocardial injury that is clearly distinct from conventional myocarditis (chapter 8).[568]

Although many of those promoting the experimental COVID injections have suggested that the risk of myocarditis is higher after COVID infection than after "vaccination," multiple studies have disproven this premise. A large population-based Israeli study revealed no increased incidence of myocarditis following COVID infections in the nearly 200,000 patients evaluated.[569] Similarly, a study conducted by Dr. Tracy Høeg and colleagues at the University of California found that males ages twelve to seventeen *were over six times more likely to be hospitalized for cardiac events* following their second COVID "vaccine" dose, than they were to be hospitalized from COVID infection, over a four-month period.[570]

In light of mounting evidence of severe adverse events, including myocarditis and sudden unexplained cardiac arrests, Denmark, Sweden, Finland, and Norway halted boosters for healthy teenagers under the age of eighteen in fall 2022. In September 2021, the United Kingdom recommended against "vaccinating" individuals under sixteen and in February 2023 *ended boosters entirely for most healthy adults under fifty*.[571] The US, in stark contrast, continues to recommend boosters for everyone aged six months and older—making America an *increasingly isolated outlier* in global public health policies.

CHILDREN ARE DIFFERENT

It's often said in medicine that "children are not just little adults"—meaning they don't necessarily benefit from the same interventions and therapeutics as their adult counterparts, simply dose-adjusted for their smaller statures and lower body weights.

Up to and even beyond puberty, children have not completed the development of various organ systems, including the brain, musculoskeletal system, reproductive system, and immune system. The risk of any intervention initiated during childhood is compounded by the recognition that health in adulthood is predicted by health in childhood and that the results of medications, vaccinations, or other therapeutics given in childhood may have profound impacts on lifespan and overall health. In addition to the risk of acute injury in children, we must be vigilant regarding the unknown potential for long-term injury. Independent of the concerns regarding the distribution and longevity of the modRNA genetic material contained in the injections, lipid nanoparticles themselves have long been known to have potential toxic effects on organs such as the liver, brain, spleen, blood, kidney, heart, colon, and bone, and can lead to deformation and inhibition of cell growth in humans and animals. The potential toxicity of nanomaterial is particularly important in children whose organ systems are not fully developed.[572]

THE PEDIATRIC BRAIN

The American Academy of Pediatrics presents increasing evidence that our brains have not reliably reached adult levels of functioning until well into the third decade of life.[573] We know that a number of major morphological and functional changes occur in the human brain during adolescence and that particularly significant changes occur in the limbic system, impacting self-control, decision-making, emotions, and risk-taking behaviors. Brain maturation is governed by multiple factors but is particularly vulnerable to pharmacotherapy and other environmental interventions during childhood.[574]

It is well-established that the prefrontal cortex is one of the last regions of the brain to reach maturation. Neuronal proliferation and "rewiring" of this critical area occurs until around age twenty-five, and neurotoxic insult may have a profoundly negative impact during this sensitive period of brain development.

Parents have reported a worrisome number of children developing debilitating headaches, profound personality and behavioral changes, sleep disturbance, memory impairment, and outright psychosis within hours or days of modRNA injection. A literature review from the first ten months of the initial "vaccine" rollout revealed reports of headache, Guillain-Barré syndrome, transverse myelitis, facial nerve palsy, small fiber neuropathy, newly developing multiple sclerosis, and multiple other neurological side effects possibly related to the COVID "vaccines'" neurological impacts on kids (chapter 9).[575]

While neurological adverse events such as headache, fatigue, muscle, and joint pains following COVID-19 "vaccination" were generally found to be mild and transient, researchers also found a greater than expected occurrence of severe neurological adverse events including cortical sinus venous thrombosis, Bell's palsy, transverse myelitis, and Guillain-Barré syndrome, as well as new-onset demyelinating brain lesions and worsening of preexisting neurological disorders such as epilepsy and multiple sclerosis (chapter 9).[576] An analysis of VAERS data revealed the incidence of new-onset seizures following COVID-19 "vaccines" was 3.191, as compared to 0.090 for influenza vaccines, representing a *thirty-five-fold increase*.[577]

MUSCULOSKELETAL SYSTEM

The musculoskeletal system is similar to the neurologic system, in that skeletal maturity is a time-dependent process that begins in childhood but is not fully complete until approximately age twenty-five. Virtually all drug classes may interrupt bone and soft-tissue development in children and induce musculoskeletal disorders, but corticosteroids, vaccines, and antibiotics are amongst the most common offending agents.[578]

Multiple studies have reported inflammatory musculoskeletal complications following modRNA injection. The spectrum of short-term inflammatory musculoskeletal manifestations after COVID-19 "vaccine" administration includes polymyalgia, polyarthritis, girdle pain and stiffness, tenosynovitis, and sacroiliitis and/or spondylitis. It is completely unknown, however, if these acute cases reflect only a transient reactogenic response or if they may lead to a structured, chronic inflammatory muscle or joint disease in the future.[579]

A systematic review and meta-analysis of clinical trials on the incidences of neuromuscular adverse events after COVID modRNA "vaccination" concluded that "adverse events were common," with nearly 40 percent of patients suffering from postinjection headache and 30 percent reporting myalgias (muscle pain).[580]

REPRODUCTIVE SYSTEM

Although puberty begins in females from the ages of eight to ten years old, they do not reach sexual maturity and full fertility until approximately age sixteen. The hormones required for initiation of puberty are released in a pulsatile fashion (in waves), and these hormone elevations remain essential for maintaining the cyclic reproductive function. Similarly, in boys puberty usually occurs ages ten to fourteen years, but full sexual maturity does not occur until seventeen to eighteen years of age. In both males and females, sequences of the somatic and hormonal changes are critical to achieve normal sexual maturation and the active functions of reproduction.

Despite being told repeatedly that the modRNA material would remain at the injection site in the deltoid muscle of the arm, biodistribution studies conducted by Pfizer, well prior to the launch, revealed the concentration of injected modRNA in multiple organ systems, including 11 percent in the reproductive system (ovaries and testes). Without a clear understanding of potential impact on future fertility, this single fact alone should have precluded the injections from being given to children. Again, independent of any risks from the modRNA itself, there is growing concern amongst scientists about potential harmful effects of lipid nanoparticles on the reproductive system specifically. A study by Wang et al. reported a multitude of toxicities in both males and females, ranging from "injured uterine and ovarian tissue" to "testicular dysgenesis syndromes."[581]

The potential for long-delayed evidence of adverse impact is one of the many reasons that vaccines are traditionally required to undergo vigorous and prolonged testing. It will likely be a full decade or more before the data will be available to fully assess the effects of the experimental modRNA COVID shots on the fertility of children who received them.

THE PREPONDERANCE OF THE EVIDENCE

In January 2023, *The Journal of the American Medical Association* (*JAMA*) published a systematic review and meta-analysis of multiple studies looking at the safety and effectiveness of the COVID modRNA injections on five- to eleven-year-old children. Two randomized clinical trials and five observational studies investigated adverse events among "vaccinated" children. The vast majority—more than 85 percent—of modRNA "vaccinated" children experienced at least one local adverse event such as injection site pain, redness, or swelling, following both the first and second injections. "Vaccination" was also associated with a higher risk of any of the adverse events compared with a placebo. Nearly half of the "vaccinated" children developed at least one systemic adverse event—including fatigue, fever, headache, myalgias, or myocarditis—following the first injection (20,369 of 55,380 [45.1 percent]), and more than half following the second injection (20,182 of 45,998 [56.4 percent]). Overall, the incidence of an adverse event severe enough that it prevented normal daily activities was 8.8 percent—*nearly one in ten children*.[582]

THE CHILDHOOD VACCINATION SCHEDULE

On May 10, 2022, despite mounting evidence of serious adverse cardiac events and dismal data on efficacy, FDA voted to expand the use of Pfizer's experimental modRNA "vaccine" to children as young as twelve, stating that the injection was safe and "offers strong protection" for younger teens. Two days later, CDC's Advisory Committee on Immunization Practices (ACIP), a group that offers guidance and recommendations to CDC, voted unanimously to approve the use of the Pfizer "vaccine" on children ages twelve to fifteen. Shortly thereafter, CDC revealed that its Vaccine Safety Technical Work Group was reviewing cases of myocarditis in teenagers and young adults who had received one of the modRNA "vaccines," adding that heart inflammation was primarily seen in adolescents and young adults, and was more likely in males, with onset of symptoms commonly four days following the second injection.

Despite these overwhelming and readily apparent safety signals, in June 2022—in what can only be described as an indefensible breach of previous vaccine review standards—FDA's vaccine advisory committee voted unanimously to *further* expand the emergency use authorization of the experimental modRNA injections to include children as young as six months. Subsequently, in October 2022, CDC's Advisory Committee on Immunization Practices (ACIP) voted to add the injections to the childhood vaccine schedule, the list of routine shots recommended for children, adolescents, and adults against common infectious diseases. The current list also includes shots for influenza, chicken pox, measles, mumps and rubella, polio, and others. Under CDC's most recent guidelines, in September 2023, healthy children aged six months to four years old, and those aged five to eleven years old are supposed to receive a primary two-dose series of either the Moderna or Pfizer-BioNTech monovalent COVID-19 "vaccine," followed by a third "updated monovalent booster." Recommendations for children twelve and up are to receive two doses of the Moderna, Pfizer, or Novavax "vaccine," followed by a monovalent "booster." While CDC does not have the authority to mandate vaccines (that decision is left up to states and local jurisdictions), the vaccine schedule clearly serves as a resource and guide for physicians, particularly pediatricians, regarding which vaccines should be administered and when. Furthermore, states generally incorporate CDC's recommendations when establishing criteria for enrollment in daycare and school. As a result of its inclusion on the childhood vaccine schedule, the COVID modRNA shot "recommendations" from CDC may well become codified within the requirements for schools, sports activities, and other parts of kids' lives. In addition, per the National Childhood Vaccine Injury Act of 1986, once a vaccine has been added to the childhood vaccine schedule, the manufacturers enjoy broad liability protection against adverse events, even if the emergency use authorization expires or is rescinded—*almost certainly the "real" reason the modRNA shots were added to the childhood schedule in the first place.*

Vaccines are not uncommonly required when they are given to protect the health of the general public by preventing disease spread. These mandated vaccines not only must be proven effective in preventing transmission of the disease but also must be supremely safe because they are given to large numbers of healthy people. On the other hand, vaccines that are given primarily to prevent serious infection or life-threatening illnesses fundamentally benefit the individual vaccine recipient, *not the population as a whole*. There is no moral or scientific rationale for mandating a "vaccine" that neither stops the individual from contracting the illness nor from transmitting it to others—yet that is precisely what has occurred with the experimental COVID injections.

PRIMUM NON NOCERE—"FIRST DO NO HARM"

As health-care practitioners, we have a fundamental obligation—moral, ethical, and legal—to act in the best interests of our patients. The four pillars of medical ethics—autonomy, beneficence, non-malevolence, and justice—require us to provide fully informed consent, eschew coercion, ensure positive impact, do no harm, and treat patients fairly. Available information on the COVID modRNA injections is woefully inadequate to provide informed consent or to conclude a positive risk-benefit calculation. Although we still have no way of knowing their long-term impacts, the data gathered to date on the COVID modRNA injections are overwhelming, and the evidence is irrefutable: *the "vaccines" aren't safe, effective, or necessary.* While the benefits for high-risk adults and the immunocompromised may have appeared compelling during the original outbreak of the Wuhan strain and subsequent Delta strains, *this was never true for children.*

Given the de minimis risk to children from COVID infection, the unassailable evidence of acute postinjection adverse events, the currently unquantified risk of medium- and long-term injury from the "vaccines," and their continually declining efficacy, the critical risk-benefit calculation clearly falls *against COVID "vaccines" for children.* Regardless of how or why these experimental injections were allowed to be released to the public, we implore the government of the Unites States, and those around the world, to immediately halt their use until further safety and efficacy studies can be conducted. *They have no place on the childhood vaccine schedule.*

CHAPTER 13

"VACCINE" MORTALITY INSIGHTS FROM AUTOPSY REPORTS

By Peter A. McCullough, MD, MPH, and
Harvey Risch, MD, PhD, et al.

Peter McCullough and Harvey Risch gratefully acknowledge collaborators and original coauthors Nicolas Hulsch, Paul Alexander, Richard Amerling, Heather Gessling, Roger Hodkinson, William Makis, and Mark Trozzi for their critical contributions to the research summarized here. Much of the information presented in this chapter was originally submitted to The Lancet *in the form of a coauthored "preprint" on July 5, 2023. However, the following day the preprint, still pending peer review, was removed from* The Lancet's *server, on the grounds later conveyed that "the study's conclusions are not supported by the study methodology." No further explanation or additional detail had been provided at the time of publication of this book.*

The first doses of the experimental COVID-19 "vaccines" were administered less than eleven months after the identification of the SARS-CoV-2 genetic sequence, representing the fastest "vaccine" development in history, with limited assurances of short- and long-term safety.[583] As of mid-2023, about 69 percent of the world population have been inoculated with at least one dose of a COVID-19 "vaccine."[584]

The preceding chapters have outlined some of the likely mechanisms of injury inflicted by the modRNA pro-vaccines. This chapter will further explore possible causal links between the COVID-19 "vaccines" and deaths—using autopsy and postmortem data.

Clustering of harms in certain organ systems, close resemblance to post-"vaccination" deaths reported through pharmacovigilance systems, and consistency of these findings with likely mechanisms of harm described in preceding chapters all strongly suggest that COVID-19 "vaccines" were the main or contributing cause of death in the large majority, if not all, of the cases examined here. Circulating spike protein, produced uncontrollably throughout the body by the experimental shots, is likely the main mechanism of harm (chapters 4, 5, 7–11).[585]

If a large number of deaths are indeed causally linked to COVID-19 "vaccination," the implications could be immense, including: the complete withdrawal of all COVID-19 "vaccines" globally; suspension of all remaining COVID-19 "vaccine" mandates and passports; loss of public trust in government and medical institutions; investigations and inquiries into the censorship, silencing, and persecution of doctors and scientists who raised these concerns; and compensation for those who were harmed as a result of the administration of COVID-19 "vaccines."

"VACCINE" TYPES INCLUDED

There are a number of different COVID-19 "vaccines," all relying on inadequately tested experimental technologies, referred to in the autopsies considered in this study. The most frequently utilized COVID-19 "vaccine" platforms include inactivated virus (Sinovac—CoronaVac), protein subunit (Novavax—NVX- CoV2373), viral vector (AstraZeneca—ChAdOx1 nCoV-19, Johnson & Johnson—Ad26.COV2.S), and modified messenger RNA (mRNA) or modRNA (Pfizer-BioNTech—BNT162b2, Moderna— mRNA-1273).[586] All utilize mechanisms that can cause serious adverse events, generally involving the uncontrolled synthesis and distribution of the spike protein as the basis of an antibody-focused immune response.

METHODS AND FINDINGS

The research described here is a meta-analysis, a type of study that analyzes multiple other studies together using statistical techniques in an effort to detect patterns and relationships that may not be readily apparent in any individual study. In this case, the meta-analysis considered autopsy and necropsy reports relating to COVID-19 "vaccination" up until May 2023. After screening 678 studies mentioning post-"vaccination" autopsies for consistency and comparability of data, forty-four papers covering a total of 325 autopsy cases and 1 necropsy case were determined to meet the criteria for inclusion in the meta-analysis.

Each case was independently reviewed by three physicians to determine whether COVID-19 "vaccination" was the direct cause of death, a contributing cause, or unrelated. A case was determined to be related if two of three reviewers agreed that death was causally connected to COVID-19 "vaccination." Through this system of independent review by three physicians, a total of 240 deaths—73.9 percent of the total—were adjudicated to be directly due to, or significantly related to, COVID-19 "vaccination." It should be noted most decisions were unanimous, with consensus regarding 203 deaths, or 62.5 percent of the cases.

The average time between "vaccination" and death was just over two weeks (14.3 days). Among deaths causally linked to the COVID-19 modRNA "vaccines," the organ systems most likely to be involved were cardiovascular (53 percent), hematological (17 percent), respiratory (8 percent), and multiple organ systems (7 percent). In the latter category, 21 cases (6.5 percent) involved three or more organ systems.

RESEARCH IN CONTEXT

To the best of our knowledge, at the time of writing this is the largest review of autopsy findings after COVID-19 "vaccination" yet conducted. Despite mounting evidence of widespread harms, detailed throughout this book, the mechanisms of death from COVID-19 "vaccination" remain largely unexplored. Further urgent investigation is needed to confirm these results and better understand the mechanisms underlying fatal outcomes from the COVID-19 shots, with the goal of risk mitigation for the large numbers of individuals who received them.

Many hypothetical causes of COVID-19 "vaccine" injuries have been offered. A growing body of research confirms that the COVID-19 spike protein, encoded in genetic instructions (modRNA or DNA) or delivered directly by the "vaccines" discussed here, is highly pathogenic in its own right (chapter 4). There is also compelling evidence of the toxicity and dangerous inflammatory properties of other "vaccine" components, such as LNPs, PEG, and the "vaccine" genetic material (modRNA) itself (chapters 1, 5, 7).

- The spike protein as well as its subunits and smaller fragments can trigger ACE2 receptor degradation and internalization, which may lead to destabilization of the renin-angiotensin system (RAS), resulting in possible inflammation, contraction of blood vessels, and blood clots.[587]
- The spike protein activates platelets, causes endothelial damage, and directly promotes arterial and venous clotting.[588]
- Immune system cells take up lipid nanoparticles (LNPs), then release them back into circulation with elevated numbers of "exosomes"—special encapsulated message pods used by cells to communicate. The exosomes contain both spike protein and microRNAs, which play a role signaling responses in recipient cells at distant sites, contributing to severe inflammation.[589]
- Long-term cancer control may be handicapped by IRF7 and IRF9 suppression, among other causal mechanisms (chapters 1, 7, 9, 10).
- COVID-19 modRNA "vaccination" has also been linked to neurodegenerative disease, myocarditis, immune thrombocytopenia (low white blood cells), Bell's palsy, liver disease, impaired adaptive immunity, impaired DNA damage response, and tumorigenesis (chapters 5–10).
- New studies have shown the modRNA "vaccines" trigger production of high levels of IgG4 antibodies, raising the possibility of immune tolerance to spike protein, immune suppression, autoimmune disease, myocarditis, and cancer growth (chapters 1, 7).[590]
- Neurotoxic effects of the spike protein include headache, tinnitus, autonomic dysfunction, and small fiber neuropathy (chapter 9).[591]
- Separately, in 2021, research linked the adenoviral vector "vaccines" (principally AstraZeneca and Johnson & Johnson) to a new clinical syndrome: "vaccine-induced immune thrombotic thrombocytopenia" (VITT), characterized by spontaneous blood clots at distant body sites that are not usually prone to clotting, and severe loss of blood cells. The precise mechanism behind VITT remains unknown, but researchers have hypothesized it is caused by post-"vaccination" antibodies against platelet factor 4 (PF4) triggering extensive platelet activation.[592]

- Myocarditis continues to be one the most widely discussed "vaccine" injuries, due in part to its notable prevalence among healthy young men, at very low risk of severe COVID-19 disease. Multiple overlapping causal mechanisms have been proposed for post-"vaccination" myocarditis (chapter 8).[593]

Biodistribution data (chapter 4) suggests that spike protein may be expressed in cells from many vital organ systems, raising significant concerns regarding the safety profile of COVID-19 "vaccines." Given the identified "vaccination" syndromes and their possible mechanisms, the frequency of adverse event reports is expected to be high, especially given the vast number of "vaccine" doses administered globally. Unfortunately, data from VAERS and other sources confirm this expectation (chapters 5, 6, 14).

Using VAERS data alone to establish a causal link between COVID-19 "vaccination" and death, however, is not possible, due to acknowledged limitations and confounding factors (chapter 6). Autopsies are one of the most powerful diagnostic tools in medicine to establish cause of death and clarify the pathophysiology of disease.[594] COVID-19 "vaccines," with plausible mechanisms of injury to the human body and a substantial number of adverse event reports, represent an exposure that may be causally linked to death in some cases, and autopsy analysis is the clearest and most direct route.

DISCUSSION

A total of 44 studies were included in the meta-analysis, covering a total of 325 autopsy cases and 1 necropsy case (heart).[595] The mean age of death was 70.4 years, and there were 139 females (42.6 percent). Most received a Pfizer/BioNTech "vaccine" (41 percent), followed by Sinovac (37 percent), AstraZeneca (13 percent), Moderna (7 percent), Johnson & Johnson (1 percent), and Sinopharm (1 percent). Among causes of "vaccine"-related death, the cardiovascular system was most frequently implicated (53 percent), followed by hematological (17 percent), respiratory (8 percent), multiple organ systems (7 percent), neurological (4 percent), immunological (3 percent), and gastrointestinal (1 percent). In 7 percent of cases, the cause of death was either unknown, non-natural (drowning, head injury, and so forth), or infection. One organ system was affected in 302 cases, two organ systems in 3 cases, three in 8 cases, and four or more in 13 cases.

The number of days from "vaccination" until death was 14.3 (mean), 3 (median) irrespective of dose; 7.8 (mean), 3 (median) after one dose; 23.2 (mean), 2 (median) after two doses; and 5.7 (mean), 2 (median) after three doses. The distribution of days from last "vaccine" administration to death is highly right skewed, showing that most of the deaths occurred within a week from last "vaccination" (see figure).

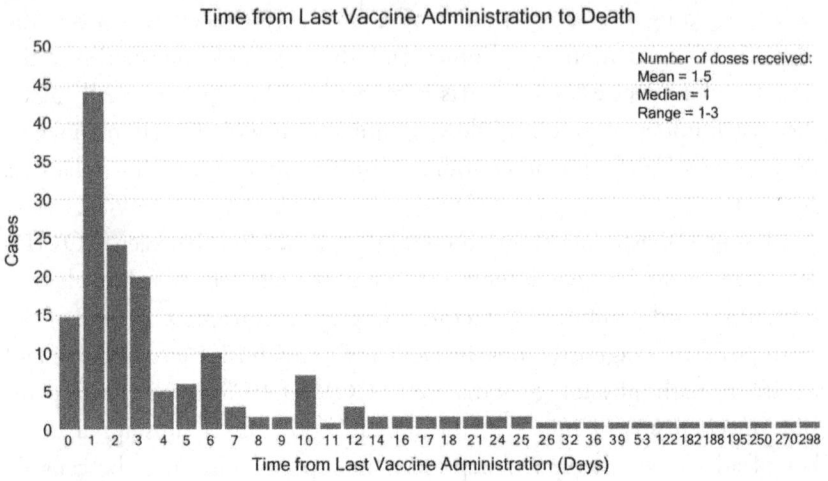

Three physicians independently adjudicated 240 deaths (73.9 percent) to be significantly linked to COVID-19 "vaccination." Among adjudicators, there was complete independent agreement (all three physicians) of "vaccination" causing or contributing to death in 203 cases (62.5 percent). The 1 necropsy case was also judged to be linked to "vaccination" with complete agreement.

As noted, the cardiovascular system was by far the most implicated organ system in death, followed by hematological, respiratory, multiple organ systems, neurological, immunological, and gastrointestinal, with three or more organ systems affected in 21 cases. These results corroborate known COVID-19 "vaccine"-induced syndromes and show significant, temporal associations between COVID-19 "vaccination" and death involving multiple organ systems, with a predominant implication of the cardiovascular and hematological systems.

Criteria of causality from an epidemiological perspective have been met, including:

- biological plausibility,
- temporal association,
- internal and external validity,
- coherence,
- analogy, and
- reproducibility with each successive report of death after COVID-19 "vaccination."

Our findings amplify concerns regarding COVID-19 "vaccine" adverse events and their mechanisms, especially those affecting the heart.[596] Further, they highlight the involvement of multiple organ systems in some of the deaths associated with COVID-19 "vaccination." This might be attributed to multisystem inflammatory syndrome (MIS), detected following COVID-19 "vaccination" in both children and adults.[597] A possible mechanism by which MIS occurs after "vaccination" may be the systemic distribution of the LNPs containing modRNA, following administration, and the consequent systemic spike protein expression and circulation resulting in system-wide inflammation.[598]

A large share of post-"vaccination" mortality was due to hematological system injuries—particularly plausible in light of VITT and pulmonary embolism reported in the literature following COVID-19 "vaccination."[599] Deaths caused by adverse effects to the respiratory system were also relatively common, in line with the possibility of acute respiratory distress syndrome (ARDS) or drug-induced interstitial lung disease (DIILD) after COVID-19 "vaccination."[600] Although less common in this study, immunological, neurological, and gastrointestinal adverse events were also reported.[601]

Most of the deployed "vaccine" platforms are associated with death, suggesting they share a common feature that causes adverse effects, most likely the toxic spike protein. Further, the large number of COVID-19 "vaccine"-induced deaths evaluated in this review is consistent with multiple papers that report excess mortality after "vaccination" (chapters 5–7).

- Spiro Pantazatos and Herve Seligmann found that all-cause mortality increased zero to five weeks postinjection in most age groups, resulting in an estimated 146,000–187,000 "vaccine"-associated deaths in the United States between February and August 2021.[602]

- These concerning results were further elucidated by Jarle Aarstad and Olav Andreas Kvitastein, who found that among thirty-one countries in Europe, a higher population COVID-19 "vaccine" uptake in 2021 was positively correlated with increased all-cause mortality in the first nine months of 2022, after controlling for alternative explanations.[603]
- Excess mortality from non-COVID-19 causes has been detected in many countries since the mass "vaccination" programs began, suggesting a common deleterious exposure among populations.[604]

Pantazatos estimated that VAERS deaths are underreported by a factor of 20.[605] If we apply this underreporting factor to the May 5, 2023, VAERS death report count of 35,324, the number of deaths in the United States *alone* becomes 706,480.[606] If this extrapolated number of deaths were to be confirmed, the COVID-19 "vaccines" would easily represent the worst man-made medical disaster in history.

CONCLUSION

In summary, we identified a large series of deaths after COVID-19 "vaccination," confirmed with autopsy and necropsy, to help the medical community better understand fatal COVID-19 "vaccine" syndromes. The consistency seen among cases in this review with known COVID-19 "vaccine" adverse events, their mechanisms, and related excess death—coupled with autopsy confirmation and expert physician death adjudication—suggests there is a high likelihood of a causal link between COVID-19 "vaccines" and death, in most cases. Even with substantial evidence, our paper cannot definitively determine causality, as we face all the limitations of systematic literature reviews, including selection bias, publication bias, and confounding variables. Further investigation is urgently required to confirm our results and better understand the mechanisms underlying the described fatal outcomes, with the goal of risk mitigation for the large numbers of individuals who have taken one or more COVID-19 "vaccines."

CHAPTER 14

"ALL HANDS ON DECK"— THE CATASTROPHE OF US LONGEVITY, AND WHAT WE CAN DO ABOUT IT

By Josh Stirling, MBA

Following the publication of the 2022 provisional life expectancy estimate by CDC in November 2023, FDA commissioner Dr. Robert M. Califf posted a thoughtful series of tweets to provide context and issue a challenge. Critically, Dr. Califf identified America's declining life expectancy as an extraordinary public health challenge, which after nearly a decade cannot be dismissed as merely a trend but is in reality a "catastrophe."[607] He further called for accountability and an "all hands on deck effort" to address the suffering and social costs portended by these ominous longevity statistics. He also challenged all of society—government, industry, and public—to get engaged to help drive toward a solution.

Dr. Califf's points are inarguable. In view of the many different factors contributing to our nation's poor health and decline in life expectancy, leaders across many institutions, including in government, health care, pharmaceutical, food, and media, as well as institutions like employers and insurers, will have to work together on real changes to arrest this tragic and worrisome trend.*

---

* An example of one such effort is the Insurance Collaboration to Save Lives, a nonprofit led by global insurance leaders, seeking to engage and empower global insurers to do exactly that—insurers can greatly mitigate excess mortality and elevated morbidity, and improve health, save lives, and save money by offering proactive, voluntary health screening, testing, and triage for at-risk policyholders. The goal of the collaboration is to "save a million lives," and it is seeking public and private partners to help. Learn more at www.insurancecollaboration.org.

WORRISOME TREND AND ALARMING ACCELERATION

Dr. Califf raised the alarm in response to CDC's annual update showing another year of below-trend life expectancy in 2022. Notably, the decline in COVID in 2022 did not lead to a full recovery in life expectancy to pre-COVID levels.[608] In fact, since 2020 the United States has suffered roughly 1.7 million more deaths than would have been expected had mortality remained at the approximate level of 2018–2019 (*Exhibit 1*), including around 600,000 not due to COVID-19.

While this scale of excess deaths is mind-numbingly large, the percentages are meaningful too. *Exhibit 2* (and many subsequent exhibits) displays the numbers of deaths compared to an index of the prior level of deaths in 2019—represented as a baseline of "1.00." Using this approach, one can readily see trends, highlighted with darker shades to indicate more extreme changes from the previous baseline. For example, in *Exhibit 2*, the index of 1.29 in fourth quarter of 2020 means that the US saw 29 percent more deaths in that period than in the fourth quarter of 2019. Looking at the most recent data, in 2023, we have seen improved mortality, but the index still shows 8 percent more deaths reported this year through the third quarter, when compared to the same months in pre-pandemic 2019.[609]

Exh. 1

U.S. Deaths by Quarter As Reported in (000s) All Ages						
Quarter	2018	2019	2020	2021	2022	2023
1	772	745	777	925	927	805
2	682	697	852	759	748	743
3	668	679	812	872	770	734
4	716	732	942	907	833	
Year	2,838	2,854	3,383	3,463	3,278	
YTD	2,122	2,121	2,441	2,556	2,445	2,282

Source: CDC as of 12/12/2023, full year 2022 n = 3278k

Exh. 2

U.S. Deaths by Quarter Indexed to 2019 All Ages						
Quarter	2018	2019	2020	2021	2022	2023
1	1.04	1.00	1.04	1.24	1.24	1.08
2	0.98	1.00	1.22	1.09	1.07	1.07
3	0.98	1.00	1.20	1.28	1.13	1.08
4	0.98	1.00	1.29	1.24	1.14	
Year	0.99	1.00	1.19	1.21	1.15	
YTD	1.00	1.00	1.15	1.20	1.15	1.08

Source: CDC as of 12/12/2023, full year 2022 n = 3278k

Again, it is critical to clarify that *COVID-19 accounts for only part of this elevated long-term mortality*. As of late 2023, CDC tallied around 1.1 million deaths attributed to COVID-19 over this whole period (2020–2023), leaving around 600,000 excess deaths. Even more alarming, mortality remains elevated even after the premature deaths of 1.7 million Americans, which, under normal circumstances, should logically be followed by a period of *lower* mortality. That we continue to see deaths continuing well above the levels seen in 2019—*in spite of expected below-normal levels of mortality post-pandemic*—is surprising and concerning.

Even more concerning is *the unusual spike in deaths reported among younger adults and the early working ages* in the third and fourth quarters of 2021, as seen in *Exhibit 3*. In that period (winter 2021–2022) the mortality for younger ages reached levels far exceeding the previous, more modest spikes seen in the first waves of the pandemic. In particular, in the third quarter of 2021, younger working ages suffered a mortality rate 59 percent higher than the same period of 2019.

Exh. 3

U.S. Deaths by Quarter
Indexed to 2019
Ages = 15-44

Quarter	2018	2019	2020	2021	2022	2023
1	1.02	1.00	1.12	1.39	1.43	1.27
2	0.99	1.00	1.32	1.38	1.27	1.24
3	0.98	1.00	1.32	1.59	1.27	1.18
4	0.94	1.00	1.27	1.45	1.25	
Year	0.98	1.00	1.26	1.45	1.30	
YTD	1.00	1.00	1.25	1.45	1.32	1.23

Source: CDC as of 12/12/2023, full year 2022 n = 209k

Exh. 4

U.S. Deaths by Quarter
Indexed to 2019
Ages = 45-64

Quarter	2018	2019	2020	2021	2022	2023
1	1.03	1.00	1.03	1.26	1.25	1.01
2	1.00	1.00	1.22	1.16	1.06	1.01
3	1.01	1.00	1.23	1.44	1.09	1.01
4	1.00	1.00	1.25	1.34	1.09	
Year	1.01	1.00	1.18	1.30	1.12	
YTD	1.01	1.00	1.16	1.29	1.13	1.01

Source: CDC as of 12/12/2023, full year 2022 n = 592k

This is highly unusual, because in contrast, in that same period, the oldest ages saw only a modest level of increase in reported deaths. The elderly eighty-five-plus populations saw only 11 percent increases in the third quarter of 2021—and even in the early COVID period, older age mortality increases *never came anywhere near the 59 percent increase* above 2019 levels suffered by younger, working ages in the third quarter of 2021 (older ages saw a peak at only 27 percent during the fourth quarter of 2020).

Tragically, mortality rates among children ages one to fourteen also spiked in the fourth quarter of 2021, followed by additional anomalous spikes in the fourth quarter of 2022 and third quarter of 2023. It is important to note that child mortality remains elevated for a variety of reasons, including heartbreaking increases in deaths due to homicide, suicide, drug overdoses, accidents, and use of firearms. However, rates of mortality due to disease have also increased among children, including diseases of the circulatory system, respiratory system, diabetes and metabolic disorders, and deaths coded as resulting from "abnormal clinical signs and symptoms," which includes a variety of codes including sudden infant death syndrome (SIDS).[610]

Exh. 5

	U.S. Deaths by Quarter Indexed to 2019 Ages = 1 to 14					
	Year					
Quarter	2018	2019	2020	2021	2022	2023
1	1.19	1.00	1.03	1.11	1.09	1.11
2	1.04	1.00	1.03	1.14	1.10	1.07
3	1.02	1.00	1.08	1.16	1.13	1.21
4	1.01	1.00	1.08	1.19	1.34	
Year	1.06	1.00	1.06	1.15	1.16	
YTD	1.08	1.00	1.05	1.13	1.11	1.13

Source: CDC as of 12/12/2023, full year 2022 n = 6k

Given the high risk posed by COVID to our most vulnerable older citizens, and the well-established, much lower risk to children and young adults, the *decrease* in mortality among the vulnerable elderly, accompanied by an *increase* among young, healthy people, is not just counterintuitive—it is shocking. Like the overall increase in mortality *despite the decrease in COVID-related mortality*, it once again suggests that *something besides COVID-19* is responsible for these unprecedented spikes and sustained plateaus in deaths among children and young adults.

The younger ages still represent few deaths as a share of the overall total population mortality, which remains dominated by the elderly. However, if these trends of elevated mortality rates persist, and reflect an *ongoing* phenomenon that will continue to impact future long-term mortality (rather than, say, passing short-term health, social, or environmental factors), this could represent a truly daunting challenge for our society.

This is due to the power of compounding, which compounds good outcomes and bad outcomes alike. If the higher number of deaths in today's younger age group persists, then over time, our younger age cohorts could see notably lower longevity than previous generations. Should the factors currently contributing to excess mortality in younger ages continue to impact the US population, the effect could be substantial. On that note, in July 2022 the US Congressional Budget Office (CBO) revised its long-term population forecasts, explaining:

> Changes to projected rates of fertility, mortality, and net immigration mean that the population will be older, smaller, and grow more slowly, on average, than CBO projected last year. CBO now expects the population to be 1.7 percent smaller (equaling 6.5 million fewer people) in 2051 than it projected last year.... Downward revisions to the size of the population age 24 or younger—stemming from reductions to the agency's projection of fertility rates—account for 66 percent of the overall reduction in the annual population estimates for the years from 2022 to 2051....[611]

Given the far higher net social cost implied by a decline in longevity among working-age people, the potential risk of such an outcome is a critical topic for social, business, and health leaders to proactively address, in hopes of mitigating the human and economic damage.

FOREIGN MORTALITY DATA

Countries with health-care provision comparable to the US also recorded an extraordinary increase in mortality in 2022, when the direct effects of the pandemic had largely subsided. Many of these excess deaths were attributed to causes besides COVID.[612]

- In 2021–2022, the United Kingdom experienced near-record excess mortality, only partially due to COVID-19, prompting the BBC to observe, "Though far below peak pandemic levels, it has prompted questions about why more people are still dying than normal.... We are still seeing more deaths overall than would be expected based on recent history. The difference in 2022—compared with 2020 and 2021—is that Covid deaths were one of several factors, rather than the main explanation for this excess."[613]
- In 2021, the German national statistics agency noted, "The number of reported Covid-19 deaths in autumn and until the end of 2021 can only in part explain the higher death figures." The

report offered several possible causes, including Germans deferring medical care, but admitted, "It is however currently not possible to quantify the contribution of individual effects." Reporting another "surprising" increase in excess mortality in 2022—almost double the initial COVID-19 wave in in 2020—a researcher from the German IFO think tank could again only concede, "The exact reasons for this are still unclear."[614]

- The French national statistics agency reported a similar phenomenon, as summarized by the newspaper *Les Echos*: "After two years of the Covid pandemic, INSEE (National Institute of Statistics and Economic Studies) experts expected to see the number of deaths return to their usual level in 2022. However, last year, the statistical institute recorded 675,000 deaths, or 53,800 more than planned. This is more than in 2020 (668,900 deaths) than in 2021 (661,600 deaths).... All of these deaths cannot be attributed to Covid since the number of deaths linked to the disease has greatly decreased in 2022: 38,300 people died of the coronavirus in 2022, against 59,100 in 2021, according to provisional figures from Public Health France." INSEE attributed some of the excess mortality in France to influenza and heat waves, but the report added: "The unknown remains the increase in deaths among those under 34, a priori less worried by influenza epidemics and heat waves."[615]

- Other countries experiencing large, unexpected increases in non-COVID mortality in 2022 included Japan, South Korea, and Australia.[616]

RECORD-SETTING DISABILITY RATES

The large rise in mortality among young, healthy people has been accompanied by an equally surprising jump in long-term disability.

As part of its monitoring of the labor force, the Bureau of Labor Statistics (BLS) surveys both working and nonworking Americans to measure disability in our country and its impact on labor force participation, meaning how many people are working or actively looking for work. Available since 2008, this monthly data is not based on payment of disability claims, but merely the reported presence of disabilities in homes surveyed by BLS.

BLS defines disability as:

> A person with a disability has at least one of the following conditions: is deaf or has serious difficulty hearing; is blind or has serious difficulty seeing even when wearing glasses; has serious difficulty concentrating, remembering, or making decisions because of a physical, mental, or emotional condition; has serious difficulty walking or climbing stairs; has difficulty dressing or bathing; or has difficulty doing errands alone such as visiting a doctor's office or shopping because of a physical, mental, or emotional condition.[617]

Since year-end 2020, the number of disabled Americans has risen by 3.9 million. Since year-end 2019 (i.e., pre-COVID), the number of disabled adult Americans has risen by 2.6 million. Today fully 12.7 percent of the adult population report a disability when surveyed—a full percentage point more today than in the decade prior to COVID. Compared to year-end 2020, the rate is now 1.3 percentage points higher, representing a substantial increase in American adults with a disability. In *Exhibit 6* we present the data series from the earliest date it was reported; the increase in disability rate in 2021 and 2022 is unprecedented, with 2023 disability now at all-time highs.[618]

Exh. 6

Morbidity leads mortality and tragically, federal labor market data shows nearly four million American adults newly self-report as suffering a disability in just the past three years. Source: Bureau of Labor Statistics, as of December 10, 2023, from St. Louis Fed, FRED https://fred.stlouisfed.org/series/LNU00074597.

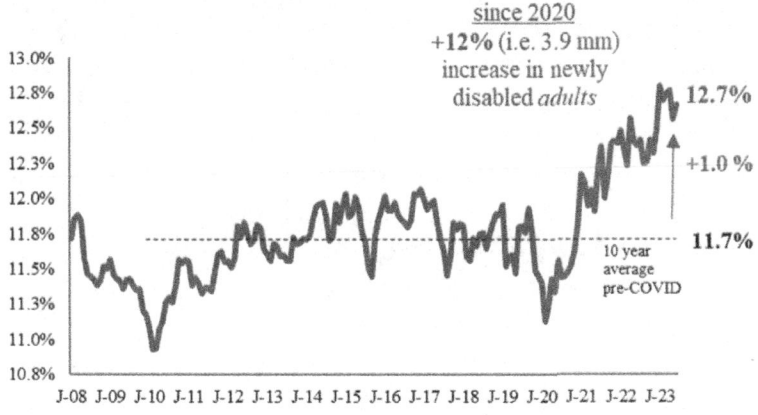

It should be emphasized that while disability *claims* can sometimes be influenced by broad economic weakness, *this* data does not reflect disability claims (public or private), but is an actual survey of workers' self-reported health. As such, this data series represents a useful aggregate metric of nearly real-time public health, rather than labor market strength (historically, economic hard times have seen an increase in formal disability claims, for obvious reasons).

It is counterintuitive and deeply concerning that the most significant increases in disability seen since 2020 came *among workers who are currently working or actively seeking work*. As noted, this trend runs sharply counter to established historical precedent, suggesting a wave of new, sometimes profound, disability among previously healthy individuals. In fact, following a sharp rise beginning in mid-2021, there has been a shocking 36 percent increase in disabilities among adults in the labor force—nearly three times the overall rate of increase in disability in the overall adult population—and disability remains at unprecedented levels in late 2023. As in the overall population, looking at the full data series shows that historically these numbers were quite stable, and an increase of this magnitude was never before seen.

Exhibit 7

Among adults in the labor force, the rate of disability is lower, but the concentrated increase since 2020 has driven this measure of health to tragic and uncharted record levels. Source: Bureau of Labor Statistics, as of December 10, 2023, from St. Louis Fed, FRED https://fred.stlouisfed.org/series/LNU01074597.

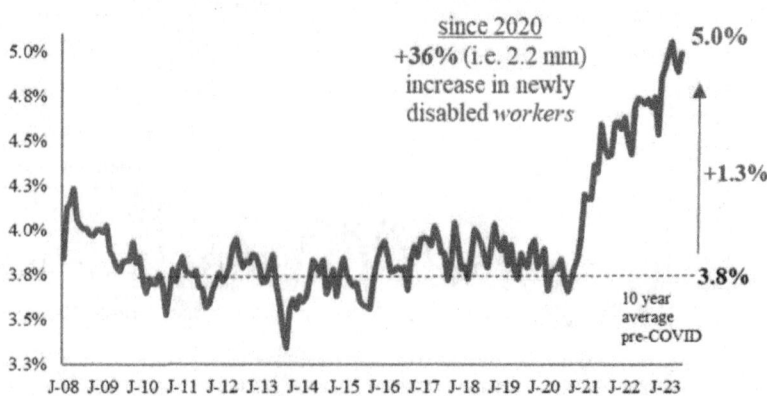

UK DISABILITY DATA

New disability benefits claims by working age people in the UK doubled from 2021 to 2022, according to the IFS think tank, which noted, "The increase in claimants is seen across medical conditions and ages, with the fastest rise among teenagers, where claim rates have tripled." IFS went on: "This sudden increase seems to be driven by a worsening of health across the population—something for which there is now accumulating evidence across a number of sources." IFS author Sam Ray-Chaudhuri stated: "Almost as remarkable as the rise in disability benefit claims itself is how widespread it is. We see a doubling in claims at essentially every age and for most major conditions, from mental illness to arthritis and back pain. Worsening health seems to be behind the rise, but precisely why health is getting worse is a puzzle of its own."[619]

Large increases in the number of people with disabilities were seen in Canada in 2021 and Australia in 2022, but interpretation is difficult due to government outreach initiatives to identify disabled people during this time, a definite confounder for these datasets.[620]

WHAT'S BEHIND THE TREND?

Parsing the factors driving elevated mortality and disability is extraordinarily challenging, as statisticians, epidemiologists, and insurance actuaries all find themselves facing the same "sea of red"—numerous, overlapping signals of increased pathologies, which they must analyze with data that is incomplete at best. Yet certain conclusions can already be drawn from mortality data.

Nearly without exception, all major contributing causes of mortality rose in 2020, and most have remained elevated *even as the death toll from COVID-19 subsided* (*Exhibits 8–35*). This is consistent with a broad systemic health factor leading to inflammation, injury, infection, and disease across many tissues, organs, and systems, but does not—as coded—reveal a pattern conforming to any single, specific, known disease as the cause. Rather, the systemic nature of the injury categories revealed by the following pages are suggestive of a systemic pathology, most likely circulatory (blood-borne). Analysis of multiple cause of death patterns from 2018 to 2023 shows a wide range of health factors contributing or linked to this rise in mortality.

A review of US deaths, highlighting the relative changes in important "contributing" causes of death, reveals the breadth of the challenge. In in the following pages, we present analyses of "Multiple Cause of Death" data, sorted by prevalence in 2022, which totals the counts of reported "contributing" factors for each death to show changes over time—rather than considering only the "underlying" cause of death as coded by CDC.

Exh. 8

U.S. Contributing Cause of Death Counts, Indexed
I00-I99 | Diseases of the circulatory system

Quarter	2018	2019	2020	2021	2022	2023
1	1.02	1.00	1.04	1.22	1.25	1.11
2	0.96	1.00	1.21	1.10	1.11	1.10
3	0.97	1.00	1.20	1.26	1.18	1.12
4	0.97	1.00	1.27	1.23	1.18	
Year	0.98	1.00	1.18	1.20	1.18	
YTD	0.99	1.00	1.15	1.19	1.18	1.11

Source: CDC as of 12/12/2023, full year 2022 n = 2868k

Exh. 9

U.S. Contributing Cause of Death Counts, Indexed
J00-J98 | Diseases of the respiratory system

Quarter	2018	2019	2020	2021	2022	2023
1	1.11	1.00	1.08	1.63	1.57	1.11
2	0.97	1.00	1.49	1.16	1.09	1.08
3	0.99	1.00	1.44	1.84	1.23	1.14
4	0.98	1.00	1.78	1.70	1.28	
Year	1.02	1.00	1.44	1.58	1.30	
YTD	1.03	1.00	1.32	1.54	1.31	1.11

Source: CDC as of 12/12/2023, full year 2022 n = 1232k

Exh. 10

U.S. Contributing Cause of Death Counts, Indexed
E00-E89 | Endocrine, nutritional & metabolic diseases

Quarter	2018	2019	2020	2021	2022	2023
1	0.99	1.00	1.07	1.49	1.53	1.31
2	0.94	1.00	1.38	1.27	1.28	1.28
3	0.95	1.00	1.41	1.55	1.36	1.31
4	0.95	1.00	1.53	1.48	1.36	
Year	0.96	1.00	1.34	1.45	1.39	
YTD	0.96	1.00	1.28	1.44	1.40	1.30

Source: CDC as of 12/12/2023, full year 2022 n = 809k

Exh. 11

U.S. Contributing Cause of Death Counts, Indexed
C00-D48 | Neoplasms (including cancers)

Quarter	2018	2019	2020	2021	2022	2023
1	1.00	1.00	1.02	1.03	1.07	1.04
2	0.99	1.00	1.02	1.03	1.03	1.04
3	1.00	1.00	1.04	1.07	1.06	1.05
4	1.00	1.00	1.05	1.06	1.06	
Year	1.00	1.00	1.03	1.05	1.05	
YTD	1.00	1.00	1.03	1.04	1.05	1.04

Source: CDC as of 12/12/2023, full year 2022 n = 728k

Exh. 12

U.S. Contributing Cause of Death Counts, Indexed
R00-ER99 | Symptoms, signs and abnormal clinical and laboratory findings, not classified elsewhere

Quarter	2018	2019	2020	2021	2022	2023
1	1.04	1.00	1.04	1.27	1.32	1.20
2	0.98	1.00	1.19	1.13	1.15	1.19
3	0.99	1.00	1.22	1.33	1.23	1.28
4	0.99	1.00	1.33	1.31	1.24	
Year	1.00	1.00	1.19	1.26	1.24	
YTD	1.00	1.00	1.15	1.24	1.24	1.22

Source: CDC as of 12/12/2023, full year 2022 n = 656k

Exh. 13

U.S. Contributing Cause of Death Counts, Indexed
G00-G98 | Diseases of the nervous system

Quarter	2018	2019	2020	2021	2022	2023
1	1.03	1.00	1.06	1.21	1.27	1.17
2	0.94	1.00	1.21	1.07	1.13	1.13
3	0.95	1.00	1.23	1.20	1.21	1.16
4	0.94	1.00	1.29	1.16	1.18	
Year	0.96	1.00	1.20	1.16	1.20	
YTD	0.97	1.00	1.16	1.16	1.20	1.15

Source: CDC as of 12/12/2023, full year 2022 n = 454k

TOXIC SHOT

Exh. 14

U.S. Contributing Cause of Death Counts, Indexed
N00-N99 | Diseases of the genitourinary system

Quarter	2018	2019	2020	2021	2022	2023
1	1.02	1.00	1.04	1.37		1.14
2	0.96	1.00	1.24	1.15	1.14	1.12
3	0.97	1.00	1.28	1.43	1.21	1.15
4	0.97	1.00	1.41	1.39	1.20	
Year	0.98	1.00	1.24	1.34	1.24	
YTD	0.99	1.00	1.18	1.32	1.25	1.14

Source: CDC as of 12/12/2023, full year 2022 n = 373k

Exh. 15

U.S. Contributing Cause of Death Counts, Indexed
A00-B99 | Certain infectious and parasitic diseases

Quarter	2018	2019	2020	2021	2022	2023
1	1.09	1.00	1.05	1.37	1.30	1.12
2	0.98	1.00	1.19	1.13	1.10	1.09
3	1.01	1.00	1.25	1.48	1.20	1.12
4	0.99	1.00	1.34	1.42	1.22	
Year	1.02	1.00	1.20	1.35	1.21	
YTD	1.03	1.00	1.16	1.33	1.21	1.11

Source: CDC as of 12/12/2023, full year 2022 n = 320k

Exh. 16

U.S. Contributing Cause of Death Counts, Indexed
K00-K92 | Diseases of the digestive system

Quarter	2018	2019	2020	2021	2022	2023
1	0.99	1.00	1.05	1.23	1.28	1.18
2	0.95	1.00	1.09	1.16	1.17	1.15
3	0.97	1.00	1.17	1.26	1.21	1.16
4	0.97	1.00	1.22	1.25	1.22	
Year	0.97	1.00	1.13	1.22	1.22	
YTD	0.97	1.00	1.10	1.22	1.22	1.17

Source: CDC as of 12/12/2023, full year 2022 n = 316k

Exh. 17

U.S. Contributing Cause of Death Counts, Indexed
D50-D89 | Diseases of blood & blood-forming organs,
and certain disorders involving immune mechanism

Quarter	2018	2019	2020	2021	2022	2023
1	1.00	1.00	1.06	1.32	1.41	1.26
2	0.97	1.00	1.18	1.18	1.24	1.25
3	0.97	1.00	1.23	1.38	1.30	1.28
4	0.97	1.00	1.31	1.33	1.27	
Year	0.98	1.00	1.19	1.30	1.31	
YTD	0.98	1.00	1.15	1.29	1.32	1.26

Source: CDC as of 12/12/2023, full year 2022 n = 119k

Exh. 18

U.S. Contributing Cause of Death Counts, Indexed
L00-L98 | Diseases of the skin & subcutaneous tissue

Quarter	2018	2019	2020	2021	2022	2023
1	0.99	1.00	1.02	1.26	1.49	1.41
2	0.97	1.00	1.15	1.21	1.36	1.38
3	0.99	1.00	1.22	1.30	1.45	1.37
4	0.97	1.00	1.26	1.36	1.41	
Year	0.98	1.00	1.16	1.28	1.43	
YTD	0.98	1.00	1.12	1.26	1.44	1.39

Source: CDC as of 12/12/2023, full year 2022 n = 38k

Exh. 19

U.S. Contributing Cause of Death Counts, Indexed
M00-M99 | Diseases of the musculoskeletal system
and connective tissue

Quarter	2018	2019	2020	2021	2022	2023
1	0.99	1.00	1.02	1.21	1.27	1.17
2	0.96	1.00	1.18	1.07	1.13	1.13
3	0.98	1.00	1.21	1.20	1.21	1.16
4	0.99	1.00	1.29	1.16	1.18	
Year	0.98	1.00	1.17	1.16	1.20	
YTD	0.98	1.00	1.13	1.16	1.20	1.15

Source: CDC as of 12/12/2023, full year 2022 n = 78k

Exh. 20

U.S. Contributing Cause of Death Counts, Indexed
Q00-Q99 | Congenital malformations, deformations, and chromosomal abnormalities

Quarter	2018	2019	2020	2021	2022	2023
1	1.02	1.00	1.02	1.01	1.10	1.10
2	0.99	1.00	1.04	1.06	1.10	1.09
3	1.00	1.00	1.07	1.14	1.18	1.02
4	0.99	1.00	1.08	1.14	1.15	
Year	1.00	1.00	1.05	1.09	1.13	
YTD	1.00	1.00	1.04	1.07	1.13	1.07

Source: CDC as of 12/12/2023, full year 2022 n = 19k

Exh. 21

U.S. Contributing Cause of Death Counts, Indexed
P00-P96 | Certain conditions originating in perinatal period

Quarter	2018	2019	2020	2021	2022	2023
1	1.05	1.00	0.99	0.97	0.98	1.01
2	0.99	1.00	0.94	0.93	0.98	0.91
3	1.08	1.00	0.94	0.96	1.05	0.91
4	1.02	1.00	0.90	0.96	1.06	
Year	1.03	1.00	0.94	0.95	1.02	
YTD	1.04	1.00	0.96	0.95	1.01	0.94

Source: CDC as of 12/12/2023, full year 2022 n = 18k

Exh. 22

U.S. Contributing Cause of Death Counts, Indexed
H00-H59 | Diseases of the eye and adjoining tissues

Quarter	2018	2019	2020	2021	2022	2023
1	0.95	1.00	0.98	1.08	1.17	1.07
2	1.05	1.00	1.31	1.01	1.15	1.16
3	1.07	1.00	1.19	1.34	1.25	1.31
4	0.98	1.00	1.33	1.09	1.09	
Year	1.01	1.00	1.20	1.12	1.16	
YTD	1.02	1.00	1.15	1.13	1.19	1.04

Source: CDC as of 12/12/2023, full year 2022 n = 3k

Exh. 23

U.S. Contributing Cause of Death Counts, Indexed
O00-O99 | Pregnancy, childbirth and the puerperium

Quarter	2018	2019	2020	2021	2022	2023
1	1.08	1.00	0.62	0.73	0.85	0.56
2	0.82	1.00	0.77	0.76	0.63	0.57
3	0.99	1.00	0.83	1.36	0.61	0.57
4	0.81	1.00	0.74	0.98	0.73	
Year	0.92	1.00	0.74	0.96	0.70	
YTD	0.96	1.00	0.74	0.96	0.69	0.57

Source: CDC as of 12/12/2023, full year 2022 n = 1k

WHAT IS THE SYSTEMIC FACTOR CAUSING HARMS?

The broad deterioration in health reflected in the preceding charts undoubtedly has many causes, but it also appears consistent with a blood-borne systemic factor affecting many different organs, interfering with numerous bodily systems, limiting the immune system, and worsening the course of underlying chronic and episodic disease. We are unlikely to determine the precise contribution of each in the near term. From the perspective of a veteran insurance executive, however, it is clear America's worsening health is due to some combination of the effects of COVID-19 itself, lockdowns, lingering "long COVID," *and unfortunately the experimental "vaccines" themselves,* all amplifying negative health trends already evident before the pandemic.

The previous chapters present a compelling case these impacts are causally related to the experimental modRNA products. In short, it appears an untested gene therapy with known toxic properties was rushed to market without standard safety testing, while ever since its introduction, public health authorities have consistently ignored data showing high rates of serious side effects, including massive disability and mortality. Yet information confirming the dangers of the modRNA "vaccines" continues to pile up, through litigation, whistleblowers, FOIA requests, and further scientific research.

HAVE WE SEEN THIS BEFORE?

Mark Twain reportedly observed, "History doesn't repeat itself, but it often rhymes." Tragically, there are far too many examples of dangerous products marketed as "miracles" that continued to be sold despite mounting evidence of harms. Examples include asbestos, tobacco, myriad forms of industrial pollution, fertilizers, and insecticides, as well as myriad pharmaceutical products like thalidomide, Vioxx, and most recently opioids, with their woeful toll of American lives (remarkably, OxyContin was first marketed as a less addictive alternative to other drugs).

Industry, government, science, and media were complicit in many cases, and in some we have proof of outright conspiracies to hide the negative effects of these products, *or even amplify them*, for profit. Only after decades of tragedy, inevitably followed by litigation and policy change, were these dangerous products finally addressed.

Asbestos provides a useful case study of a long-term product liability catastrophe with many authors. The hazards of asbestos were well known in the 1930s yet were hidden from workers and consumers by government, corporations, academia, and mass media deeply invested in the success of this "wonder material" for insulation and fire protection applications. Through their complicity, those in positions of authority profited from the preventable deaths and injuries of millions of Americans. Further, the decades-long delay in legal accountability led to widespread bankruptcies and job losses across the industrial heartland, and—last but certainly not least—an "extinction-level event" for the US liability insurance industry in the 1980s.

WHY DOES THIS KEEP HAPPENING?

This troubling pattern of negligence and malfeasance naturally raises critical questions about the systemic frailties that continue to enable it. Many different explanations can be advanced, often pointing to overlapping factors. An economist would likely blame market failure, lack of consumer choice, and inadequate communication of the actual risks and benefits of the product, allowing the company responsible to evade responsibility and push the long-term costs of future harms onto the rest of society. A sociologist might add that many large organizations—public, private, and government—make decisions based on internal dynamics that may have nothing to do with their stated mission or how their actions affect others. A trial lawyer could remind us that these negative tendencies are given free rein when the law limits plaintiffs' right to seek legal redress with regulatory preemption, limits on liability, or outright immunity. Ethicists rightly note that media, scientists, and regulators are not independent of commercial interests.

Most businesses are decent, most government regulators are diligent and attentive, and most journalists and academics remain committed to the truth. However, history shows that the public can be harmed when the natural checks and balances between these groups break down, hollowing out a system based on healthy confrontation and replacing it with complicit collaboration. This appears to be precisely what has happened with the COVID-19 "vaccines," typified, for example, by the unprecedented liability shield granted to Pfizer, outlined in chapter 2; FDA "moving the goalposts" to get Pfizer's product authorized, detailed in chapter 3; the unprecedented collusion of Big Tech, media companies, and government to censor dissenting opinions about "vaccine" safety or efficacy, described in chapter 5; and the secret subordination of medical professional societies to CDC dictates on COVID-19 and the "vaccines," documented in chapter 11.

A CALL TO ACTION FROM INSURANCE

As an insurance leader, with a career's worth of interest in catastrophic risk management failures in product liability, when I heard leading doctors (including my co-authors) trying to warn the public, and saw the institutional barriers being placed in their way, I immediately saw parallels to past catastrophic product liability disasters, *and particularly those such as asbestos, which very nearly destroyed the casualty insurance industry in the twentieth century.* My concern grew with the strange patterns in mortality data in 2021, once again suggesting the Cassandras might be right.

Trying to come to grips with the scale of this tragedy, I felt an obligation to help, drawing on my business background and familiarity with past insurance industrywide calamities. Working with other insurance leaders and our team of life and health insurance actuaries, in consultation with medical experts and scientists, we analyzed the data, then cooperated with government regulators to study the problem and work toward a solution.

As a result, I was asked to share our team's findings as part of Senator Johnson's briefing at the US Capitol in December 2022. Included in nearly seventy pages of analysis were data published by the Office of National Statistics in the United Kingdom, which when analyzed *showed mortality rates among "vaccinated" deteriorating faster than among the "unvaccinated."*

I then explained to the senator's panel that if the findings from the ONS's data were extrapolated to the United States, the elevated mortality rate among the "vaccinated" could help explain a large share of the recent unexplained rise in excess deaths—this simple math would imply that hundreds of thousands of American deaths may have been caused by the "vaccines." Again, we are unlikely to ever know the precise extent of "vaccine"-related injuries and deaths. But every week since Senator Johnson's event seems to bring more confirmation of their baneful effect on human health, and every quarter, more population-level data showing unprecedented negative public health trends.

On a more hopeful note, three relatively recent events point to changes in the legal and regulatory landscape, potentially opening a new chapter in the COVID-19 saga:

1. The State of Missouri litigating against federal government COVID-related censorship;
2. The State of Florida requesting FDA withdraw the COVID-19 "vaccines" for safety; and
3. The State of Texas suing Pfizer for fraud in selling the COVID-19 "vaccine."

It is also noteworthy that, according to one recent survey by Rasmussen, *fully 54 percent of Americans believe the "vaccine" caused widespread death and disability.* This daunting figure, alongside continuing low uptake of the monovalent COVID-19 "booster" in winter 2023–2024 (foreword, chapter 3), suggests that public understanding has, once again, substantially outstripped concerted official attempts to mold and suppress it.

FACING REALITY

These data and other encouraging trends give some cause for comfort. However, we must still face a new, long-term reality, of poor—and possibly worsening—public health. The American population, already displaying negative health trends before the COVID-19 pandemic, now faces the prospect of even worse health, due to all the factors mentioned above, including the "vaccines" themselves.

Regardless of cause, elevated mortality and disability present a clear moral, medical, economic, and administrative challenge requiring immediate, urgent attention. Above all, leaders in business and government need to advance proactive strategies to help people take control of their health, targeted to the lasting impacts of both COVID-19 and the "vaccines," with their shared common pathogenic agent, the spike protein (chapter 4).

Fortunately, we can use low-cost blood testing to screen the population at large scale to identify patients and community members who have suffered the greatest exposure to this systemic risk factor, and who are thus more likely to be at higher risk of heart attack, stroke, pulmonary embolism, blood clots, or serious kidney, liver, or other disease. Governments, health systems, employers, and private insurers of all kinds, will realize financial benefit from rolling out proactive screening to identify individuals at high risk, *and can potentially help save millions of lives.*

For example, a simple low-cost cardiac and circulatory panel (including hsCRP, NT ProBnP, and D-Dimer) is effective for identifying inflammation and injury to the heart, blood, and related organs, helping identify people at high risk of cardiovascular events including heart attack and stroke. Other low-cost tests, including A1C, vitamin D, and homocysteine, can help individuals cost-effectively identify key changes to nutrition and lifestyle to improve their overall immune, heart, and kidney health, and reduce their risk of diabetes and other long-term chronic diseases.

Using commonly available tests, already on the shelves of every lab today, a blood work panel costing around one hundred dollars could help countless Americans and world citizens live longer, healthier lives and reduce the toll of unnecessary, premature death. Technical innovation can doubtless bring this cost far lower, while advancing our knowledge of systemic harms and potential therapeutics.

If business leaders, government and health-care workers can put the rancorous debates of the COVID-19 era behind them, and focus instead on helping millions of Americans address the health challenges they face today, we can still change the downward trend in longevity lamented by Dr. Califf, and reduce the unprecedented excess morbidity and mortality we have experienced in recent years. This insight—that the path forward for post-COVID health care is screening, testing, and triage to help the most at-risk improve their health—led to the launch of the Insurance Collaboration to Save Lives, a nonprofit with the goal of saving a million lives through insurance-led health initiatives; the ICSL had no role in funding or publishing this book.

ENDNOTES

Foreword

1. World Health Organization, *Ebola Outbreak 2014–2016—West Africa*, accessed July 25, 2023, https://www.who.int/emergencies/situations/ebola-outbreak-2014-2016-West-Africa.
2. World Health Organization, *Middle East Respiratory Syndrome Coronavirus—Oman*, accessed July 25, 2023, https://www.who.int/emergencies/disease-outbreak-news/item/2023-DON436.
3. "MERS-CoV, SARS-CoV, SARS-CoV-2 Agent Information Sheet," Research Occupational Health Program (ROHP), Boston University, accessed July 25, 2023, https://www.bu.edu/research/ethics-compliance/safety/rohp/agent-information-sheets/coronaviruses-agent-information-sheet/.
4. John P. A. Ioannidis, "A Fiasco in the Making? As the Coronavirus Pandemic Takes Hold, We Are Making Decisions without Reliable Data," STAT News, March 17, 2020, https://www.statnews.com/2020/03/17/a-fiasco-in-the-making-as-the-coronavirus-pandemic-takes-hold-we-are-making-decisions-without-reliable-data/.
5. US Department of Health and Human Services, Centers for Disease Control and Prevention, *Past Seasons Estimated Influenza Disease Burden*, October 18, 2022, https://www.cdc.gov/flu/about/burden/past-seasons.html.
6. Jason Oke and Carl Heneghan, "Global Covid-19 Case Fatality Rates," Centre for Evidence-Based Medicine, April 29, 2020, https:/www.cebm.net/covid-19/global-covid-19-case-fatality-rates/
7. Angelo Maria Pezzullo et al., "Age-Stratified Infection Fatality Rate of COVID-19 in the Non-elderly Informed from Pre-vaccination National Seroprevalence Studies," medRxiv preprint, last modified October 13, 2022, https://doi: 10.1101/2022.10.11.22280963.
8. Shawn Johnson, "Top US Health Official Rips Ron Johnson's Coronavirus Comments," Wisconsin Public Radio, March 20, 2020, https://www.wpr.org/top-us-health-official-rips-ron-johnsons-coronavirus-comments.
9. Ibid.
10. Editorial Board, "Francis Collins Has Regrets, But Too Few," *Wall Street Journal*, December 29, 2023, https://www.wsj.com/articles/francis-collins-covid-lockdowns-braver-angels-anthony-fauci-great-barrington-declaration-f08a4fcf?-mod=RSSMSN.

11 Oxfam, "The Inequality Virus," January 2021, https://oxfamilibrary.openrepository.com/bitstream/handle/10546/621149/bp-the-inequality-virus-250121-en.pdf.

12 Pharmaceuticals and Medical Devices Agency of Japan, *SARS-CoV-2 mRNA Vaccine (BNT162, PF-07302048)*, accessed July 25, 2023, https:/www.pmda.go.jp/drugs/2021/P20210212001/672212000_30300AMX00231_I100_1.pdf.

13 Aaron Siri, "Why a Judge Ordered FDA to Release Covid-19 Vaccine Data Pronto," Bloomberg Law News, last modified January 18, 2022, https://news.bloomberglaw.com/health-law-and-business/why-a-judge-ordered-fda-to-release-covid-19-vaccine-data-pronto.

14 Qiuyue Ma et al., "Global Percentage of Asymptomatic SARS-CoV-2 Infections among the Tested Population and Individuals with Confirmed COVID-19 Diagnosis," *JAMA Network* 4, no. 12 (December 14, 2021): e2137257, https://doi: 10.1001/jamanetworkopen.2021.37257.

15 US Census Bureau, "Population and Housing Unit Estimates," accessed July 25, 2023, https://www.census.gov/programs-surveys/popest.html; World Health Organization, "Coronavirus (COVID-19) Dashboard," accessed July 25, 2023, https://covid19.who.int/.

16 Lance Ignon, "USC Study: Mandatory Business Closures Drove the Economic Decline during COVID-19 Pandemic," University of Southern California, Sol Price School of Public Policy, January 25, 2023, https://priceschool.usc.edu/news/covid-cost-gdp-adam-rose-usc-price/.

17 National Childhood Vaccine Injury Act of 1986, 42 U.S.C. §§ 300aa-1-300aa-34 (1986), via Cornell Law School, accessed July 25, 2023, https://www.law.cornell.edu/uscode/text/42/300aa-1.

18 "Table 4: CICP Claims Compensated (Fiscal Years 2010–2023)," Health Resources and Services Administration, last updated December 1, 2023, https://www.hrsa.gov/cicp/cicp-data/table-4.

19 Lev Facher, "Biden Pledged to 'Follow the Science.' But Experts Say He's Sometimes Fallen Short," STAT News, last modified September 1, 2021, https://www.statnews.com/2021/09/01/biden-pledged-follow-the-science-but-hes-fallen-short/; US Department of Health and Human Services, Centers for Disease Control and Prevention, "Safety of COVID-19 Vaccines," March 7, 2023, https://www.cdc.gov/coronavirus/2019-ncov/vaccines/safety/safety-of-vaccines.html; LaShawn Hudson, "CDC Director on Combating the COVID-19 Pandemic: 'No One is Safe Until Everyone Is Safe,'" WABE, December 20, 2021, https://www.wabe.org/cdc-director-on-leading-the-agency-and-combating-the-covid-19-pandemic-no-one-is-safe-until-everyone-is-safe/; Peter A. McCullough, MD, MPH® (@P_McCulloughMD), X (Twitter), December 13, 2022, https://twitter.com/P_McCulloughMD/status/1602778814836260867; Aditi Sangal et al., "Biden: 'This Is a Pandemic of the Unvaccinated,'" CNN, September 24, 2021, https://edition.cnn.com/us/

live-news/coronavirus-pandemic-vaccine-updates-09-24-21/h_0f8fab1a204b-09d660a23aa3c1e32954; Azmi Haroun and Hilary Brueck, "CDC Director Says Data 'Suggests That Vaccinated People Do Not Carry the Virus,'" Business Insider, March 30, 2021, https://www.businessinsider.com/cdc-director-data-vaccinated-people-do-not-carry-covid-19-2021-3; Calvin Woodward and Hope Yen, "AP FACT CHECK: Biden Goes Too Far in Assurances on Vaccines," AP News, July 22, 2021, https://apnews.com/article/joe-biden-business-health-government-and-politics-coronavirus-pandemic-46a270ce0f681caa7e4143e2ae9a0211.

20 Senator Ron Johnson, letter to Francis Collins, director, National Institutes of Health; Rochelle Walensky, director Centers for Disease Control and Prevention; and Janet Woodcock, acting commissioner, Food and Drug Administration, July 13, 2021, https://www.ronjohnson.senate.gov/services/files/17788FED-A947-4143-8C1B-95C59E60EE87.

21 "Reuters Fact Check: VAERS Data Does Not Prove Thousands Died from Receiving COVID-19 Vaccines," Reuters, April 8, 2021, https://www.reuters.com/article/factcheck-vaers-deaths-idUSL1N2LV0NY; Bayliss Wagner, "Fact Check: Vaccine Adverse Reporting System Isn't Proof of COVID-19 Vaccine Deaths," *USA Today*, June 28, 2021, https://www.usatoday.com/story/news/factcheck/2021/06/28/fact-check-covid-19-vaers-death-reports-not-verified/7587577002/.

22 Kat Eschner, "The Long Shadow of the 1976 Swine Flu Vaccine 'Fiasco,'" *Smithsonia*n, February 6, 2017, https://www.smithsonianmag.com/smart-news/long-shadow-1976-swine-flu-vaccine-fiasco-180961994/; "Ex-CDC Head Recalls '76 Swine Flu Outbreak," CNN, April 30, 2009, https://edition.cnn.com/2009/HEALTH/04/30/swine.flu.1976/index.html.

23 See VAERS database query: United States Department of Health and Human Services (DHHS), Public Health Service (PHS), US Department of Health and Human Services, Centers for Disease Control and Prevention (CDC), Food and Drug Administration (FDA), Vaccine Adverse Event Reporting System (VAERS), 1990–4/23/2021, CDC WONDER On-line Database, accessed April 23, 2021, http://wonder.cdc.gov/vaers.html. Query criteria—Vaccine Products: COVID-19 Vaccine (COVID19); COVID-19-2 (COVID-192). Group By: Month Received. State/Territory: All locations. Event Category: All Events. Show Totals: True. Show Zero Values: False; VAERS database query: United States Department of Health and Human Services (DHHS), Public Health Service (PHS), Centers for Disease Control (CDC), Food and Drug Administration (FDA), Vaccine Adverse Event Reporting System (VAERS) 1990–4/23/2021, CDC WONDER On-line Database, accessed on April 23, 2021, http://wonder.cdc.gov/vaers.html. Query criteria—Vaccine Products: COVID-19 Vaccine (COVID19); COVID-19-2 (COVID-192). Group By: Month Received. State/Territory: All locations. Event Category: Death. Show Totals: True. Show Zero Values: False.

24 *See* VAERS database query: United States Department of Health and Human Services (DHHS), Public Health Service (PHS), Centers for Disease Control (CDC) / Food and Drug Administration (FDA), Vaccine Adverse Event Reporting System (VAERS) 1990–7/24/2023, CDC WONDER On-line Database, accessed on July 24, 2023, http://wonder.cdc.gov/vaers.html. Query criteria—Vaccine Products: COVID-19 Vaccine (COVID19); COVID-19-2 (COVID-192). Group By: Month Received. State/Territory: All locations. Event Category: All Events. Show Totals: True. Show Zero Values: False; VAERS database query: United States Department of Health and Human Services (DHHS), Public Health Service (PHS), Centers for Disease Control (CDC) / Food and Drug Administration (FDA), Vaccine Adverse Event Reporting System (VAERS) 1990–7/24/2023, CDC WONDER On-line Database. accessed on July. 24, 2023, http://wonder.cdc.gov/vaers.html. Query criteria—Vaccine Products: COVID-19 Vaccine (COVID19); COVID-19-2 (COVID-192). Group By: Month Received. State/Territory: All locations. Event Category: Death. Show Totals: True. Show Zero Values: False.
25 "Aaron Siri," Campfire Wiki, January 24, 2022, https://www.campfire.wiki/doku.php?id=aaron_siri; "Legal Action: V-Safe," Informed Consent Action Network, October 18, 2022, https://icandecide.org/article/v-safe/; Aaron Siri, "V-Safe Part 7: CDC Deceived the Public with Limited Release of V-Safe Check-the-Box Data Until Forced to Release It All," *Injecting Freedom by Aaron Siri* (Substack), February 14, 2023, https://aaronsiri.substack.com/p/v-safe-part-7-cdc-deceived-the-public; Aaron Siri, "V-Safe Part 6: A First Look at What the V-Safe Check-the-Box Data Reveals," *Injecting Freedom by Aaron Siri* (Substack), February 8, 2023, https://aaronsiri.substack.com/p/v-safe-part-6-a-first-look-at-what.
26 "COVID 19: Virus Deaths vs. Vaccine Deaths," Rasmussen Reports, March 31, 2023, https://www.rasmussenreports.com/public_content/politics/public_surveys/covid_19_virus_deaths_vs_vaccine_deaths.
27 Senator Ron Johnson, "Investigating the Federal Government's Failed Response to Covid-19 and Demanding Transparency and Accountability through Congressional Oversight," ronjohnson.senate.gov/, https://www.ronjohnson.senate.gov/covid.
28 Ibid.
29 Ibid.
30 Ibid.
31 Ibid.
32 Peter A. McCullough, Harvey Risch, et al., "Multifaceted Highly Targeted Sequential Multidrug Treatment of Early Ambulatory High-Risk SARS-CoV-2 Infection (COVID-19)," *Reviews in Cardiovascular Medicine* 21, no. 4 (2020): 517–530, https://doi: 10.31083/j.rcm.2020.04.264.
33 Johnson, "Investigating the Federal Government's Failed Response to Covid-19 and Demanding Transparency and Accountability through Congressional Oversight."

34 Nick Arama, "CNN Tries to Flip the Script on Hotez-RFK Jr. Debate, but It Doesn't Go Well," RedState.com, last modified June 19, 2023, https://redstate.com/nick-arama/2023/06/19/cnn-tries-to-flip-the-script-on-hotez-rfk-jr-debate-but-it-doesnt-go-well-n764005.

Introduction: An Urgent Call

35 Isobel Freund et al., "RNA Modifications Modulate Activation of Innate Toll-Like Receptors," *Genes* (Basel) 10, no. 2 (February 2019): 92, doi: 10.3390/genes10020092.

36 Kuei-Meng Wu, "A New Classification of Prodrugs: Regulatory Perspectives," *Pharmaceuticals* (Basel) 2 (2009): 77–81, doi: 10.3390/ph2030077.

37 Marco Cosentino and Franca Marino, "Understanding the Pharmacology of COVID-19 mRNA Vaccines: Playing Dice with the Spike?" *International Journal of Molecular Sciences* 23, no. 18 (September 17, 2022): 10881, doi: 10.3390/ijms231810881; Helene Banoun, "mRNA: Vaccine or Gene Therapy? The Safety Regulatory Issues," *International Journal of Molecular Sciences* 24, no. 13 (June 22, 2023): 10514, doi: 10.3390/ijms241310514.

38 *The Pfizer Papers: Pfizer's Crimes against Humanity*, ed. DailyClout LLC (October 15, 2024), Kindle, https://www.amazon.com/ Pfizer-Papers-Pfizers-Against-Humanity/dp/1648210376.

39 Pfizer Documents Investigation Team and Amy Kelly, *War Room/DailyClout Pfizer Documents Analysis Volunteers' Reports eBook: Find Out What Pfizer, FDA Tried to Conceal*, ed. DailyClout LLC (B0BSK6LV5D: January 16, 2023), Kindle, https://www.amazon.com/DailyClout-Documents-Analysis-Volunteers-Reports-ebook/dp/B0BSK6LV5D/; *The Pfizer Papers: Pfizer's Crimes against Humanity*, ed. DailyClout LLC (October 15, 2024), Kindle, https://www.amazon.com/Pfizer-Papers-Pfizers-Against-Humanity/dp/1648210376/.

40 Pfizer Documents Investigation Team and Amy Kelly, *War Room/DailyClout Pfizer Documents Analysis Volunteers' Reports eBook: Find Out What Pfizer, FDA Tried to Conceal*, ed. DailyClout LLC (B0BSK6LV5D: January 16, 2023), Kindle, https://www.amazon.com/DailyClout-Documents-Analysis-Volunteers-Reports-ebook/dp/B0BSK6LV5D/; *The Pfizer Papers: Pfizer's Crimes against Humanity*, ed. DailyClout LLC (October 15, 2024), Kindle, https://www.amazon.com/Pfizer-Papers-Pfizers-Against-Humanity/dp/1648210376/.

41 Nazeeh Hanna et al., "Detection of Messenger RNA COVID-19 Vaccines in Human Breast Milk," *Journal of the American Medical Association Pediatrics* 176, no. 12 (September 26, 2022): 12681270, doi:10.1001/jamapediatrics.2022.3581; Kevin McKernan et al., "Sequencing of Bivalent Moderna and Pfizer mRNA Vaccines Reveals Nanogram to Microgram Quantities of Expression Vector dsDNA Per Dose," OSF Preprints, updated April 11, 2023, doi: 10.31219/osf.io/b9t7m.

42 "Florida State Surgeon General Calls for Halt in the Use of COVID-19 mRNA Vaccines," Floridahealth.gov, press release, January 3, 2024, https://www.floridahealth.gov/newsroom/2024/01/20240103-halt-use-covid19-mrna-vaccines.pr.html.
43 Marcia Angell, *The Truth about the Drug Companies: How They Deceive Us and What to Do about It* (New York: Random House Trade Paperbacks, August 9, 2005), https://www.amazon.com/Truth-About-Drug-Companies-Deceive/dp/0375760946.
44 Abigail Zuger, MD, "A Drumbeat on Profit Takers," *New York Times*, March 20, 2012, https://www.nytimes.com/2012/03/20/science/a-drumbeat-on-profit-takers.html.
45 Philipp Schmid and Cornelia Betsch, "Effective Strategies for Rebutting Science Denialism in Public Discussions," *Nature Human Behavior* 3, no. 9 (September 2019): 931–939, doi: 10.1038/s41562-019-0632-4.
46 Peter McCullough, Harvey Risch, et al., "Pathophysiological Basis and Rationale for Early Outpatient Treatment of SARS-CoV-2 (COVID-19) Infection," *American Journal of Medicine* 134, no. 1 (January 2021): 16–22, doi: 10.1016/j.amjmed.2020.07.003.

Chapter 1: The COVID-19 modRNA Shots Are Not Real Vaccines

47 US Department of Health and Human Services, Centers for Disease Control and Prevention, *Immunization: The Basics*, September 1, 2021, https://www.cdc.gov/vaccines/vac-gen/imz-basics.htm; US Food and Drug Administration letter to Coalition Advocating for Adequately Licensed Medicines (CAALM), August 23, 2021, https://www.documentcloud.org/documents/23599242-fda-response-to-caalm.
48 *Immunization: The Basics.*
49 Roy M. Anderson, "The Concept of Herd Immunity and the Design of Community-Based Immunization Programmes," *Vaccine* 10 (1992): 928–935, doi: 10.1016/0264-410x(92)90327-g.
50 Jennifer M. Dan et al., "Immunological Memory to SARS-CoV-2 Assessed for Up to 8 Months after Infection," *Science* 371, no. 6529 (February 5, 2021), doi: 10.1126/science.abf4063; Alison Tarke et al., "Negligible Impact of SARS-CoV-2 Variants on CD4 (+) and CD8 (+) T Cell Reactivity in COVID-19 Exposed Donors and Vaccinees," bioRxiv, https://pubmed.ncbi.nlm.nih.gov/33688655/.
51 Yonatan Woodbridge et al., "Viral Load Dynamics of SARS-CoV-2 Delta and Omicron Variants Following Multiple Vaccine Doses and Previous Infection," *Nature Communication* 13, no. 6706 (November 7, 2022); Sivan Gazit et al., "Severe Acute Respiratory Syndrome Coronavirus 2 (SARS-CoV-2) Naturally Acquired Immunity versus Vaccine-Induced Immunity, Reinfections versus Breakthrough Infections: A Retrospective Cohort Study," *Clinical Infectious Diseases* 75, no. 1 (July 1, 2022): e545–e551, doi: 10.1093/cid/ciac262.
52 The Centers for Disease Control and Prevention, *Our Shot to End the Pandemic—Interpretive Summary*, July 23, 2021, https://archive.cdc.gov/www_cdc_gov/coronavirus/2019-ncov/covid-data/covidview/past-reports/07232021.html.

53. European Parliament, *Special Committee on COVID-19 Pandemic*, video, October 10, 2022, https://multimedia.europarl.europa.eu/en/webstreaming/special-committee-on-covid-19-pandemic_20221010-1430-COMMITTEE-COVI.
54. Fernando P. Polack et al., "Safety and Efficacy of the BNT162b2 mRNA Covid-19 Vaccine," *New England Journal of Medicine* 383, no. 27 (December 10, 2020): 2603–2615, doi: 10.1056/NEJMoa2034577.
55. US Department of Health and Human Services, Centers for Disease Control and Prevention, "CDC Real-World Study Confirms Protective Benefits of COVID mRNA Vaccines," press release, March 29, 2021, https://www.cdc.gov/media/releases/2021/p0329-COVID-19-Vaccines.html.
56. Byram W. Bridle, "5 Factors That Could Dictate the Success or Failure of the COVID-19 Vaccine Rollout," The Conversation, February 10, 2021, https://theconversation.com/5-factors-that-could-dictate-the-success-or-failure-of-the-covid-19-vaccine-rollout-152856; Geert Vanden Bossche to the Oregon State Legislature, "The Science behind the Catastrophic Consequences of Thoughtless Human Intervention in the Covid-19 Pandemic," March 13, 2021, https://olis.oregonlegislature.gov/liz/2021R1/Downloads/FloorLetter/3166.
57. Sheryl Gay Stolberg, "B.1.1.7 Variant Most Common Source of New Infections, CDC Says," *New York Times*, April 7, 2021, https://www.nytimes.com/2021/04/07/us/covid-variant-infection.html.
58. David W. Eyre et al., "Effect of Covid-19 Vaccination on Transmission of Alpha and Delta Variants," *New England Journal of Medicine* 386 (2022):744–756, https://www.nejm.org/doi/full/10.1056/NEJMoa2116597 doi: 10.1056/NEJMoa2116597; Annelies Wilder-Smith, "What Is the Vaccine Effect on Reducing Transmission in the Context of the SARS-CoV-2 Delta Variant?" *The Lancet Infectious Diseases* 22, no. 2 (February 2022): 152–153, doi: 10.1016/S1473-3099(21)00690-3.
59. Smriti Mallapaty, "COVID Vaccines Cut the Risk of Transmitting Delta—but Not for Long," *Nature*, October 5, 2021, https://www.nature.com/articles/d41586-021-02689-y; Annika Singanayagam et al., "Community Transmission and Viral Load Kinetics of the SARS-CoV-2 Delta (B.1.617.2) Variant in Vaccinated and Unvaccinated Individuals in the UK: A Prospective, Longitudinal, Cohort Study," *The Lancet Infectious Diseases* 22 (2022): 183–95, doi: 10.1016/S1473-3099(21)00648-4; Charlotte B. Acharya, "Viral Load among Vaccinated and Unvaccinated, Asymptomatic and Symptomatic Persons Infected with the SARS-CoV-2 Delta Variant," *Open Forum Infectious Disease* 9, no. 5 (May 2022): ofac135, doi: 10.1093/ofid/ofac135; Liesl Hagan et al., "Outbreak of SARS-CoV-2 B.1.617.2 (Delta) Variant Infections among Incarcerated Persons in a Federal Prison—Texas, July–August 2021," US Department of Health and Human Services, Centers for Disease Control and Prevention, *Morbidity and Mortality Weekly Report* (*MMWR*) 70 (2021): 1349–1354, doi: 10.15585/mmwr.mm7038e3.

60 Catherine M. Brow et al., "Outbreak of SARS-CoV-2 Infections, Including COVID-19 Vaccine Breakthrough Infections, Associated with Large Public Gatherings—Barnstable County, Massachusetts, July 2021," US Department of Health and Human Services, Centers for Disease Control and Prevention, *Morbidity and Mortality Weekly Report* (*MMWR*) 70, no. 31 (August 6, 2021):1059–1062, doi: 10.15585/mmwr.mm7031e2; Holly Ellyatt, "Why Are Covid Cases So High When Millions Are Fully Vaccinated? Blame the Delta Variant, Experts Say," CNBC, September 10, 2021, https://www.cnbc.com/2021/09/10/why-are-covid-cases-so-high-when-vaccination-is-widespread.html; Günter Kampf, "The Epidemiological Relevance of the COVID-19-Vaccinated Population Is Increasing," *The Lancet Regional Health Europe* 11, no. 100272 (December 2021), doi: 10.1016/j.lanepe.2021.100272.

61 Madeline Holcombe and Christina Maxouris, "Fully Vaccinated People Who Get a COVID-19 Breakthrough Infection Can Transmit the Virus, CDC Chief Says," CNN, August 6, 2021, https://www.cnn.com/2021/08/05/health/us-coronavirus-thursday/index.html; Josh Moody, "Colleges Requiring a Coronavirus Vaccine for Fall," *US News & World Report*, August 12, 2021, https://www.usnews.com/education/best-colleges/articles/colleges-requiring-a-coronavirus-vaccine-for-fall-what-to-know.

62 S. V. Subramanian et al., "Increases in COVID-19 Are Unrelated to Levels of Vaccination across 68 Countries and 2947 Counties in the United States," *European Journal of Epidemiology* 36, no. 12 (2021): 1237–1240, doi: 10.1007/s10654-021-00808-7.

63 Nabin K. Shrestha et al., "Effectiveness of the Coronavirus Disease 2019 (COVID-19) Bivalent Vaccine," *Open Forum Infectious Disease*, April 19, 2023, doi: 10.1101/2022.12.17.22283625.

64 US Department of Health and Human Services, Centers for Disease Control and Prevention, *Immunization: The Basics*, July 6, 2012, https://web.archive.org/web/20130707100647/https:/www.cdc.gov/vaccines/vac-gen/imz-basics.htm.

65 US Department of Health and Human Services, Centers for Disease Control and Prevention, *Immunization: The Basics*, August 26, 2013 (last reviewed May 16, 2018), https://web.archive.org/web/20210826113846/https:/www.cdc.gov/vaccines/vac-gen/imz-basics.htm.

66 Polack et al., "Safety and Efficacy of the BNT162b2 mRNA Covid-19 Vaccine."

67 US Department of Health and Human Services, US Army Contracting Command, Technical Direction Letter for Medical CRBN Defense Consortium (MCDC), Request for Prototype Proposals (RPP) 20-11, Objective PRE-20-11 for "COVID-19 Pandemic—Large Scale Vaccine Manufacturing Demonstration" (Pfizer, Inc.), July 21, 2020, https://www.hhs.gov/sites/default/files/pfizer-inc-covid-19-vaccine-contract.pdf.

68 US Department of Health and Human Services, Centers for Disease Control and Prevention, *Immunization: The Basics*, last reviewed September 1, 2021.

69 US Food and Drug Administration letter to Coalition Advocating for Adequately Licensed Medicines (CAALM), August 23, 2021, https:// www.documentcloud.org/documents/23599242-fda-response-to-caalm.

70 S. N. Meydani and W. K. Ha, "Immunologic Effects of Yogurt," *American Journal of Clinical Nutrition* 7 (2000): 861–872, https://doi: 10.1093/ajcn/71.4.861; Roghayeh Shahbazi et al., "Anti-Inflammatory and Immunomodulatory Properties of Fermented Plant Foods," *Nutrients* 13, no. 5 (2021): 1516, https://doi: 10.3390/nu13051516.

71 Laith A. Abu-Raddad et al., "Severity of SARS-CoV-2 Reinfections as Compared with Primary Infections," *New England Journal of Medicine* 385 (December 23, 2021): 2487–2489, https://doi: 10.1056/NEJMc2108120; Jennifer M. Dan et al., "Immunological Memory to SARS-CoV-2 Assessed for Up to 8 Months After Infection."

72 Vladimir N. Uversky et al., "IgG4 Antibodies Induced by Repeated Vaccination May Generate Immune Tolerance to the SARS-CoV-2 Spike Protein," *Vaccines* (Basel) 11, no. 5 (May 17, 2023): 991, doi: 10.3390/vaccines11050991.

73 Thomas C. William and Wendy A. Burgers, "SARS-CoV-2 Evolution and Vaccines: Cause for Concern?" *Lancet Respiratory Medicine* 9, no. 4 (April 2021): 333–335, doi: 10.1016/S2213-2600(21)00075-8.

74 S. Dokka et al., "Oxygen Radical-Mediated Pulmonary Toxicity Induced by Some Cationic Liposomes," *Pharmacological Research* 17, no. 5 (May 2000): 521–525, doi: 10.1023/a:1007504613351; Ranit Kedmi et al., "The Systemic Toxicity of Positively Charged Lipid Nanoparticles and the Role of Toll-Like Receptor 4 in Immune Activation," *Biomaterials* 31, no. 26 (September 2010): 6867–6875, doi: 10.1016/j.biomaterials.2010.05.027; Maja Sedic et al., "Safety Evaluation of Lipid Nanoparticle-Formulated Modified mRNA in the Sprague-Dawley Rat and Cynomolgus Monkey," *Veterinary Pathology* 55, no. 2 (2018): 341–354, doi: 10.1177/0300985817738095; Hongtao Lv et al., "Toxicity of Cationic Lipids and Cationic Polymers in Gene Delivery," *Journal of Controlled Release* 114, no. 1 (August 10, 2006): 100–109, doi: 10.1016/j.jconrel.2006.04.014; Mario C. Filion and Nigel C. Phillips, "Toxicity and Immunomodulatory Activity of Liposomal Vectors Formulated with Cationic Lipids toward Immune Effector Cells," *Biochimica et Biophysica Acta* 1329, no. 2 (October 23, 1997): 345–356, doi: 10.1016/s0005-2736(97)00126-0.

75 Wim H. De Jong and Paul J. Borm, "Drug Delivery and Nanoparticles: Applications and Hazards," *International Journal of Nanomedicine* 3 (June 2008): 133–149, doi: 10.2147/ijn.s596; Yechezkel Barenholz, "Liposome Application: Problems and Prospects," *Current Opinion in Colloid and Interface Science* 6, no. 1 (2001): 66–77, doi.org/10.1016/S1359-0294(00)00090-X; Banu S. Zolnik et al., "Nanoparticles and the Immune System," *Endocrinology* 151, no. 2 (February 1, 2010): 458–65, doi: 10.1210/en.2009-1082; Sebastien Spagnou et al., "Lipidic Carriers of siRNA: Differences in the Formulation, Cellular Uptake, and Delivery with Plasmid DNA," *Biochemistry* 43, no. 42 (2004): 13348–56, doi: 10.1021/bi048950a; Saghir Akhtar and Ibrahim Benter,

"Toxicogenomics of Non-viral Drug Delivery Systems for RNAi: Potential Impact on siRNA-Mediated Gene Silencing Activity and Specificity," *Advanced Drug Delivery Review* 59, nos. 2–3 (March 30, 2007): 164–82, doi: 10.1016/j.addr.2007.03.010; Mario C. Filion and Nigel C. Phillips, "Major Limitations in the Use of Cationic Liposomes for DNA Delivery," *International Journal of Pharmaceutics* 162, nos. 1–2 (1998): 159–70, doi: 10.1016/S0378-5173(97)00423-7.

76 Damian Garde, "Ego, Ambition, and Turmoil: Inside One of Biotech's Most Secretive Startups," STAT News, September 13, 2016, https://www.statnews.com/2016/09/13/moderna-therapeutics-biotech-mrna/.

Chapter 2: A Government Prototype Rushed to Market without Adequate Testing

77 Katalin Karikó et al., "Suppression of RNA Recognition by Toll-Like Receptors: The Impact of Nucleoside Modification and the Evolutionary Origin of RNA," *Immunity* 23, no. 2 (August 2005): 165–75, doi: 10.1016/j.immuni.2005.06.008.

78 Arthur Allen, "For Billion-Dollar COVID Vaccines, Basic Government-Funded Science Laid the Groundwork," *Scientific American*, November 18, 2020, https://www.scientificamerican.com/article/for-billion-dollar-covid-vaccines-basic-government-funded-science-laid-the-groundwork/; Elie Dolgin, "The Tangled History of mRNA Vaccines," *Nature*, September 21, 2021, https://www.nature.com/articles/d41586-021-02483-w; Enyue Fang et al., "Advances in COVID-19 mRNA Vaccine Development," *Signal Transduction and Targeted Therapy* 7 (March 23, 2022): 94, https://doi: 10.1038/s41392-022-00950-y; Xucheng Hou et al., "Lipid Nanoparticles for mRNA Delivery," *Nature Reviews Materials* 6 (2021): 1078–1094, https://www.nature.com/articles/s41578-021-00358-0; Stew Magnuson, "Early DARPA Pandemic Research Investments Paying Off," *National Defense*, July 30, 2020, https://www.nationaldefensemagazine.org/articles/2020/7/30/early-darpa-pandemic-research-investments-paying-off; Paul Sonne, "How a Secretive Pentagon Agency Seeded the Ground for a Rapid Coronavirus Cure," *Washington Post*, July 30, 2021, https://www.washingtonpost.com/national-security/how-a-secretive-pentagon-agency-seeded-the-ground-for-a-rapid-coronavirus-cure/2020/07/30/ad1853c4-c778-11ea-a9d3-74640f25b953_story.html.

79 Defense Advanced Research Projects Administration (DARPA), "Removing the Viral Threat: Two Months to Stop Pandemic X from Taking Hold," February 6, 2017, https://www.darpa.mil/news-events/2017-02-06a; Defense Advanced Research Projects Administration, "ADEPT: PROTECT," 2020, https://www.darpa.mil/attachments/ADEPTVignetteFINAL.pdf; Hussain S. Lalani et al., "US Public Investment in Development of mRNA Covid-19 Vaccines: Retrospective Cohort Study," *BMJ* 380 (2023): e073747, doi: 10.1136/bmj-2022-073747; Nick Paul Taylor, "Pentagon Tasks Pfizer with Radically Rethinking Vaccine Development," Fierce

Pharma, December 9, 2013, https://www.fiercepharma.com/r-d/pentagon-tasks-pfizer-radically-rethinking-vaccine-development.

80. Mark Terry, "JPM17: Secretive Moderna Finally Unveils Pipeline, Financials," BioSpace, January 11, 2017, https://www.biospace.com/article/jpm17-secretive-moderna-finally-unveils-pipeline-financials-/; National Institutes of Health, *Decades in the Making: mRNA COVID-19 Vaccines*, https://covid19.nih.gov/nih-strategic-response-covid-19/decades-making-mrna-covid-19-vaccines.

81. Mario Gaviria et al., "A Network Analysis of COVID-19 mRNA Vaccine Patents," *Nature Biotechnology* 39 (May 12, 2021): 546–548, doi: 10.1038/s41587-021-00912-9.

82. "ADEPT: PROTECT"; Alexander Tin, "Moderna Offers NIH Co-ownership of COVID Vaccine Patent amid Dispute with Government," CBS News, November 15, 2021, https://www.cbsnews.com/news/moderna-covid-vaccine-patent-dispute-national-institutes-health/.

83. DCMA/Moderna, "Contract W911QY20C0100," KEI Online.org, August 9, 2020, https://www.keionline.org/misc-docs/DOD-Moderna-Contract-W911QY20C0100-9Aug2020-SEC.pdf.

84. Defense Acquisition University, Other Transactions website, https://aaf.dau.edu/aaf/contracting-cone/ot/.

85. Defense Acquisition University, Other Transactions website, https://aaf.dau.edu/aaf/contracting-cone/ot/.

86. US Dist. Court for the Eastern Dist. of Texas, Beaumont Division, United States of America Ex Rel. Brook Jackson, Plaintiff v. Ventavia Research Group, Llc; Pfizer Inc.; Icon Plc, Defendants, Case No. 1:21-CV-00008-MJT, "Pfizer's Motion to Dismiss Relator's Amended Complaint and Memorandum of Law in Support," April 22, 2022, https://bailiwicknewsarchives.files.wordpress.com/2022/10/2022.04.22-pfizer-motion-to-dismiss.pdf.

87. US District Court for the Eastern District of Texas, Beaumont Division, United States of America Ex Rel. Brook Jackson, Plaintiff v. Ventavia Research Group, LLC; Pfizer Inc.; Icon Plc, Defendants, Case No. 1:21-CV-00008-MJT, "The United States' Statement of Interest Supporting Dismissal of the Amended Complaint," October 4, 2022, https://bailiwicknewsarchives.files.wordpress.com/2022/10/2022.10.04-jackson-v.-ventavia-us-gov-intervene.pdf.

88. Judicial Watch, "JW v. HHS Biodistribution Prod 4 02418 Pgs 671–701," Judicial Watch, Document Archives, December 13, 2022, https://www.judicialwatch.org/documents/jw-v-hhs-biodistribution-prod-4-02418-pgs-671-701/.

89. BARDA/Moderna, "Contract 75A50120C00034," KEI Online.org, February 8, 2021, https://www.keionline.org/misc-docs/HHS-BARDA-Moderna-Contract-75A50120C00034-16April2020-Version8Feb2021.pdf.

90. Yousef Haik and Eleni Polymenopoulou, "COVID-19 Vaccines and Their Pitfalls in Informed Consent," UC Law Science and Technology Journal 12, no. 2: 3, https://repository.uclawsf.edu/hastings_science_technology_law_journal/vol12/iss2/3/.

91 "42 U.S. Code § 247d–6d–Targeted Liability Protections for Pandemic and Epidemic Products and Security Countermeasures," US Code Title 42, Chapter 6A, Subchapter II, Part B, https://www.law.cornell.edu/uscode/text/42/247d-6d; Cornell Law School Legal Information Institute; Health and Human Services. "Declaration under the Public Readiness and Emergency Preparedness Act for Medical Countermeasures Against COVID-19," *Federal Register*, March 17, 2020, https://www.federalregister.gov/documents/2020/03/17/2020-05484/declaration-under-the-public-readiness-and-emergency-preparedness-act-for-medical-countermeasures.

92 Paul D. Thacker, "Covid-19: Researcher Blows the Whistle on Data Integrity Issues in Pfizer's Vaccine Trial," *BMJ* 375 (2021): n2635, doi: 10.1136/bmj.n2635.

93 "Mother of Maddie de Garay, Speaks Out about Her 13 Year Old Daughter's Life Altering Injuries from Pfizer's Covid Vaccine," TrialSite News, December 11, 2021, https://www.trialsitenews.com/a/mother-of-maddie-de-garay-speaks-out-about-her-13-year-old-daughters-life-altering-injuries-from-pfizers-covid-vaccine.

94 Elke Bodderas, "The Many Inconsistencies of the Pfizer Approval Study," *Die Welt*, February 23, 2023, https://www.welt.de/politik/deutschland/plus243820767/Corona-Impfstoff-Die-vielen-Ungereimtheiten-der-Pfizer-Zulassungsstudie.html.

95 US Food and Drug Administration, *Summary Basis for Regulatory Action—Comirnaty, BioNTech Manufacturing GmbH, in Partnership with Pfizer, Inc.*, November 8, 2021, https://www.fda.gov/media/151733/download.

96 Maryanne Demasi, "From FDA to MHRA: Are Drug Regulators for Hire?" *BMJ* 377 (2022): o1538, https://doi: 10.1136/bmj.o1538; Christina Jewett, "FDA's Drug Industry Fees Fuel Concerns over Influence," *New York Times*, September 15, 2022, https://www.nytimes.com/2022/09/15/health/fda-drug-industry-fees.html.

97 Cassie Frank et al., "Era of Faster FDA Drug Approval Has Also Seen Increased Black-Box Warnings and Market Withdrawals," *Health Affairs* 33, no. 8 (2014): 1453–1459, doi: 10.1377/hlthaff.2014.0122.

98 Marc Rodwin et al., "Institutional Corruption and the Pharmaceutical Policy," *Journal of Law, Medicine, and Ethics* 41, no. 3 (2013): 544–552, https://ethics.harvard.edu/news/institutional-corruption-and-pharmaceutical-policy.

99 Charles Piller, "FDA's Revolving Door," *Science*, July 5, 2018, https://www.science.org/content/article/fda-s-revolving-door-companies-often-hire-agency-staffers-who-managed-their-successful; Karen Hobert Flynn, "For Big Pharma, the Revolving Door Keeps Spinning," The Hill, July 11, 2019, https://thehill.com/blogs/congress-blog/politics/452654-for-big-pharma-the-revolving-door-keeps-spinning/.

100 Sheila Kaplan, "Elizabeth Warren Calls on Former F.D.A. Chief to Quit Pfizer Board," *New York Times*, July 2, 2019, https://www.nytimes.com/2019/07/02/health/elizabeth-warren-scott-gottlieb-pfizer.html.

101 Sydney Lupkin, "A Look at How the Revolving Door Spins from FDA to Industry," NPR, September 28, 2016, https://www.npr.org/sections/health-

shots/2016/09/28/495694559/a-look-at-how-the-revolving-door-spins-from-fda-to-industry.

102 Stephanie L. Kuschel et al., "Analysis of Conflicts of Interest in Pharmaceutical Payments Made to Food and Drug Administration Physician Advisers after Dermatologic Drug Approval," *Journal of the American Academy of Dermatology* 81, no. 6 (December 2019): 1419–1420, doi.org/10.1016/j.jaad.2019.05.059.

103 Charles Piller, "Hidden Conflicts? Pharma Payments to FDA Advisers after Drug Approval Spark Ethical Concerns," *Science*, July 6, 2018, https://www.science.org/content/article/hidden-conflicts-pharma-payments-fda-advisers-after-drug-approvals-spark-ethical.

104 Maryanne Demasi, "FDA Oversight of Clinical Trials Is 'Grossly Inadequate,' Say Experts," *BMJ* 379 (2022): o2628, doi: 10.1136/bmj.o2628.

105 Charles Piller, "Official Inaction," *Science*, October 1, 2020, https://www.science.org/content/article/fda-s-own-documents-reveal-agency-s-lax-slow-and-secretive-oversight-clinical-research.

106 Gardiner Harris and Eric Koli, "Lucrative Drug, Danger Signals and the F.D.A.," *New York Times*, June 10, 2006, https://www.nytimes.com/2005/06/10/business/lucrative-drug-danger-signals-and-the-fda.html.

107 Snigdha Prakash and Vikki Valentine, "Timeline: The Rise and Fall of Vioxx," NPR, November 10, 2007, https://www.npr.org/2007/11/10/5470430/timeline-the-rise-and-fall-of-vioxx; Harlan M. Krumholz et al., "What Have We Learnt from Vioxx?" *BMJ* 334 (2007): 120, doi: 10.1136/bmj.39024.487720.68; Eric J. Topol, MD, "Failing the Public Health: Rofecoxib, Merck, and the FDA," *New England Journal of Medicine* 351, no. 17 (2004): 1707–1709, doi: 10.1056/NEJMp048286; Richard Horton, "Vioxx, the Implosion of Merck, and Aftershocks at the FDA," *Lancet* 364 (2004): 1995–1996, doi: 10.1016/S0140-6736(04)17523-5.

108 Ed Silverman, "Pill for Women's Libido Carries Sobering Risk," STAT News, September 6, 2015, https://www.statnews.com/pharmalot/2015/09/06/pill-for-womens-libido-carries-sobering-risk/; Loes Jaspers et al., "Efficacy and Safety of Flibanserin for the Treatment of Hypoactive Sexual Desire Disorder in Women," *JAMA Internal Medicine* 176, no. 4 (2016): 453–462, doi: 10.1001/jamainternmed.2015.8565; Abby Miller and Susan K. Flinn, "Keep Passing on the Pink Pill: DON'T 'Get Addyi Now'!" National Women's Health Network, January 24, 2019, https://www.thefreelibrary.com/Keep+Passing+on+the+Pink+Pill%3a+DON%27T+"Get+Addyi+Now"!-a0562137991.

109 Ed Silverman, "Behind the Sarepta Drug Approval Was Intense FDA Bickering," STAT News, September 19, 2016, https://www.statnews.com/pharmalot/2016/09/19/sarepta-fda-duchenne-behind-the-decision/; Toni Clarke and Natalie Grover, "Bowing to Pressure, FDA Approves Sarepta's Duchenne Drug," Reuters, September 19, 2016, https://www.reuters.com/article/us-sarepta-fda/bowing-to-pressure-fda-approves-sareptas-duchenne-drug-idUSKCN11P1HK.

110 Robin Foster, "Congressional Report Slams FDA, Drugmaker Over Approval of Alzheimer's Drug," *US News*, December 29, 2022, https://www.usnews.com/news/health-news/articles/2022-12-29/congressional-report-slams-fda-drugmaker-over-approval-of-alzheimers-drug-aduhelm; David S. Knopman et al., "Failure to Demonstrate Efficacy of Aducanumab: An Analysis of the EMERGE and ENGAGE Trials as Reported by Biogen, December 2019," *Alzheimer's & Dementia* 17, no. 4 (April 2021): 696–701, doi: 10.1002/alz.12213.

111 Chris McGreal, "Biden Urged Not to Give Top FDA Job to Official Over Her Role in Opioid Crisis," *The Guardian*, January 28, 2021, https://www.theguardian.com/us-news/2021/jan/28/fda-janet-woodcock-opioids-biden; Andrew Kolodny, "How FDA Failures Contributed to the Opioid Crisis," *AMA Journal of Ethics* 22, no. 8 (2020): e743–750, doi: 10.1001/amajethics.2020.743.

Chapter 3: Introduction to *The Pfizer Papers: Pfizer's Crimes Against Humanity*

112 *The Pfizer Papers: Pfizer's Crimes against Humanity*, ed. DailyClout LLC (October 15, 2024), Kindle, https://www.amazon.com/Pfizer-Papers-Pfizers-Against-Humanity/dp/1648210376/

Chapter 4: The Spike Protein Is Harmful by Itself

113 Jop De Vrieze, "Suspicions Grow That Nanoparticles in Pfizer's COVID-19 Vaccine Trigger Rare Allergic Reactions," *Science*, December 20, 2020, https://www.science.org/content/article/suspicions-grow-nanoparticles-pfizer-s-covid-19-vaccine-trigger-rare-allergic-reactions; Anthony L. Komaroff, "Why Are mRNA Vaccines So Exciting?," Harvard Health Letter, November 1, 2021, https://www.health.harvard.edu/blog/why-are-mrna-vaccines-so-exciting-2020121021599; Matthew T. J. Halma et al., "Strategies for the Management of Spike Protein-Related Pathology," *Microorganisms* 11, no. 5 (May 20, 2023): 1308, doi: 10.3390/microorganisms11051308.

114 Linda Wastila to the US Food and Drug Administration, "Citizen Petition Requesting That the FDA Require That the Vaccine Manufacturers Provide the FDA with the Data Outlined in the Petition Before Approval of Any COVID-19 Vaccine," June 1, 2021, https://www.regulations.gov/document/FDA-2021-P-0521-0001.

115 Sandhya Bansal et al., "Cutting Edge: Circulating Exosomes with COVID Spike Protein Are Induced by BNT162b2 (Pfizer-BioNTech) Vaccination Prior to Development of Antibodies: A Novel Mechanism for Immune Activation by mRNA Vaccines," *Journal of Immunology* 207 (2021): 2405–10, doi: 10.4049/jimmunol.2100637; Tudor Emmanuel Fertig et al., "Vaccine mRNA Can Be Detected in Blood at 15 Days Post-Vaccination," *Biomedicines* 10, no. 7 (July 2022): 1538, doi: 10.3390/biomedicines10071538; Jose Alfredo Samaniego Castruita et al., "SARS-CoV-2 Spike mRNA

Vaccine Sequences Circulate in Blood Up to 28 Days after COVID-19 Vaccination," *APMIS* 131, no. 3 (March 2023): 128–132, doi: 10.1111/apm.13294.

116 Bansal et al., "Cutting Edge: Circulating Exosomes with COVID Spike Protein Are Induced by BNT162b2 (Pfizer-BioNTech) Vaccination Prior to Development of Antibodies."

117 Fertig et al., "Vaccine mRNA Can Be Detected in Blood at 15 Days Post-Vaccination"; Jose Alfredo Samaniego Castruita et al., "SARS-CoV-2 Spike mRNA Vaccine Sequences Circulate in Blood Up to 28 Days after COVID-19 Vaccination."

118 Judicial Watch, "JW v HHS FDA Pfizer BioNTech Vaccine prod 3 02418," March 21, 2022, https://www.judicialwatch.org/documents/jw-v-hhs-fda-pfizer-biontech-vaccine-prod-3-02418/

119 European Medicines Agency, Committee for Medicinal Products for Human Use (CHMP), "Comirnaty Assessment Report COVID-19 Vaccine Comirnaty," EMA/707383/2020 Corr.2, February 19, 2021, https://www.ema.europa.eu/en/documents/assessment-report/comirnaty-epar-public-assessment-report_en.pdf.

120 European Medicines Agency, Committee for Medicinal Products for Human Use, "Moderna Assessment Report COVID-19 Vaccine Moderna," EMA/15689/2021 Corr.1.1, https://www.ema.europa.eu/en/documents/assessment-report/spikevax-previously-covid-19-vaccine-moderna-epar-public-assessment-report_en.pdf.

121 Ministry of Health, Labour and Welfare of Japan, *SARS-CoV-2 mRNA Vaccine (BNT162, PF-07302048): Summary Text of the Pharmacokinetic Study*, https://www.docdroid.net/xq0Z8B0/pfizer-report-japanese-government-pdf.

122 Nazeeh Hanna et al., "Detection of Messenger RNA COVID-19 Vaccines in Human Breast Milk," research letter, *JAMA Network Pediatrics* 176, no. 12 (2022): 1268–1270, doi: 10.1001/jamapediatrics.2022.3581.

123 Lobelia Samavati and Bruce D. Uhal, "ACE2, Much More Than Just a Receptor for SARS-COV-2," *Frontiers in Cellular and Infection Microbiology* 10 (June 5, 2020), doi: 10.3389/fcimb.2020.00317.

124 Balamurali K. Ambati et al., "MSH3 Homology and Potential Recombination Link to SARS-Cov-2 Furin Cleavage Site," *Frontiers in Virology* 10 (February 21, 2022), https://doi.org.10.3389/fviro.2022.834808.

125 Lael M. Yonker et al., "Circulating Spike Protein Detected in Post–COVID-19 mRNA Vaccine Myocarditis," *Circulation* 147, no. 11 (2023), https://doi.org.10.1161/CIRCULATIONAHA.122.061025.

126 Yongjun Sui et al., "SARS-CoV-2 Spike Protein Suppresses ACE2 and Type I Interferon Expression in Primary Cells From Macaque Lung Bronchoalveolar Lavage," *Frontiers in Immunology* 12 (June 4, 2021), https://doi.org.10.3389/fimmu.2021.658428; Aval B. Gussow et al., "Genomic Determinants of Pathogenicity in SARS-CoV-2 and Other Human Coronaviruses," *PNAS* 117, no. 26 (June 10, 2020): 15193–15199, https://doi.org.10.1073/pnas.2008176117; Ahmed M. Almehdi et al., "SARS-CoV-2 Spike

Protein: Pathogenesis, Vaccines, and Potential Therapies," *Infection* 49, no. 5 (October 2021): 855–876, doi: org.10.1007/s15010-021-01677-8.

127 Yuyang Lei et al., "SARS-CoV-2 Spike Protein Impairs Endothelial Function via Downregulation of ACE 2," *Circulation Research* 128, no. 9 (2021): 1323–1326, doi: org.10.1161/CIRCRESAHA.121.318902.

128 Si Zhang et al., "SARS-CoV-2 Binds Platelet ACE2 to Enhance Thrombosis in COVID-19," *Journal of Hematology & Oncology* 13 no. 120 (2020): 120, doi: org.10.1186/s13045-020-00954-7.

129 Yasushi Matsuzawa et al., "Impact of Renin–Angiotensin–Aldosterone System Inhibitors on COVID-19," *Hypertension Research* 45, no. 7 (2022): 1147–1153, doi: org.10.1038/s41440-022-00922-3.

130 Cosima T. Baldari et al., "Emerging Roles of SARS-CoV-2 Spike-ACE2 in Immune Evasion and Pathogenesis," *Trends in Immunology* 44 no. 6 (June 2023), doi: org.10.1016/j.it.2023.04.001.

131 Xiang Gao et al., "Spike-Mediated ACE2 Down-Regulation Was Involved in the Pathogenesis of SARS-CoV-2 Infection," *Journal of Infection* 85, no. 4 (October 2022), 418–427, doi: org.10.1016/j.jinf.2022.06.030.

132 Elisa Avolio et al., "The SARS-CoV-2 Spike Protein Disrupts Human Cardiac Pericytes Function through CD147 Receptor-Mediated Signalling: A Potential Non-infective Mechanism of COVID-19 Microvascular Disease," *Clinical Science* 135, no. 24. (December 22, 2021): 2667–2689, doi: org.10.1042/CS20210735.

133 Norma Maugeri et al., "Unconventional CD147-Dependent Platelet Activation Elicited by SARS-CoV-2 in COVID-19," *Journal of Thrombosis and Haemostasis* 20, no. 2. (October 28, 2021): 434–448, doi: org.10.1111/jth.15575.

134 Ken Shirato and Takako Kizaki, "SARS-CoV-2 Spike Protein S1 Subunit Induces Pro-inflammatory Responses via Toll-Like Receptor 4 Signaling in Murine and Human Macrophages," *Heliyon* 7, no. 2 (February 2, 2021):e06187, doi. org.10.1016/j.heliyon.2021.e06187.

135 "Coronavirus Spike Protein Activated Natural Immune Response, Damaged Heart Muscle Cells," *DAIC*, July 27, 2022, https://www.dicardiology.com/content/coronavirus-spike-protein-activated-natural-immune-response-damaged-heart-muscle-cells.

136 Shahanshah Khan et al., "SARS-CoV-2 Spike Protein Induces Inflammation via TLR2-Dependent Activation of the NF-κB Pathway," *eLife* 10 (December 6, 2021): e68563, doi: org.10.7554/eLife.68563.

137 Pei-Shan Sung et al., "CLEC5A and TLR2 Are Critical in SARS-CoV-2-Induced NET Formation and Lung Inflammation," *Journal of Biomedical Science* 29, no. 52 (2022), doi: 10.1186/s12929-022-00832-z.

138 Roberto Carnevale et al., "Toll-Like Receptor 4-Dependent Platelet-Related Thrombosis in SARS-CoV-2 Infection," *Circulation Research* 132, no. 3 (2023): 290–305, doi: 10.1161/CIRCRESAHA.122.321541.

139 Fabricia L. Fontes-Dantas, "SARS-CoV-2 Spike Protein Induces TLR4-Mediated Long-Term Cognitive Dysfunction Recapitulating Post-COVID-19 Syndrome in Mice," *Cell Reports* 42, no. 3 (March 2023):112189, doi: 10.1016/j.celrep.2023.112189.

140 Yi Zheng et al., "SARS-CoV-2 Spike Protein Causes Blood Coagulation and Thrombosis by Competitive Binding to Heparan Sulfate," *International Journal of Biological Macromolecules* 193 (December 15, 2021): 1124–1129, doi: 10.1016/j.ijbiomac.2021.10.112.

141 Lize M. Grobbelaar et al., "SARS-CoV-2 Spike Protein S1 Induces Fibrin(ogen) Resistant to Fibrinolysis: Implications for Microclot Formation in COVID-19," *Bioscence Reports* 41, no. 8 (August 27, 2021): BSR20210611, doi: 10.1042/BSR20210611.

142 Celine Boschi et al., "SARS-CoV-2 Spike Protein Induces Hemagglutination: Implications for COVID-19 Morbidities and Therapeutics and for Vaccine Adverse Effects," *International Journal of Biological Macromolecules* 23, no. 24 (2022): 15480, doi: 10.3390/ijms232415480.

143 Tianyang Li et al., "Platelets Mediate Inflammatory Monocyte Activation by SARS-CoV-2 Spike Protein," *Journal of Clinical Investigation* 132, no. 4 (February 15, 2022): e150101, https://doi.org.10.1172/JCI150101.

144 Scot B. Biering et al., "SARS-CoV-2 Spike Triggers Barrier Dysfunction and Vascular Leak via Integrins and TGF-β Signaling," *Nature Communications* 13 (2022): 7630, https://doi.org.10.1038/s41467-022-34910-5; Juan Pablo Robles et al., "The Spike Protein of SARS-CoV-2 Induces Endothelial Inflammation through Integrin α5β1 and NF-κB Signaling," *JBC* 298, no. 3 (March 2022):3, 101695, https://doi.org.10.1016/j.jbc.2022.101695.

145 Michael Mörz, "A Case Report: Multifocal Necrotizing Encephalitis and Myocarditis after BNT162b2 mRNA Vaccination against COVID-19," *Vaccines* 10, no. 10 (2022): 1651, doi: 10.3390/vaccines10101651.

146 Junyoung Oh et al., "SARS-CoV-2 Spike Protein Induces Cognitive Deficit and Anxiety-Like Behavior in Mouse via Non-cell Autonomous Hippocampal Neuronal Death," *Scientific Reports* 12, no. 5496 (2022), doi: 10.1038/s41598-022-09410-7.

Chapter 5: Debunking the CDC's Bad Science

147 Apoorva Mandavilli, "Your Coronavirus Test Is Positive. Maybe It Shouldn't Be," *New York Times,* August 29, 2020, https://www.nytimes.com/2020/08/29/health/coronavirus-testing.html; Oyungerel Byambasuren et al., "Estimating the Extent of Asymptomatic COVID-19 and Its Potential for Community Transmission: Systematic Review and Meta-Analysis," *JAMMI* 5, no. 4 (December 2020): 223–234, doi: 10.3138/jammi-2020-0030.

148 "COVID-19 Treatment Studies for Hydroxychloroquine," accessed April 2023, https://c19hcq.org/.

149 Can Li et al., "Intravenous Injection of Coronavirus Disease 2019 (COVID-19) mRNA Vaccine Can Induce Acute Myopericarditis in Mouse Model," *Clinical Infectious Diseases* 74, no. 11 (June 1, 2022): 1933–1950, doi: 10.1093/cid/ciab707; JoEllen. Wolicki, "Vaccine Administration," in *Epidemiology and Prevention of Vaccine-Preventable Diseases*, US Department of Health and Human Services, Centers for Disease Control and Prevention, accessed July 17, 2021, https://www.cdc.gov/vaccines/pubs/pinkbook/vac-admin.html; Kirk U. Knowlton, "Editorial: Insights from a Murine Model of Coronavirus Disease 2019 (COVID-19) mRNA Vaccination-Induced Myopericarditis: Could Accidental Intravenous Vaccine Injection Induce Myopericarditis?" *Clinical Infectious Diseases* 74 no. 11 (June 10, 2022): 1951–1952, doi: 10.1093/cid/ciab741.

150 Max Schmeling et al., "Batch-Dependent Safety of the BNT162b2 mRNA COVID-19 Vaccine," *European Journal of Clinical Investigation* 53, no. 8 (March 30, 2023), doi: 10.1111/eci.13998; Yihua Bruce Yu et al., "All Vials Are Not the Same: Potential Role of Vaccine Quality in Vaccine Adverse Reactions," *Vaccine* 39, no. 45 (2021): 6565–6569, doi: 10.1016/j.vaccine.2021.09.065.

151 Peter Doshi, "Will Covid-19 Vaccines Save Lives? Current Trials Aren't Designed to Tell Us," *BMJ* 371 (2020): m4037, doi: 10.1136/bmj.m4037.

152 Tanya R. Myers et al., "The V-Safe after Vaccination Health Checker: Active Vaccine Safety Monitoring during CDC's COVID-19 Pandemic Response," *Vaccine* 41, no. 7 (2023): 1310–1318, doi: 10.1016/j.vaccine.2022.12.031.

153 Hannah G. Rosenblum, MD, et al., "Safety of mRNA Vaccines Administered during the Initial 6 Months of the US COVID-19 Vaccination Program an Observational Study of Reports to the Vaccine Adverse Event Reporting System and V-Safe," *Lancet Infectious Disease* 22, no. 6 (June 2022): 802–812, doi: 10.1016/S1473-3099(22)00054-8.

154 "Aaron Siri," Campfire Wiki, January 24, 2022, https://www.campfire.wiki/doku.php?id=aaron_siri.

155 "Legal Action: V-Safe," ICAN, October 18, 2022, https://icandecide.org/article/v-safe/.

156 Aaron Siri, "V-Safe Part 7: CDC Deceived the Public With Limited Release of V-Safe Check-the-Box Data Until Forced to Release It All," *Injecting Freedom* (Substack), February 14, 2023, https://aaronsiri.substack.com/p/v-safe-part-7-cdc-deceived-the-public.

157 Aaron Siri, "V-Safe Part 6: A First Look at What the V-Safe Check-the-Box Data Reveals," *Injecting Freedom* (Substack), February 8, 2023, https://aaronsiri.substack.com/p/v-safe-part-6-a-first-look-at-what.

158 Organic Consumers Association, "Zogby Poll: 15% of American Adults Diagnosed with New Condition after COVID Vaccine," July 29, 2022, https://organicconsumers.org/15-of-american-adults-diagnosed-with-new-condition-after-covid-vaccine-zogby-survey-finds/.

159 Theresa Andrasfay, PhD, et al., "Reductions in 2020 US Life Expectancy Due to COVID-19 and the Disproportionate Impact on the Black and Latino Populations," *PNAS* 118, no. 5 (January 14, 2021): e2014746118, doi: 10.1073/pnas.2014746118.

160 Gerard J. Nuovo et al., "Endothelial Cell Damage Is the Central Part of COVID-19 and a Mouse Model Induced by Injection of the S1 Subunit of the Spike Protein," *Annals of Diagnostic Pathology* 51, no. 151682, (April 2021), doi: 10.1016/j.anndiagpath.2020.151682.

161 Mario Dioguardi et al., "Innate Immunity in Children and the Role of ACE2 Expression in SARS-CoV-2 Infection," *Pediatric Reports* 13, no. 3 (July 2021): 363–382, doi: 10.3390/pediatric13030045.

162 Joseph Fraiman et al., "Serious Adverse Events of Special Interest following mRNA COVID-19 Vaccination in Randomized Trials in Adults," *Vaccine* 40, no. 40 (September 22, 2022): 5798–5805, doi: 10.1016/j.vaccine.2022.08.036; Arne Burckhardt, "Histopathological Reevaluation Serious Adverse Events and Deaths Following COVID-19 Vaccination," Conference Presentation: Pandemic Strategies, Lessons, and Consequences, January 21–22, 2023, Rumble video, https://rumble.com/v290q9s-histopathological-reevaluation-serious-adverse-events-and-deaths-following-.html.

163 McKenzie Beard, "COVID-19 Is No Longer a Pandemic of the Unvaccinated," *Washington Post*, November 23, 2022, https://www.washingtonpost.com/politics/2022/11/23/vaccinated-people-now-make-up-majority-covid-deaths/; Sarah Tanveer et al., "Transparency of COVID-19 Vaccine Trials: Decisions without Data," *BMJ Evidence Based Medicine* 27, no. 4 (August 9, 2021), doi: 10.1136/bmjebm-2021-111735; Peter Doshi et al., "Covid-19 Vaccines and Treatments: We Must Have Raw Data, Now," *BMJ* 376 (January 19, 2022): o102, doi: 10.1136/bmj.o102.

164 Jeffrey K. Aronson et al., "The Use of Mechanistic Evidence in Drug Approval," *Journal of Evaluation in Clinical Practice* 24, no. 5 (October 2018): 1166–1176, doi: 10.1111/jep.12960.

165 "FDA Records Show a Significant Number of mRNA Test Rats Born with Skeletal Deformations," Judicial Watch, December 13, 2022, https://www.judicialwatch.org/mrna-test-rats-born-with-skeletal-deformations/.

166 "A Study of mRNA-1647 Cytomegalovirus Vaccine in Healthy Participants 9 to 15 Years of Age and Participants 16 to 25 Years of Age," Clinicaltrials.gov, https://classic.clinicaltrials.gov/ct2/show/NCT05575492; Derek Lowe, "Moderna's Upcoming Clinical Trials," *Science*, April 21, 2021, https://www.science.org/content/blog-post/moderna-s-upcoming-clinical-trials.

167 "Charles River Biodistribution Study," Judicial Watch, August 17, 2022, https://www.judicialwatch.org/documents/jw-v-hhs-biodistribution-prod-4-02418/.

168 "Pages 671–701," Judicial Watch, December 13, 2022, https://www.judicialwatch.org/documents/jw-v-hhs-biodistribution-prod-4-02418-pgs-671-701/.

169 Andreas M. Reichmuth et al., "mRNA Vaccine Delivery Using Lipid Nanoparticles," *Therapeutic Delivery* 7, no. 6 (2016): 319–34, doi: 10.4155/tde-2016-0006; Seyed Moein Moghimi and Dmitri Simberg, "Pro-inflammatory Concerns with Lipid Nanoparticles," *Molecular Therapy* 30, no. 6 (June 2022): 2109–2110, doi: 10.1016/j.ymthe.2022.04.011; Sonia Ndeupen et al., "The mRNA-LNP Platform's Lipid Nanoparticle Component Used in Preclinical Vaccine Studies Is Highly Inflammatory," *iScience* 24, no. 103479 (December 17, 2021), doi: 10.1016/j.isci.2021.103479.

170 Rave Harpaz et al., "Signaling COVID-19 Vaccine Adverse Events," *Drug Safety* 45 (2022): 765–80, doi: 10.1007/s40264-022-01186-z.

171 Philip C. Huang et al., "Cov19VaxKB: A Web-based Integrative COVID-19 Vaccine Knowledge Base," *Vaccine X* (April 2021): 100139, doi: 10.1016/j.jvacx.2021.100139.

172 Zachary Stieber, "CDC Finds Hundreds of Safety Signals for Pfizer and Moderna COVID-19 Vaccines," *Epoch Times*, January 3, 2023, https://www.theepochtimes.com/exclusive-cdc-finds-hundreds-of-safety-signals-for-pfizer-and-moderna-covid-19-vaccines_4956733.html.

173 JW v. HHS.

174 Ibrahim Chahoud et al., "Dose-Response Relationships of Rat Fetal Skeleton Variations: Relevance for Risk Assessment," *Environmental Research* 109, no. 7 (October 2009): 922–929, doi: 10.1016/j.envres.2009.07.013.

175 US Department of Health and Human Services, Centers for Disease Control and Prevention, "New CDC Data: COVID-19 Vaccination Safe for Pregnant People," media statement, August 11, 2021, https://www.cdc.gov/media/releases/2021/s0811-vaccine-safe-pregnant.html.

176 Ah Khan Syed, "Release the V-Safe Pregnancy Data—Now," *Akrmedic's blog* (Substack), October 15, 2022, https://www.arkmedic.info/p/release-the-v-safe-pregnancy-data; Nevio Cimolai, "Do RNA Vaccines Obviate the Need for Genotoxicity Studies?" *Mutagenesis* 35, no. 6 (November 20, 2020): 509–510, doi: 10.1093/mutage/geaa028.

177 Ah Khan Syed, "BNT162b2 Cumulative Review from Pharmacovigilance Database for Clinical Trial C4591001 FDA-CBER-2021-5683-0779745. Cumulative Review and Summary of Relevant Cases Reported in Pfizer's Pharmacovigilance (Safety) Database from the Time of Drug Product Development to 28-FEB-2021," *Akrmedic's blog* (Substack), February 26, 2023, https://arkmedic.substack.com/p/the-miscarriage-of-medicine; Sonia Elijah, "Pfizer's Pregnancy & Lactation Cumulative Review Reveals Damning Data," TrialSiteNews, April 22, 2023, https://www.trialsitenews.com/a/pfizers-pregnancy-lactation-cumulative-review-reveals-damning-data-2b15c969. Pfizer Documents Investigation Team and Amy Kelly, *War Room/DailyClout Pfizer Documents Analysis Volunteers' Reports eBook: Find Out What Pfizer, FDA Tried to Conceal*, ed. DailyClout LLC (B0BSK6LV5D: January 16, 2023), Kindle, https://www.amazon.com/DailyClout-Documents-Analysis-Volunteers-Reports-ebook/dp/B0BSK6LV5D/; *The Pfizer Papers: Pfizer's Crimes against Humanity*, ed. DailyClout LLC (October 15,

2024), Kindle, https://www. amazon.com/Pfizer-Papers-Pfizers-Against-Humanity/dp/1648210376/.
178 Syed, "Release the V-Safe Pregnancy Data—Now."; Sonia Elijah, "EMA's failure to pull COVID 19 jabs even though risk-benefit balance nullified," Children's Health Defense Europe, February 19, 2023, https://childrenshealthdefense.eu/eu-affairs/emas-failure-to-pull-covid-19-jabs-even-though-risk-benefit-balance-nullified/; Pfizer Documents Investigation Team and Amy Kelly, *War Room/DailyClout Pfizer Documents Analysis Volunteers' Reports eBook: Find Out What Pfizer, FDA Tried to Conceal*, ed. DailyClout LLC (B0BSK6LV5D: January 16, 2023), Kindle, https://www.amazon.com/DailyClout-Documents-Analysis-Volunteers-Reports- ebook/dp/B0BSK6LV5D/; *The Pfizer Papers: Pfizer's Crimes against Humanity*, ed. DailyClout LLC (October 15, 2024), Kindle, https://www. amazon.com/Pfizer-Papers-Pfizers-Against-Humanity/dp/1648210376/.
179 "When Is a DSMB Needed?" UNC School of Medicine, North Carolina Translational and Clinical Sciences Institute, accessed September 2023, https://tracs.unc.edu/index.php/services/regulatory/data-and-safety-monitoring-board/when-is-a-dsmb-needed.
180 Ross Lazarus et al., "Electronic Support for Public Health–Vaccine Adverse Event Reporting System," Harvard Pilgrim Healthcare, 2011, https://digital.ahrq.gov/sites/default/files/docs/publication/r18hs017045-lazarus-final-report-2011.pdf.
181 Ibid; Tom T. Shimabukuro et al., "Safety Monitoring in the Vaccine Adverse Event Reporting System (VAERS)," *Vaccine*, 33, no. 36 (2015): 4398–4405, https://doi.org.10.1016/j.vaccine.2015.07.035; Weigong Zhou et al., "Surveillance Summaries, Surveillance for Safety after Immunization: Vaccine Adverse Event Reporting System (VAERS)—United States, 1991–2001", *Morbidity and Mortality Weekly Reports (MMWR)* 52, no. SS-1 (January 24, 2003): 1–24, US Department of Health and Human Services, Centers for Disease Control, https://pubmed.ncbi.nlm.nih.gov/12825543/.
182 Patrick R. Funk et al., "Benefit-Risk Assessment of COVID-19 Vaccine, mRNA (Comirnaty) for Age 16–29 Years," *Vaccine* 40, no. 19 (2022), 2781–2789, https://doi.org.10.1016/j.vaccine.2022.03.030.
183 Bette Korber et al., "Tracking Changes in SARS-CoV-2 Spike: Evidence that D614G Increases Infectivity of the COVID-19 Virus," *Cell* 182, no. 4 (2020): 812–827, .e19, doi: 10.1016/j.cell.2020.06.043; Yixuan J. Hou et al., "SARS-CoV-2 D614G Variant Exhibits Efficient Replication Ex Vivo and Transmission in Vivo," *Science* 370, no. 6523 (2020): 1464–1468, doi: 10.1126/science.abe8499.
184 Moriah Bergwerk et al., "Covid-19 Breakthrough Infections in Vaccinated Health Care Workers," *New England Journal of Medicine* 385, no. 16 (2021): 1474–1484, doi: 10.1056/NEJMoa2109072; Anyin Feng et al., "Modelling COVID-19 Vaccine Breakthrough Infections in Highly Vaccinated Israel—The Effects of Waning Immunity and Third Vaccination Dose," *PLOS*, November 9, 2022, doi: 10.1371/journal.pgph.0001211; Tal Brosh-Nissimov et al., "BNT162b2 Vaccine Breakthrough:

Clinical Characteristics of 152 Fully Vaccinated Hospitalized COVID-19 Patients in Israel," *Clinical Microbiology and Infection* 27, no. 11 (2021): 1652–1657, doi: 10.1016/j.cmi.2021.06.036.

185 American Society for Microbiology, "How Dangerous Is the Delta Variant (B.1.617.2)?" July 30, 2021, https://asm.org/Articles/2021/July/How-Dangerous-is-the-Delta-Variant-B-1-617-2.

186 Owen Dyer, "Covid-19: Delta Infections Threaten Herd Immunity Vaccine Strategy," *BMJ* 374 (2021): n1933, doi: 10.1136/bmj.n1933; Delphine Planas et al., "Reduced Sensitivity of SARS-CoV-2 Variant Delta to Antibody Neutralization," *Nature* 596 (2021): 276–280, doi: 10.1038/s41586-021-03777-9.

187 Emma C. Wall et al., "Neutralising Antibody Activity against SARS-CoV-2 VOCs B.1.617.2 and B.1.351 by BNT162b2 Vaccination," *Lancet* 397, no. 10292 (June 2021): 2331–2333, doi: 10.1016/S0140-6736(21)01290-3.

188 Beard, "COVID-19 Is No Longer a Pandemic of the Unvaccinated."

189 Zachary Stieber, "CDC Finds Hundreds of Safety Signals for Pfizer and Moderna COVID-19 Vaccines," *The Defender*, January 3, 2023, https://childrenshealthdefense.org/defender/cdc-safety-signals-pfizer-moderna-covid-vaccines-et/.

190 Zachary Stieber, "CDC Officials Make False Statements about Possible COVID-19 Vaccine Side Effects," *Epoch Times*, April 26, 2023, https://www.theepochtimes.com/health/exclusive-cdc-finds-hundreds-of-safety-signals-for-pfizer-and-moderna-covid-19-vaccines_4956733.html.

191 Abraham Shulman et al., "Neuroinflammation and Tinnitus," *Current Topics in Behavioral Neurosciences* 51 (2021): 161–174, doi: 10.1007/7854_2021_238.

192 Ramsi A. Woodcock et al., "Preliminary Evidence of a Link between COVID-19 Vaccines and Otologic Symptoms," medRxiv preprint, February 24, 2022, doi.org: 10.1101/2022.02.23.22271144.

193 Jennifer Henderson, "Vaccine Researcher Who Developed Tinnitus after COVID Shot Calls for Further Study," MedPage Today, March 9, 2022, https://www.medpagetoday.com/special-reports/exclusives/97592.

194 S. J. Evans et al., "Use of Proportional Reporting Ratios (PRRs) for Signal Generation from Spontaneous Adverse Drug Reaction Reports," *Pharmacoepidemiology and Drug Safety* 10, no. 6 (October–November 2001): 483–6, doi: 10.1002/pds.677; US Department of Health and Human Services, *VAERS Data User Guide*, November 2020, https://vaers.hhs.gov/docs/VAERSDataUseGuide_November2020.pdf; National Institutes of Health, *NIA Adverse Event and Serious Adverse Event Guidelines*, September 2019, https://www.nia.nih.gov/sites/default/files/2017-06/nia_ae_and_sae_guidelines.docx; US Department of Health and Human Services, Centers for Disease Control and Prevention, *Vaccine Adverse Event Reporting System (VAERS), Standard Operating Procedures for COVID-19*, VAERS Team: Immunization Safety Office, Division of Healthcare Quality Promotion National Center for Emerging and Zoonotic Infectious Diseases and Centers for Disease Control and Prevention,

January 2021, https://www.cdc.gov/vaccinesafety/pdf/VAERS-v2-SOP.pdf; Frederick Varricchio et al., "Understanding Safety Information from the Vaccine Adverse Event Reporting System," *Pediatric Infectious Disease Journal* 23, no. 4 (April 2004): 287–94, doi: 10.1097/00006454-200404000-00002.

195 Jessica Freeborn, "Misfolded Spike Protein Could Explain Complicated COVID-19 Symptoms," Medical News Today, May 26, 2022, https://www.medicalnewstoday.com/articles/misfolded-spike-protein-could-explain-complicated-covid-19-symptoms.

196 George Tetz et al., "Prion-Like Domains in Spike Protein of SARS-CoV-2 Differ across Its Variants and Enable Changes in Affinity to ACE2," *Microorganisms* 10, no. 2 (2022): 280, doi: 10.3390/microorganisms10020280.

197 Sofie Nyström and Per Hammarström, "Amyloidogenesis of SARS-CoV-2 Spike Protein," *Journal of the American Chemical Society*, 144, no. 20. (2022): 8945–8950, doi: 10.1021/jacs.2c03925.

198 Emily Henderson, "Researchers Discover Possible Connection between Harmful Amyloid Production and COVID-19 Spike Protein," News Medical, May 19, 2022, https://www.news-medical.net/news/20220519/Researchers-discover-possible-connection-between-harmful-amyloid-production-and-COVID-19-symptoms.aspx

199 Zhouyi Rong et al., "SARS-CoV-2 Spike Protein Accumulation in the Skull-Meninges-Brain Axis: Potential Implications for Long-Term Neurological Complications in post-COVID-19," bioRxiv preprint, April 5, 2023, doi: 10.1101/2023.04.04.535604; Omid Tavassoly et al., "Seeding Brain Protein Aggregation by SARS-CoV-2 as a Possible Long-Term Complication of COVID-19 Infection," *ACS Chemical Neuroscience* 11, no. 22 (2020): 3704–3706, doi: 10.1021/acschemneuro.0c00676; Burkhard, "Histopathological Reevaluation Serious Adverse Events and Deaths Following COVID-19 Vaccination."

200 Steven J. Hatfill, "Significance of the SARS-CoV-2 Spike Protein 'Superantigen' Sequence in the mRNA Vaccines," *JPANDS* 27, no. 2 (2022): 52–55, https://www.jpands.org/vol27no2/hatfill2.pdf.

201 Joseph A. Bellanti, *Immunology III* (Philadelphia: WB Saunders Co., 1985), https://www.amazon.com/Immunology-III-Joseph-Bellanti/dp/0721616682.

202 Jackson S. Turner et al., "SARS-CoV-2 Infection Induces Long-Lived Bone Marrow Plasma Cells in Humans," *Nature* 595 (2021): 421–425, doi: 10.1038/s41586-021-03647-4.

203 Robert Hart, "More Infectious and Airborne Covid-19 Mutant Replaced Wuhan Virus to Dominate Worldwide, Study Finds," *Forbes*, November 13, 2020, https://www.forbes.com/sites/roberthart/2020/11/13/more-infectious-and-airborne-covid-19-mutant-replaced-wuhan-virus-to-dominate-worldwide-research-finds/.

204 Muriel Aguilar-Bretones et al., "Impact of Antigenic Evolution and Original Antigenic Sin on SARS-CoV-2 Immunity," *Journal of Clinical Investigation* 133, no. 1 (January 3, 2023): e162192, doi: 10.1172/JCI162192.

205 Sivan Gazit et al., "Severe Acute Respiratory Syndrome Coronavirus 2 (SARS-CoV-2) Naturally Acquired Immunity versus Vaccine-induced Immunity, Reinfections versus

Breakthrough Infections: A Retrospective Cohort Study," *Clinical Infectious Diseases* 75, no. 1 (August 24, 2022): e545-e551, doi: 10.1093/cid/ciac262; Thaddeus Bartter et al., "We Must Stop Ignoring Natural Immunity," *BMJ* 374 (2021): n2101, doi: 10.1136/bmj.n2101; Alec Schemmel, "New Study Indicates Natural Immunity Offers Greater Protection from COVID-19 Than Vaccines," KATV, June 20, 2022, https://katv.com/news/nation-world/new-study-indicates-natural-immunity-offers-greater-protection-from-covid-19-than-vaccines-new-england-journal-medicine-coronavirus-hybrid; Yair Goldberg et al., "Protection and Waning of Natural and Hybrid Immunity to SARS-CoV-2," *New England Journal of Medicine* 386 (2022): 2201–2212, https://www.nejm.org/doi/full/10.1056/NEJMoa2118946.

206 Beard, "COVID-19 Is No Longer a Pandemic of the Unvaccinated."

207 Ruth Link-Gelles, US Food and Drug Administration, VRBPAC meeting, "COVID-19 Vaccine Coverage & Effectiveness during Omicron for Children and Adolescents," June 14, 2022, https://www.cdc.gov/vaccines/acip/meetings/downloads/slides-2022-06-17-18/03-covid-link-gelles-508.pdf.

208 Nabin K. Shrestha et al., "Effectiveness of the Coronavirus Disease 2019 (COVID-19) Bivalent Vaccine," *Open Forum Infectious Diseases,* April 19, 2023, doi: 10.1101/2022.12.17.22283625.

209 Noa Dagan et al., "BNT162b2 mRNA Covid-19 Vaccine in a Nationwide Mass Vaccination Setting," *New England Journal of Medicine* 384 (2021): 1412–1423, doi: 10.1056/NEJMoa2101765; Noam Barda et al., "Safety of the BNT162b2 mRNA Covid-19 Vaccine in a Nationwide Setting," *New England Journal of Medicine* 385 (2021): 1078–1090, doi: 10.1056/NEJMoa2110475.

210 Hanne-Dorthe Emborg et al., "Vaccine Effectiveness of the BNT162b2 mRNA COVID-19 Vaccine against RT-PCR Confirmed SARS-CoV-2 Infections, Hospitalisations and Mortality in Prioritised Risk Groups," medRxiv preprint, 2021: 2021.05.27.21257583, doi: 10.1101/2021.05.27.21257583.

211 Richard L. Ward et al., "Minimum Infective Dose of Animal Viruses," *Critical Reviews in Environmental Control* 14, no. 4 (1984): 297–310, doi: 10.1080/10643388409381721; Saber Yezli et al., "Minimum Infective Dose of the Major Human Respiratory and Enteric Viruses Transmitted Through Food and the Environment," *Food and Environmental Virology* 3, no. 1 (March, 2011): 1–30, doi: 10.1007/s12560-011-9056-7.

212 Takuya Sekine et al., "Robust T Cell Immunity in Convalescent Individuals with Asymptomatic or Mild COVID-19," *Cell* 183, no. 1 (October 1 2020): 158–168.e14, doi: 10.1016/j.cell.2020.08.017; Zhongfang Wang et al., "Exposure to SARS-CoV-2 Generates T-cell Memory in the Absence of a Detectable Viral Infection," *Nature Communications* 12 (2021): 1724, doi: 10.1038/s41467-021-22036-z.

213 Allison J. Greaney et al., "Antibodies Elicited by mRNA-1273 Vaccination Bind More Broadly to the Receptor Binding Domain Than Do Those from SARS-CoV-2

Infection," *Science Translational Medicine* 13, no. 600 (June 30, 2021), doi: 10.1126/scitranslmed.abi9915.

214 Yair Goldberg et al., "Similarity of Protection Conferred by Previous SARS-CoV-2 Infection and by BNT162b2 Vaccine: A 3-Month Nationwide Experience From Israel," *American Journal of Epidemiology* 191, no. 8 (August 2022): 1420–1428, doi: 10.1093/aje/kwac060.

215 Victoria Jane Hall et al., "SARS-CoV-2 Infection Rates of Antibody-Positive Compared with Antibody-Negative Health-Care Workers in England: Large, Multicenter, Prospective Cohort Study (SIREN)," *Lancet* 397, no. 10283 (April 2021): 1459–1469, doi: 10.1016/S0140-6736(21)00675-9.

216 Nabin K. Shrestha et al., "Necessity of Coronavirus Disease 2019 (COVID-19) Vaccination in Persons Who Have Already Had COVID-19," *Clinical Infectious Diseases* 75, no. 1 (July 1, 2022): e662–e671, doi: 10.1093/cid/ciac022.

217 Turner et al, "SARS-CoV-2 Infection Induces Long-Lived Bone Marrow Plasma Cells in Humans."

218 Andrew D. Redd et al., "CD8+ T-cell Responses in Covid-19 Convalescent Individuals Target Conserved Epitopes from Multiple Prominent SARS-CoV-2 Circulating Variants," *Open Forum Infectious Diseases* 8 (2021): ofab143, doi: 10.1093/ofid/ofab143; Alison Tarke et al., "Impact of SARS-CoV-2 variants on the total CD4+ and CD8+ T cell reactivity in infected or vaccinated individuals," *Cell Reports Medicine* 2, no. 7 (July 20, 2021): 100355, doi: 10.1016/j.xcrm.2021.100355.

219 National Institutes of Health, "Lasting Immunity Found after Recovery from COVID-19," January 26, 2021, https://www.nih.gov/news-events/nih-research-matters/lasting-immunity-found-after-recovery-covid-19#main-content.

220 Jennifer M. Dan et al., "Immunological Memory to SARS-CoV-2 Assessed for Up to 8 Months after Infection," *Science* 371 (2021): eabf4063, doi: 10.1126/science.abf4063.

221 US Department of Health and Human Services, Centers for Disease Control and Prevention, "COVID-19 Vaccine Breakthrough Infections Reported to CDC—United States, January 1–April 30, 2021," *Morbidity and Mortality Weekly Report (MMWR)* 70, no. 21 (2021): 792–793, doi: 10.15585/mmwr.mm7021e3.

222 Alyson M. Cavanaugh, et al., "Reduced Risk of Reinfection with SARS-CoV-2 after COVID-19 Vaccination—Kentucky, May–June, 2021," *Morbidity and Mortality Weekly Report (MMWR)* 70, no. 32 (2021): 1081–3, US Department of Health and Human Services, Centers for Disease Control and Prevention,doi: 10.15585/mmwr.mm7032e1.

223 Cristina Menni et al., "Vaccine Side-Effects and SARS-CoV-2 Infection after Vaccination in Users of the COVID Symptom Study App in the UK: A Prospective Observational Study," *Lancet Infectious Diseases* 21 (2021): 939–49, doi: 10.1016/S1473-3099(21)00224-3.

224 Alexander G. Mathioudakis et al., "Self-Reported Real-World Safety and Reactogenicity of Covid-19 Vaccines: A Vaccine Recipient Survey," *Life* (Basel) 11 (2021): 249, doi: 10.3390/life11030249.

225 Peter W. Marks et al., "Urgent Need for Next-Generation COVID-19 Vaccines," *Journal of the American Medical Association* 329, no. 1 (2023): 19–20, doi: 10.1001/jama.2022.22759.

226 Alice Park, "Data Doesn't Support New COVID-19 Booster Shots for Most, Says Vaccine Expert," *Time*, January 11, 2023, https://time.com/6246525/bivalent-booster-not-very-effective-paul-offit/.

227 Emily Bell, "The Fact Check Industry," *Columbia Journalism Review*, Fall 2019, https://www.cjr.org/special_report/fact-check-industry-twitter.php.

228 "Trusted News Initiative (TNI) to Combat Spread of Harmful Vaccine Disinformation and Announces Major Research Project," BBC, December 10, 2020, https://www.bbc.com/mediacentre/2020/trusted-news-initiative-vaccine-disinformation.

229 America First Legal, "AFL Lawsuit Uncovers More Audacious CDC Documents Revealing the Biden Administration's Blatant Complicity with Big Tech to Push Disinformation and Suppress and Censor Free Speech," September 6, 2022, https://aflegal.org/afl-lawsuit-uncovers-more-audacious-cdc-documents-revealing-the-biden-administrations-blatant-complicity-with-big-tech-to-push-disinformation-and-suppress-and-censor-free-speech/.

230 America First Legal, "AFL Lawsuit Uncovers More Damning CDC Documents Revealing Twitter's 'Partner Support Portal' for COVID-19 Related Censorship and the U.S. Government's Advancement of 'Social Inoculation' Against the 'Infodemic,'" December 6, 2022, https://aflegal.org/afl-lawsuit-uncovers-more-damning-cdc-documents-revealing-twitters-partner-support-portal-for-covid-19-related-censorship-and-the-u-s-governments-advancement-of/.

231 Rebecca Coombes and Madlen Davies, "Facebook versus the *BMJ*: When Fact Checking Goes Wrong," *BMJ* 376 (2022): o95, doi: 10.1136/bmj.o95.

232 America First Legal, "AFL Releases More CDC Documents Revealing Bizarre 'Equity' Agenda in COVID-19 Vaccination and Slides Discussing the Policy Objective of Injecting Children Even When 'Parent Is Not Present,'" December 15, 2022, https://aflegal.org/afl-releases-more-cdc-documents-revealing-bizarre-equity-agenda-in-covid-19-vaccination-and-slides-discussing-the-policy-objective-of-injecting-children-even-when-parent-is/.

Chapter 6: Safety Signals from the Vaccine Adverse Event Reporting System (VAERS)

233 Medicines and Healthcare Products Regulatory Agency (MHRA), "Coronavirus vaccine—Summary of Yellow Card Reporting," March 8, 2023, https://www.gov.uk/government/publications/coronavirus-covid-19-vaccine-adverse-reactions/coronavi-

rus-vaccine-summary-of-yellow-card-reporting; Therapeutic Goods Administration (TGA), Database of Adverse Events Notification, February 16, 2023, https://www.tga.gov.au/safety/safety/safety-monitoring-daen-database-adverse-event-notifications/database-adverse-event-notifications-daen; European Medicines Agency, "EudraVigilance—European Database of Suspected Adverse Drug Reaction Reports," accessed August 7, 2023, https://www.adrreports.eu/en/index.html.

234 US Food and Drug Administration, "Moderna COVID-19 Vaccine: Moderna COVID-19 Vaccine (2023-2024 Formula) Authorized for Individuals 6 Months Through 11 Years of Age," November 1, 2023, https://www.fda.gov/emergency-preparedness-and-response/coronavirus-disease-2019-covid-19/moderna-covid-19-vaccines.

235 Stephanie Seneff et al., "Innate Immune Suppression by SARS-CoV-2 mRNA Vaccinations: The Role of G-Quadruplexes, Exosomes, and MicroRNAs," *Food and Chemical Toxicology* 164 (June 2022):113008, doi: 10.1016/j.fct.2022.113008; Michael Repajic et al., "Bell's Palsy after Second Dose of Pfizer COVID-19 Vaccination in a Patient with History of Recurrent Bell's Palsy," *Brain Behavior & Immunity Health* 13. (2021): 100217, doi: 10.1016/j.bbih.2021.100217; Natalija Novak et al., "Adverse Rare Events to Vaccines for COVID-19: From Hypersensitivity Reactions to Thrombosis and Thrombocytopenia," *International Reviews of Immunology* 41, no. 4 (July 2021): 1–10, doi: 10.1080/08830185.2021.1939696; Kerry J. Welsh et al., "Thrombocytopenia Including Immune Thrombocytopenia after Receipt of mRNA COVID-19 Vaccines Reported to the Vaccine Adverse Event Reporting System (VAERS)," *Vaccine*, 39, no. 25 (June 2021): 3329–3332, doi: 10.1016/j.vaccine.2021.04.054; Prashant K. Minocha et al., "Recurrence of Acute Myocarditis Temporally Associated with Receipt of the mRNA Coronavirus Disease 2019 (COVID-19) Vaccine in a Male Adolescent," *Journal of Pediatrics* 238 (June 21, 2021): 32103, doi: 10.1016/j.jpeds.2021.06.035; Nicola Klein, "Rapid Cycle Analysis (RCA) to Monitor the Safety of COVID-19 Vaccines in Near Real-Time within the Vaccine Safety Datalink: Guillain-Barré Syndrome (GBS)," US Department of Health and Human Services, Centers for Disease Control and Prevention, Kaiser Permanente Vaccine Study Center, Kaiser Permanente Northern California, Marshfield Clinic Research Institute, Vaccine Safety Datalink—Immunization Safety Office, July 2021, https://www.cdc.gov/vaccines/acip/meetings/downloads/slides-2021-07/03-COVID-Klein-508.pdf; Michelle Trimboli et al., "Guillain-Barré Syndrome following BNT162b2COVID-19 Vaccine," *Neurological Sciences* 42, no. 11 (November 2021): 4401–4402, doi: 10.1007/s10072-021-05523-5; Waqar Waheed et al., "Post COVID-19 Vaccine Small Fiber Neuropathy," *Muscle & Nerve* 64, no. 1 (July 2021): e1–e2, doi: 10.1002/mus.27251; Edward Eid et al., "Herpes Zoster Emergence following mRNA COVID-19 Vaccine," *Journal of Medical Virology* 93, no. 9 (September 2021): 5231–5232, doi: 10.1002/jmv.27036; Eric Tano et al., "Perimyocarditis in Adolescents after

Pfizer-BioNTech COVID-19 Vaccine," *Journal of Pediatric Infectious Disease Society* 10, no. 10 (November 2021): 962–966, doi: 10.1093/jpids/piab060; George A. Diaz et al., "Myocarditis and Pericarditis after Vaccination for COVID-19," *JAMA Network* 326, no. 12 (September 2021): 1210–1212, doi: 10.1001/jama.2021.13443; Shinichi Matsuzaki et al., "COVID-19 mRNA Vaccine-Induced Pneumonitis," *Internal Medicine* 61, no. 1 (January 2022): 81–86, doi: 10.2169/internalmedicine.8310-21; Johad Khoury et al., "COVID-19 Vaccine—Long Term Immune Decline and Breakthrough Infections," *Vaccine* 39, no. 48 (November 2021): 6984-6989, doi: 10.1016/j.vaccine.2021.10.038; W-J A. Lee, "COVID-19 Vaccine-Associated Optic Neuritis," *QJM* 115, no. 10 (October 25, 2022): 683–685, doi: 10.1093/qjmed/hcac208; Amani Elimam and Sarah Al-Dhahir, "Pfizer COVID-19 Vaccine-Induced Peritonitis," *Clinical Medicine* (London) 22 (Suppl 4) (July 2022): 53, doi: 10.7861/clinmed.22-4-s53; Lene H. Garvey and Shuaib Nasser, "Anaphylaxis to the First COVID-19 Vaccine: Is Polyethyleneglycol (PEG) the Culprit?" *British Journal of Anaesthesia* 126, no. 3 (March 2021): e106–e108, doi: 10.1016/j.bja.2020.12.020; Wafa Bouleftour et al., "COVID-19 Vaccine-Related Adverse Events in Solid Cancer Patients Treated with Immunotherapy," *Cancer Investigation* 40, no. 9 (October 2022): 760–766, doi: 10.1080/07357907.2022.2121966; W. Sriwijitalai and V. Wiwanitkit, "COVID-19 Vaccine, Myocardial Infarction and Kounis Syndrome," *QJM* 115, no. 3 (March 2022):193, doi: 10.1093/qjmed/hcac016; Ameena Shafiq et al., "Neurological Immune-Related Adverse Events after COVID-19 Vaccination: A Systematic Review," *Journal of Clinical Pharmacology* 62, no. 3 (March 2022): 291–303, doi: 10.1002/jcph.2017; Joel Reis et al., "Pemphigus Foliaceous after mRNA COVID-19 Vaccine," *European Journal of Dermatology* 32, no. 3 (May 2022): 428–429, doi: 10.1684/ejd.2022.4294; T. Michel et al., "Acute Macular Neuroretinopathy after COVID-19 Vaccine," *Journal of French Ophthalmology* 45, no. 7 (September 2022): e299–e302, doi: 10.1016/j.jfo.2022.01.022; Ji Young Park et al., "Clinical Characteristics of Patients with COVID-19 Vaccine-Related Pneumonitis: A Case Series and Literature Review," *Korean Journal of Internal Medicine*, 37, no. 5 (September 2022): 989–1001, doi: 10.3904/kjim.2022.072; Rossella Talotta and Earle S. Robertson, "Antiphospholipid Antibodies and Risk of Post-COVID-19 Vaccination Thrombophilia: The Straw That Breaks the Camel's Back?" *Cytokine & Growth Factor Reviews* 60: 52–60, doi: 10.1016/j.cytogfr.2021.05.001; Iftach Sagy et al., "New-Onset Systemic Lupus Erythematosus following BNT162b2 mRNA COVID-19 Vaccine: A Case Series and Literature Review," *Rheumatology International* 42, no. 12 (December 2022): 2261–2266, doi: 10.1007/s00296-022-05203-3; Matthew W. Schelke et al., "Post-COVID-19 Vaccine Small-Fiber Neuropathy and Tinnitus Treated with Plasma Exchange," *Muscle & Nerve* 66, no. 4 (October 2022): E21–E23, doi: 10.1002/mus.27696; Rujittika Mungmunpuntipantip and Viroj Wiwanitkit, "Adrenal Haemorrhage and COVID-19 Vaccine-Induced Immune Thrombotic

Thrombocytopenia: Correspondence," *QJM* 115, no. 12 (December 2022): 875, doi: 10.1093/qjmed/hcac006; Emna Hammami et al., "Acquired Thrombotic Thrombocytopenic Purpura after BNT162b2 COVID-19 Vaccine: Case Report and Literature Review," *Laboratory Medicine* 53, no. 6 (November 2022): e145–e148, doi: 10.1093/labmed/lmac016; L. deMontjoye et al., "Eosinophilic Cellulitis after BNT162b2mRNA Covid-19 Vaccine," *Journal of the European Academy of Dermatology and Venereology* 36, no. 1 (January 2022): e26–e28, doi: 10.1111/jdv.17685; Bassem Awada et al., "Inverse Lichen Planus Post Oxford-AstraZeneca COVID-19 Vaccine," *Journal of Cosmetic Dermatology* 21, no. 3 (January 2022): 883–885, doi: 10.1111/jocd.14738; Shereen Teymour et al., "Erythema Nodosum after Moderna mRNA-1273 COVID-19 Vaccine," *Dermatologic Therapy* 35, no. 4 (April 2022): e15302, doi: 10.1111/dth.15302; Soo Jin Lee et al., "COVID-19 Vaccine-Induced Multisystem Inflammatory Syndrome with Polyserositis Detected by FDG PET/CT," *Clinical Nuclear Medicine* 47, no. 5 (May 2022): e397–e398, doi: 10.1097/RLU.0000000000004094; Alrashdi N. Mousa et al., "Systemic Lupus Erythematosus with Acute Pancreatitis and Vasculitic Rash following COVID-19 Vaccine: A Case Report and Literature Review," *Clinical Rheumatology* 41, no. 5 (May 2022): 1577–1582, doi: 10.1007/s10067-022-06097-z; Walter D. Cardona Maya et al., "Re: The Impact of COVID-19 Vaccine on Sperm Quality," *European Urology* 82, no. 3 (September 2022): 327–328, doi: 10.1016/j.eururo.2022.06.021; Anna Luo and Amanda Oakley, "Cutaneous Adverse Reactions following the Pfizer/BioNTech COVID-19 Vaccine," *Australasian Journal of Dermatology* 63, no. 3 (August 2022): e247–e250, doi: 10.1111/ajd.13859; Alexis Hilts et al.,"A Clinical Case of COVID-19 Vaccine-Associated Guillain-Barré Syndrome," *American Journal of Case Reports* 10, no. 23 (August 2022): e936896, doi: 10.12659/AJCR.936896; Alba López-Valle et al., "Cutaneous Reaction to BNT162b2 mRNA COVID-19 Vaccine," *International Journal of Dermatology* 60, no. 7 (July 2021): 891–892, doi: 10.1111/ijd.15575; Rujittika Mungmunpuntipantip and Viroj Wiwanitki, "Superior Vena Cava Syndrome and COVID-19 Vaccine Reaction," *Journal of Emergency Medicine* 63, no. 6 (December 2022): 811, doi: 10.1016/j.jemermed.2022.09.034; F-Z. Agharbi et al., "Bullous Pemphigoid Induced by the AstraZeneca COVID-19 Vaccine," *Annales de Dermatologie et de Vénéréologie* 149, no. 1 (March 2022): 56–57, doi: 10.1016/j.annder.2021.07.008; Vanessa Juddoo et al., "Erythema Nodosum Triggered by BNT162b2 mRNA COVID-19 Vaccine," *Vaccine* 40, no. 19 (April 26, 2022): 2650–2651, doi: 10.1016/j.vaccine.2022.03.052; Mehmet Fatih Atak et al., "Pigmented Purpuric Dermatosis after BNT162B2 mRNA COVID-19 Vaccine Administration," *Journal of Cosmetic Dermatology* 21, no. 2 (February 2022): 435–437, doi: 10.1111/jocd.14607; Ahmed M. Eldokla and Mohammed T. Numan, "Postural Orthostatic Tachycardia Syndrome after mRNA COVID-19 Vaccine," *Clinical Autonomic Research* 32, no. 4 (August 2022): 307–311, doi: 10.1007/s10286-022-00880-3; Israel Potasman, "Secondary

Syphilis Unmasked by BNT162b2 mRNA COVID-19 Vaccine," *Israel Medical Association Journal* 24, no. 5 (May 2022): 337–338, https://ima-files.s3.amazonaws.com/377838_79093ae9-3ede-44b8-b7fa-9b17fa5f08d0.pdf; Daisuke Ikechi et al., "A Case of Suspected COVID-19 Vaccine-Related Thrombophlebitis," *Internal Medicine* 61, no. 10 (May 15, 2022): 1631, doi: 10.2169/internalmedicine.8767-21; E. Bleve et al., "COVID-19 Vaccine and Autoimmune Diabetes in Adults: Report of Two Cases," *Journal of Endocrinological Investigation* 45, no. 6 (June 2022): 1269–1270, doi: 10.1007/s40618-022-01796-5; Mayuko Yamamoto et al., "Persistent Varicella Zoster Virus Infection following mRNA COVID-19 Vaccination Was Associated with the Presence of Encoded Spike Protein in the Lesion," *Journal of Cutaneous Immunology and Allergy* 6 (2023): 18–23, doi: 10.1002/cia2.12278.

236 World Health Organization, "Minimum Requirements for a Functional Pharmaco-Vigilance System," 2010, https://who-umc.org/media/1483/pv_minimum_requirements_2010_2.pdf; World Health Organization, "What Is Pharmacovigilance?," https://www.who.int/teams/regulation-prequalification/regulation-and-safety/pharmacovigilance.

237 "H.R. 5546—National Childhood Vaccine Injury Act of 1986," Congress.gov website, https://www.congress.gov/bill/99th- congress/house-bill/5546.

238 "Vaccine Adverse Event Reporting System (VAERS)." https://vaers.hhs.gov.

239 Ross Lazarus et al., "Electronic Support for Public Health–Vaccine Adverse Event Reporting System," Harvard Pilgrim Healthcare, 2011, https://digital.ahrq.gov/sites/default/files/docs/publication/r18hs017045-lazarus-final-report-2011.pdf; Shimabukuro et al., "Safety Monitoring in the Vaccine Adverse Event Reporting System (VAERS)," *Vaccine* 33, no. 36 (2015): 4398–4405, doi: 10.1016/j.vaccine.2015.07.035; Waigong Zhou et al., "Surveillance for Safety after Immunization: Vaccine Adverse Event Reporting System (VAERS)—United States, 1991–2001," *Morbidity and Mortality Weekly Report (MMWR)*, 52, no. SS-1 (January 24, 2003), 1–24, US Department of Health and Human Services, Centers for Disease Control and Prevention, https://www.cdc.gov/mmwr/PDF/ss/ss5201.pdf.

240 Steve Kirsch, "Why Won't the CDC or FDA Reveal the VAERS URF?" TrialSiteNews, October 25, 2021, https://www.trialsitenews.com/a/why-wont-the-cdc-or-fda-reveal-the-vaers-urf.

241 Susan Wollersheim, MD, "FDA Review of Efficacy and Safety of Pfizer-BioNTech COVID-19 Vaccine Emergency Use Authorization Request," US Food and Drug Administration, Vaccines and Related Biological Products Advisory Committee Meeting, Office of Vaccines Research and Review Division of Vaccines and Related Products Applications, December 10, 2020, https://www.fda.gov/media/144337/download.

242 Lazarus et al., "Electronic Support for Public Health–Vaccine Adverse Event Reporting System"; Shimabukuro et al., "Safety Monitoring in the Vaccine Adverse Event Reporting System (VAERS)"; Zhou et al., "Surveillance Summaries, Surveillance for

Safety after Immunization: Vaccine Adverse Event Reporting System (VAERS)—United States, 1991–2001."

243 Zachary Stieber, "FDA Refuses to Provide Key COVID-19 Vaccine Safety Analyses," *Epoch Times,* September 10, 2022, https://www.theepochtimes.com/audio/exclusive-fda-refuses-to-provide-key-covid-19-vaccine-safety-analyses_4722586.html; US Food and Drug Administration, *Good Pharmacovigilance Practices and Pharmacoepidemiologic Assessment,* March 2005, https://www.fda.gov/regulatory-information/search-fda-guidance-documents/good-pharmacovigilance-practices-and-pharmacoepidemiologic-assessment; S. Rosenthal and R. Chen, "The Reporting Sensitivities of Two Passive Surveillance Systems for Vaccine Adverse Events," *American Journal of Public Health* 85, no. 12 (December 1995): 1706–9, doi: 10.2105/ajph.85.12.1706.

244 S. J. W. Evans et al., "Use of Proportional Reporting Ratios (PRRs) for Signal Generation from Spontaneous Adverse Drug Reaction Reports," *Pharmacoepidemiology & Drug Safety* 10, no. 6 (October–November 2001): 483–6, doi: 10.1002/pds.677; US Department of Health and Human Services, "VAERS Data User Guide," November 2020, https://vaers.hhs.gov/docs/VAERSDataUseGuide_November2020.pdf; National Institutes of Health, "NIA Adverse Event and Serious Adverse Event Guidelines," September 2019, https://www.nia.nih.gov/sites/default/files/2018-09/nia-ae-and-sae-guidelines-2018.pdf; "Vaccine Adverse Event Reporting System (VAERS), Standard Operating Procedures for COVID-19," US Department of Health and Human Services, Centers for Disease Control and Prevention, VAERS Team: Immunization Safety Office, Division of Healthcare Quality Promotion National Center for Emerging and Zoonotic Infectious Diseases and Centers for Disease Control and Prevention, January 29, 2021, https://www.cdc.gov/vaccine-safety/pdf/VAERS-v2-SOP.pdf; Frederick Varricchio et al., "Understanding Safety Information from the Vaccine Adverse Event Reporting System," *Pediatric Infectious Disease Journal* 23, no. 4 (April 2004): 287–94, doi: 10.1097/00006454-200404000-00002; Jessica Rose, "Critical Appraisal of VAERS Pharmacovigilance: Is the U.S. Vaccine Adverse Events Reporting System (VAERS) a Functioning Pharmacovigilance System?" *Science, Public Health Policy & the Law,* October 2021, v3: 100–129, https://cf5e727d-d02d-4d71-89ff-9fe2d3ad957f.filesusr.com/ugd/adf864_0490c898f7514d-f4b6fbc5935da07322.pdf; Jessica Rose, "A Report on the US Vaccine Adverse Events Reporting System (VAERS) of the COVID-19 Messenger Ribonucleic Acid (mRNA) Biologicals," *Science, Public Health Policy & the Law,* May 2021, v2: 59–80, https://cf5e727d-d02d-4d71-89ff-9fe2d3ad957f.filesusr.com/ugd/adf864_a0a813acbfd-c4534a8cb50cf85193d49.pdf.

245 Angela K. Shen et al., "The Lyme Disease Vaccine—a Public Health Perspective," *Clinical Infectious Diseases* 52, no. SS-3 (February 2011): s247–s252, doi: 10.1093/cid/ciq115.

246 Kathleen Stratton et al., eds., "Immunization Safety Review: Hepatitis B Vaccine and Demyelinating Neurological Disorders," Institute of Medicine (US), Immunization Safety Review Committee (Washington, DC: National Academies Press, 2002), PMID: 25057609, doi: 10.17226/10393.

247 World Health Organization, "Porcine Circoviruses and Rotavirus Vaccines," 2010, https://www.who.int/groups/global-advisory-committee-on-vaccine-safety/topics/rotavirus-vaccines/porcine-circoviruses; AAP, "AAP Updates Guidelines on Rotavirus Vaccination," *Amer Fam Phys*, 2010, 81(4): 552-553; https://www.aafp.org/pubs/afp/issues/2010/0215/p552.html; US Department of Health and Human Services, Centers for Disease Control and Prevention, "Withdrawal of Rotavirus Vaccine Recommendation," *Morbidity and Mortality Weekly Report (MMWR)* 70, no. 31 (August 6, 2021): 1059–1062; Umesh D. Parashar et al., "Prevention of Rotavirus Gastroenteritis among Infants and Children: Recommendations of the Advisory Committee on Immunization Practices (ACIP)," *Morbidity and Mortality Weekly Report (MMWR)* 55, no. RR-12 (August 11, 2006): 1–13, US Department of Health and Human Services, Centers for Disease Control and Prevention,; Umesh D. Parashar et al., "Prevention of Rotavirus Gastroenteritis among Infants and Children: Recommendations of the Advisory Committee on Immunization Practices (ACIP)," *Morbidity and Mortality Weekly Report (MMWR)*, 58, no. RR-02 (February 6, 2009): 1–25, US Department of Health and Human Services, Centers for Disease Control and Prevention; "Withdrawal of Rotavirus Vaccine Recommendation," *Morbidity and Mortality Weekly Report (MMWR)* 48, no. 43 (November 5, 1999): 1007, US Department of Health and Human Services, Centers for Disease Control and Prevention, https://www.cdc.gov/mmwr/preview/mmwrhtml/mm4843a5.htm; US Department of Health and Human Services, Centers for Disease Control and Prevention, "Intussusception among recipients of rotavirus vaccine—United States, 1998–1999," *Morbidity and Mortality Weekly Report (MMWR)* 48, no. 27 (July 16, 1999): 577–581, https://www.cdc.gov/mmwr/PDF/wk/mm4827.pdf; Manish M. Patel et al., "Intussusception and Rotavirus Vaccination: A Review of the Available Evidence," *Expert Review of Vaccines* 8 no. 11 (November 2009): 1555–1564, doi: 10.1586/erv.09.106; Jacqueline E. Tate et al., "Trends in Intussusception Hospitalizations among US Infants, 1993–2004: Implications for Monitoring the Safety of the New Rotavirus Vaccination Program," *Pediatrics* 121, no. 5 (May 2008): e1125–1132, doi: 10.1542/peds.2007-1590; Trudy V. Murphy et al., Rotavirus Intussusception Investigation Team, "Intussusception among Infants Given an Oral Rotavirus Vaccine," *New England Journal of Medicine* 344, no. 8 (February 2021): 564–572, doi: 10.1056/NEJM200102223440804; Lynn R. Zanardi et al., "Intussusception among Recipients of Rotavirus Vaccine: Reports to the Vaccine Adverse Event Reporting System," *Pediatrics* 107, no. 6 (June 2001): E97, doi: 10.1542/peds.107.6.e97; Piotr Kramarz et al., "Population-Based Study of Rotavirus Vaccination and Intussusception," *Pediatric Infectious Disease Journal* 20, no.

4 (April 2001): 410–416, doi: 10.1097/00006454-200104000-00008; Margaret B. Rennels, "The Rotavirus Vaccine Story: A Clinical Investigator's View," *Pediatrics* 106: 123–5, doi: 10.1542/peds.106.1.123.
248 Pricilla Velentgas et al., "Risk of Guillain-Barré Syndrome after Meningococcal Conjugate Vaccination," *Pharmacoepidemiology & Drug Safety* 21, no. 12 (December 2012): 1350–8, doi: 10.1002/pds.3321.
249 Jonathan Duffy et al., Vaccine Safety Datalink, "Narcolepsy and Influenza A(H1N1) Pandemic 2009 Vaccination in the United States," *Neurology* 83, no. 20 (November 2014): 1823–30, doi: 10.1212/WNL.0000000000000987; Daniel Weibel et al., "Narcolepsy and Adjuvanted Pandemic Influenza A(H1N1) 2009 Vaccines—Multi-country Assessment," *Vaccine* 26, no. 41 (October 2018): 6202–6211, doi: 10.1016/j.vaccine.2018.08.008.
250 US Department of Health and Human Services, Centers for Disease Control and Prevention, "Selected Adverse Events Reported After COVID-19 Vaccination," updated September 12, 2023, https://www.cdc.gov/coronavirus/2019-ncov/vaccines/safety/adverse-events.html.
251 Tom Shimabukuro, "US Department of Health and Human Services, Centers for Disease Control and Prevention, COVID-19 Vaccine Task Force," Advisory Committee on Immunization Practices (ACIP), COVID-19 Vaccine Safety Updates, June 23, 2021, https://www.cdc.gov/vaccines/acip/meetings/downloads/slides-2021-06/03-COVID-Shimabukuro-508.pdf.
252 John R. Su, "Myopericarditis following COVID-19 Vaccination: Updates from the Vaccine Adverse Event Reporting System (VAERS)," ACIP Presentation, October 21, 2021, US Department of Health and Human Services, Centers for Disease Control and Prevention, Vaccine Safety Team, COVID-19 Vaccine Task Force, https://www.cdc.gov/vaccines/acip/meetings/downloads/slides-2021-10-20-21/07-COVID-Su-508.pdf.
253 U.S Department of Health and Human Services, Centers for Disease Control and Prevention, September 12, 2023, https://www.cdc.gov/coronavirus/2019-ncov/vaccines/safety/myocarditis.html.
254 A. Patricia Wodi et al., "Advisory Committee on Immunization Practices Recommended Immunization Schedule for Children and Adolescents Aged 18 Years or Younger—United States, 2023," *Morbidity and Mortality Weekly Report (MMWR)*, 72, no. 6 (February 10, 2023): 137–140, US Department of Health and Human Services, Centers for Disease Control and Prevention, https://www.cdc.gov/mmwr/volumes/72/wr/mm7206a1.htm.
255 US Department of Health and Human Services, Centers for Disease Control and Prevention, "2020-2021 Flu Season Summary," July 20, 2021, https://www.cdc.gov/flu/season/faq-flu-season-2020-2021.htm.

256 US Department of Health and Human Services, Centers for Disease Control and Prevention, *Selected Adverse Events Reported after COVID-19 Vaccination*, March 7, 2023, https://www.cdc.gov/coronavirus/2019-ncov/vaccines/safety/adverse-events.html.

257 Mikiko Watanabe et al., "Central Obesity, Smoking Habit, and Hypertension Are Associated with Lower Antibody Titres in Response to COVID-19 mRNA Vaccine," *Diabetes Metabolism Research and Reviews* 38, no. 1 (January 2022): e3465, doi: 10.1002/dmrr.3465; Julia Hippisley-Cox et al., "Risk Prediction of Covid-19 Related Death and Hospital Admission in Adults after Covid-19 Vaccination: National Prospective Cohort Study," *BMJ* 374, n2244, doi: 10.1136/bmj.n2244.

258 Sir Austin Bradford Hill, "The Environment and Disease: Association or Causation?" *Proceedings of the Royal Society of Medicine* 58, no. 5 (May 1965): 295–300, https://www.ncbi.nlm.nih.gov/pmc/articles/PMC1898525/pdf/procrsmed00196-0010.pdf.

259 John P. A. Ioannidis, "Reconciling Estimates of Global Spread and Infection Fatality Rates of COVID-19: An Overview of Systematic Evaluations," *European Journal of Clinical Investigations* 51, no. 5 (May 2021): e13554, doi: https://doi.org/10.1111/eci.13554; John P. A. Ioannidis, "Infection Fatality Rate of COVID-19 Inferred from Seroprevalence Data," *Bulletin of the World Health Organization* 99, no. 1 (January 2021): 19–33F, doi: 10.2471/BLT.20.265892.

260 Menegale F, Manica M, Zardini A, Guzzetta G, Marziano V, d'Andrea V, Trentini F, Ajelli M, Poletti P, Merler S. Evaluation of Waning of SARS-CoV-2 Vaccine-Induced Immunity: A Systematic Review and Meta-analysis. JAMA Netw Open. 2023 May 1;6(5):e2310650. doi: 10.1001/jamanetworkopen.2023.10650. PMID: 37133863; PMCID: PMC10157431.

261 Roya Hosseini and Nayere Askari, "A Review of Neurological Side Effects of COVID-19 Vaccination," *European Journal of Medical Research* 28, no. 102 (February 25, 2023, doi: 10.1186/s40001- 023-00992-0; Kunal Ajmera et al., "Gastrointestinal Complications of COVID-19 Vaccines," *Cureus* 14, no. 4 (April 12, 2022): e24070, doi: 10.7759/cureus.24070.

262 Jessica Rose, "A Report on the US Vaccine Adverse Events Reporting System (VAERS) of the COVID-19 Messenger Ribonucleic Acid (mRNA) Biologicals," *Science, Public Health Policy, & the Law* 2 (May 2021): 59–80, https://cf5e727d-d02d-4d71-89ff-9fe2d3ad957f.filesusr.com/ugd/adf864_a0a813acbfdc4534a8cb50cf85193d49.pdf.

263 Berkeley Lovelace Jr., "CDC Advisers Weigh Delaying Covid Shot to 8 Weeks," NBC News, February 4, 2022, https://www.nbcnews.com/health/health-news/covid-vaccine-cdc-advisers-weigh-delaying-second-shot-eight-weeks-rcna14905.

264 Indroneal Banerjee et al., "Determination of Cell Types and Numbers during Cardiac Development in the Neonatal and Adult Rat and Mouse," *American Journal of Physiology–Heart and Circulatory Physiology* 293, no. 3 (September 2007): H1883–91, doi: 10.1152/ajpheart.00514.2007; Alida L. P. Caforio et al., "Current State of Knowledge on Aetiology, Diagnosis, Management, and Therapy of Myocarditis:

A Position Statement of the European Society of Cardiology Working Group on Myocardial and Pericardial Diseases," *European Heart Journal*, 34, no. 33 (2013): 2636–2648, doi: 10.1093/eurheartj/eht210. 2648a-2648d; Leslie T. Cooper Jr., "Myocarditis," *New England Journal of Medicine* 360, no. 15 (April 9 2009): 1526–38, doi: 10.1056/NEJMra0800028; Valerio De Paris et al., "Pathophysiology," chapter 3 in *Dilated Cardiomyopathy: From Genetics to Clinical Management*, Gianfranco Sinagra et al., eds. (New York: Springer; 2019), doi: https://pubmed.ncbi.nlm.nih.gov/32091721/; Terri Lampejo et al., "Acute Myocarditis: Aetiology, Diagnosis and Management," *Clinical Medical Journal* 21, no. 5 (2021): e505–e510, doi: 10.7861/clinmed.2021-0121; Peter Libby et al., "The Myocardium: More Than Myocytes," *Journal of the American College of Cardiology* 74, no. 25 (December 24, 2019): 3136–3138, doi: 10.1016/j.jacc.2019.10.031.

265 Sabesan Mythili and Narasimhan Malathi, "Diagnostic Markers of Acute Myocardial Infarction," *Biomedical Reports* 3, no. 6 (2015): 743–748, doi: 10.3892/br.2015.500; Robb D. Kociol et al., "Recognition and Initial Management of Fulminant myocarditis: A Scientific Statement from the American Heart Association," *Circulation* 141, no. 6 (2020): e69–e92, doi: 10.1161/cir.0000000000000745; Jan Krejci et al., "Inflammatory Cardiomyopathy: A Current View on the Pathophysiology, Diagnosis, and Treatment," *Biomedical Research International*, 2016: 4087632, doi: 10.1155/2016/4087632; Giovanni Peretto et al., "Arrhythmias in Myocarditis: State of the Art," *Heart Rhythm* 16, no. 5 (May 2019): 793–801, doi: 10.1016/j.hrthm.2018.11.024; Fatih Mehmet Ucar et al., "Evaluation of Tp-e Interval, Tp-e/QT Ratio and Tp-e/QTc Ratio in Patients with Acute Myocarditis," *BMC Cardiovascular Disorders* 19 no. 1 (October 22, 2019): 232, doi: 10.1186/s12872-019-1207-z.

266 Keyur B. Shah et al., "Amyloidosis and the Heart: A Comprehensive Review," *Archives of Internal Medicine*, 166, no. 17 (2006): 1805–1813, doi: 10.1001/archinte.166.17.1805; Ana Martinez-Naharro et al., "Cardiac Amyloidosis," *Clinical Medicine* 18, no. Suppl 2 (April 2018): s30–s35, doi: 10.7861/clinmedicine.18-2-s30; Douglas B. Kell et al., "A Central Role for Amyloid Fibrin Microclots in Long COVID/PASC: Origins and Therapeutic Implications," *Biochemical Journal* 479, no. 4 (February 25, 2022): 537–559, doi: 10.1042/BCJ20220016; Issa Pour-Ghaz et al., "A Review of Cardiac Amyloidosis: Presentation, Diagnosis, and Treatment," *Current Problems in Cardiolo* 47, no. 12 (August 20, 2022): 101366, doi: 10.1016/j.cpcardiol.2022.101366.

267 Mirren Charnley et al., "Neurotoxic Amyloidogenic Peptides in the Proteome of SARS-COV2: Potential Implications for Neurological Symptoms in COVID-19," *Nature Communications* 13, no. 1 (June 2022): 3387, doi: 10.1038/s41467-022-30932-1; George Tetz and Victor Tetz, "Prion-Like Domains in Spike Protein of SARS-CoV-2 Differ across Its Variants and Enable Changes in Affinity to ACE2," *Microorganisms* 10, no. 2 (2022): 280, doi: 10.3390/microorganisms10020280.

268 Rose J. A Report on the U.S. Vaccine Adverse Events Reporting System (VAERS) of the COVID-19 Messenger Ribonucleic Acid (mRNA) Biologicals. Science, Public Health Policy and the Law. 2021 May 01; v2.2019-2024, https://publichealthpolicyjournal.com/a-report-on-the-u-s-vaccine-adverse-events-reporting-system-vaers-of-the-covid-19-messenger-ribonucleic-acid-mrna-biologicals/

269 Josh Guetzkow, "FOIA'd Contracts Show CDC Expected Up to 1,000 VAERS Reports per Day for COVID Vaccines," *Jackanapes Junction* (Substack), December 10, 2022, https://jackanapes.substack.com/p/foiad-contracts-show-cdc-expected.

270 Salman M. Toor et al., "T-cell Responses and Therapies against SARS-CoV-2 Infection," *Immunology* 162, no. 1 (January 2021): 30–43, doi: 10.1111/imm.13262; Davide Robbiani et al., "Convergent Antibody Responses to SARS-CoV-2 in Convalescent Individuals," *Nature* 584, no. 7821 (2020): 437–442, doi: 10.1038/s41586-020-2456-9; Baoqing Sun et al., "Kinetics of SARS-CoV-2 Specific IgM and IgG Responses in COVID-19 Patients," *Emerging Microbes & Infections* 9, no. 1 (2020): 940–948, doi: 10.1080/22221751.2020.1762515; Nina Le Bert et al., "SARS-CoV-2-Specific T Cell Immunity in Cases of COVID-19 and SARS, and Uninfected Controls," *Nature* 584, no. 7821 (2020): 457–462, doi: 10.1038/s41586-020-2550-z; Jose Mateus et al., "Selective and Cross-Reactive SARS-CoV-2 T Cell Epitopes in Unexposed Humans," *Science* 370, no. 6512 (August 2020): 89–94, doi: 10.1126/science.abd3871; Marc Lipsitch et al., "Cross-Reactive Memory T Cells and Herd Immunity to SARS-CoV-2," *Nature Reviews Immunology* 20, no. 11 (October 2020): 709–713, doi: 10.1038/s41577-020-00460-4.

Chapter 7: Immunological Harms of the COVID-19 "Vaccines"

271 Stephen J. Thomas et al., "Safety and Efficacy of the BNT162b2 mRNA Covid-19 Vaccine through 6 Months," *New England Journal of Medicine* 385 (November 2021): 1761–1773, doi: 10.1056/NEJMoa2110345.

272 Peter J. Halfmann et al., "SARS-CoV-2 Omicron Virus Causes Attenuated Disease in Mice and Hamsters," *Nature* 603 (January 2022): 687–692, doi: 10.1038/s41586-022-04441-6; Yingguang Liu, "Attenuation and Degeneration of SARS-CoV-2 Despite Adaptive Evolution," *Cureus* 15, no. 1 (January 3, 2023): e33316, doi: 10.7759/cureus.33316.

273 David M. Morens, Gregory K. Folkers, and Anthony A. Fauci, "The Concept of Classical Herd Immunity May Not Apply to COVID-19," *Journal of Infectious Diseases* 226, no. 2 (July 15, 2022): 195–198, doi: 10.1093/infdis/jiac109.

274 Velislava N. Petrova and Colin A. Russell, "The Evolution of Seasonal Influenza Viruses," *Nature Reviews Microbiology* 16 (January 2018): 47–60, doi: 10.1038/nrmicro.2017.118; Samuel Cordey et al., "Rhinovirus Genome Evolution during Experimental Human Infection," *PLOS One* 5, no. 5 (May 11, 2010): e10588, doi: 10.1371/journal.pone.0010588.

275 Hiam Chemaitelly et al., "Protection from Previous Natural Infection Compared with mRNA Vaccination against SARS-CoV-2 Infection and Severe COVID-19 in Qatar: A Retrospective Cohort Study," *Lancet Microbe* 3, no. 12 (November 11, 2022): e944–e955, doi: 10.1016/s2666-5247(22)00287-7; Laith J. Abu-Raddad et al., "Severity of SARS-CoV-2 Reinfections as Compared with Primary Infections," *New England Journal of Medicine* 385, no. 26 (December 23, 2021): 2487–2489, doi: 10.1056/NEJMc2108120; Angela L. Rasmussen and Saskia V. Popescu, "SARS-CoV-2 Transmission without Symptoms," *Science* 371, no. 6535 (2021): 1206–1207, doi: 10.1126/science.abf9569.

276 Juan F. Delgado et al., "SARS-CoV-2 Spike Protein Vaccine-Induced Immune Imprinting Reduces Nucleocapsid Protein Antibody Response in SARS-CoV-2 Infection," *Journal of Immunology Research*, 2022 (July 29, 2022): 8287087, doi: 10.1155/2022/8287087.

277 Michael W. Russell and Jiri Mestecky, "Mucosal Immunity: The Missing Link in Comprehending SARS-CoV-2 Infection and Transmission," *Frontiers in Immunology* 13 (August 17, 2022), doi: 10.3389/fimmu.2022.957107.

278 Claire Donnelly and Meghna Chakrabarti, "The Science and Politics of Natural Immunity," WBUR, March 8, 2023, https://www.wbur.org/onpoint/2023/03/08/understanding-the-impact-of-natural-immunity-to-covid-19-on-u-s-health-and-politics.

279 Manish Sagar et al., "Recent Endemic Coronavirus Infection Is Associated with Less-Severe COVID-19," *Journal of Clinical Investigation* 131, no. 1 (2021): e143380, doi: 10.1172/JCI143380.

280 Gabriella Pugliese et al., "Obesity and Infectious Diseases: Pathophysiology and Epidemiology of a Double Pandemic Condition," *International Journal of Obesity* 46, no. 3 (March 2022): 449–465, doi: 10.1038/s41366-021-01035-6; Mohan K. Tummala et al., "Clinical Immunology: Immune Senescence and the Acquired Immune Deficiency of Aging," in *Brocklehurst's Textbook of Geriatric Medicine and Gerontology*, 7th ed., eds. Howard M. Fillit et al. (Philadelphia: Saunders Elsevier, 2010): 82–90, doi: 10.1016/B978-1-4160-6231-8.10013-3.

281 Sunny Singhal et al., "Clinical Features and Outcomes of COVID-19 in Older Adults: A Systematic Review and Meta-Analysis," *BMC Geriatrics* 21, no. 321 (May 19, 2021), doi: 10.1186/s12877-021-02261-3.

282 Ursula Wiedermann et al., "Primary Vaccine Failure to Routine Vaccines: Why and What to Do?" *Human Vaccines & Immunotheraputics* 12, no. 1 (January 2016): 239–243, doi: 10.1080/21645515.2015.1093263.

283 Supinda Bunyavanich et al., "Nasal Gene Expression of Angiotensin-Converting Enzyme 2 in Children and Adults," *Journal of the American Medical Association* 323, no. 23 (May 20, 2020): 2427–2429, doi: 10.1001/jama.2020.8707.

284 Bernadette Schurink et al., "ACE2 Protein Expression during Childhood, Adolescence, and Early Adulthood," *Pediatrics and Developmental Pathology* 25, no. 4 (July–August, 2022): 404–408, doi: 10.1177/10935266221075312.

285 Chemaitelly et al., "Protection from Previous Natural Infection Compared with mRNA Vaccination against SARS-CoV-2 Infection and Severe COVID-19 in Qatar: A Retrospective Cohort Study."

286 Paula Span, "Can Long-Term Care Employers Require Staff Members to Be Vaccinated?" *New York Times,* March 5, 2021, https://www.nytimes.com/2021/03/05/health/coronavirus-vaccination-elder-facilities.html.

287 Megan Schwarz et al., "T Cell Immunity Is Key to the Pandemic Endgame: How to Measure and Monitor It," *Current Research in Immunology* 3 (September 1, 2022): 215–221, doi: 10.1016/j.crimmu.2022.08.004.

288 Nabin K. Shrestha et al., "Effectiveness of the Coronavirus Disease 2019 (COVID-19) Bivalent Vaccine," Open Forum Infectious Diseases, April 19, 2023, doi: 10.1101/2022.12.17.22283625.

289 Te Whatu Ora, Health New Zealand, "COVID-19 Case Demographics for New Zealand," accessed August 5, 2023, https://www.tewhatuora.govt.nz/our-health-system/data-and-statistics/covid-vaccine-data; "Timeline: The Year of Covid-19 in New Zealand," Radio New Zealand, updated March 24, 2023, https://www.rnz.co.nz/news/national/437359/timeline-the-year-of-covid-19-in-new-zealand; "First Batch of COVID-19 Vaccine Arrives in NZ," Beehive.govt.nz, February 15, 2021, https://www.beehive.govt.nz/release/first-batch-covid-19-vaccine-arrives-nz; Te Whatu Ora, Health New Zealand, "COVID-19 Cases by Vaccination Status," accessed August 5, 2023, https://www.tewhatuora.govt.nz/our-health-system/data-and-statistics/covid-19-data/covid-19-case-demographics.

290 "COVID-19 Data and Statistics," Covid19.govt.nz, accessed August 5, 2023, https://covid19.govt.nz/news-and-data/covid-19-data-and-statistics/.

291 Mark J. Mulligan et al., "Phase I/II Study of COVID-19 RNA Vaccine BNT162b1 in Adults," *Nature* 586 (August 20, 2020): 589–593, doi: 10.1038/s41586-020-2639-4.

292 Pascal Irrgang et al., "Class Switch toward Noninflammatory, Spike-Specific IgG4 Antibodies after Repeated SARS-CoV-2 mRNA Vaccination," *Science of Immunology* 8, no. 79 (2023): eade2798, doi: 10.1126/sciimmunol.ade2798.

293 Vladimir N. Uversky et al., "IgG4 Antibodies Induced by Repeated Vaccination May Generate Immune Tolerance to the SARS-CoV-2 Spike Protein," *Vaccines* (Basel) 11, no. 5 (May 17, 2023): 991, doi: 10.3390/vaccines11050991.

294 Maria K. Smatti et al., "Viral-Induced Enhanced Disease Illness," *Frontiers in Microbiology* 9 (December 5, 2018): 2991, doi: 10.3389/fmicb.2018.02991.

295 Rachael Kathleen Raw et al., "Previous COVID-19 Infection, but Not Long-COVID, Is Associated with Increased Adverse Events following BNT162b2/Pfizer Vaccination,"

Journal of Infection 83, no. 3 (September 2021): 381–412, doi: 10.1016/j.jinf.2021.05.035.
296 US Food and Drug Administration, "Vaccines and Related Biological Products Advisory Committee," FDA Briefing Document, Pfizer-BioNTech COVID-19 Vaccine, December 10, 2020, https://www.fda.gov/media/144245/download.
297 Ali Zhang et al., "Original Antigenic Sin: How First Exposure Shapes Lifelong Anti-Influenza Virus Immune Responses," *Journal of Immunology* 202, no. 2 (January 15, 2019): 335–340, doi: 10.4049/jimmunol.1801149; Priyadharshini Devarajan and Susan L. Swain, "Original Antigenic Sin: Friend or Foe in Developing a Broadly Cross-Reactive Vaccine to Influenza?" *Cell Host & Microbe* 25, no. 3 (March 13, 2019): 354–355, doi: 10.1016/j.chom.2019.02.009; Mee Sook Park et al., "Original Antigenic Sin Response to RNA Viruses and Antiviral Immunity," *Immune Network* 16, no. 5 (October 25, 2016): 261–270, doi: 10.4110/in.2016.16.5.261; Ralph A. Tripp and Ultan F. Power, "Original Antigenic Sin and Respiratory Syncytial Virus Vaccines," *Vaccines* 7, no. 3 (2019): 107, doi: 10.3390/vaccines7030107; Muriel Aguilar-Bretones et al., "Impact of Antigenic Evolution and Original Antigenic Sin on SARS-CoV-2 Immunity," *Journal of Clinical Investigations*, 133, no. 1 (January 3, 2023): e162192, doi: 10.1172/JCI162192.
298 Marie Tré-Hardy et al., "Reactogenicity, Safety and Antibody Response, after One and Two Doses of mRNA-1273 in Seronegative and Seropositive Healthcare Workers," *Journal of Infection*, 83, no. 2 (August 2021): 237–279, doi: 10.1016/j.jinf.2021.03.025; Alexander G. Mathioudakis et al., "Self-Reported Real-World Safety and Reactogenicity of COVID-19 Vaccines: A Vaccine Recipient Survey," *Life* (Basel) 11, no. 3 (March 17, 2021): 249, doi: 10.3390/life11030249; Florian Krammer et al., "Antibody Responses in Seropositive Persons after a Single Dose of SARS-CoV-2 mRNA Vaccine," *New England Journal of Medicine* 384, no. 14 (April 2021): 1372–1374, doi: 10.1056/NEJMc2101667; Raw et al., "Previous COVID-19 Infection, but Not Long-COVID, Is Associated with Increased Adverse Events following BNT162b2/Pfizer Vaccination."
299 Elizabeth Cairns, "The T-Cell Test Bronze Goes to Qiage," Evaluate.com, December 2, 2021, https://www.evaluate.com/vantage/articles/news/policy-and-regulation-snippets/t-cell-test-bronze-goes-qiagen.

Chapter 8: Cardiac and Cardiovascular Damage from the modRNA "Vaccines"

300 Centers for Disease Control and Prevention, "Myocarditis and Pericarditis after mRNA COVID-19 Vaccination," September 12, 2023, https://www.cdc.gov/coronavirus/2019-ncov/vaccines/safety/myocarditis.html.

301 Yuyang Lei et al., "SARS-CoV-2 Spike Protein Impairs Endothelial Function via Downregulation of ACE 2," *Circulation Research* 128, no. 9 (2021): 1323–1326, doi: 10.1161/CIRCRESAHA.121.318902.

302 Elisa Avolio et al., "The SARS-CoV-2 Spike Protein Disrupts Human Cardiac Pericytes Function through CD147 Receptor-Mediated Signalling: A Potential Non-infective Mechanism of COVID-19 Microvascular Disease," *Clinical Science* 135, no. 24 (December 22, 2021): 2667–2689, doi: 10.1042/CS20210735.

303 "Coronavirus Spike Protein Activated Natural Immune Response, Damaged Heart Muscle Cells," *DAIC*, July 27, 2022, https://www.dicardiology.com/content/coronavirus-spike-protein-activated-natural-immune-response-damaged-heart-muscle-cells.

304 Aram J. Krauson et al., "Duration of SARS-CoV-2 mRNA Vaccine Persistence and Factors Associated with Cardiac Involvement in Recently Vaccinated Patients," *NPJ Vaccines*, 8, no. 1 (September 27, 2023): 141, doi: 10.1038/s41541-023-00742-7.

305 Lael M. Yonker et al., "Circulating Spike Protein Detected in Post–COVID-19 mRNA Vaccine Myocarditis," *Circulation*, 147, no. 11 (March 14, 2023): 867–875, doi: 10.1161/CIRCULATIONAHA.122.061025.

306 Biykem Bozkurt et al., "Myocarditis with COVID-19 mRNA Vaccines," *Circulation* 144, no. 6 (August 10, 2021): 471–484, doi: 10.1161/CIRCULATIONAHA.121.056135.

307 Jason P. Block et al., "Cardiac Complications after SARS-CoV-2 Infection and mRNA COVID-19 Vaccination—PCORnet, United States, January 2021–January 2022," *Morbidity and Mortality Weekly Report (MMWR)* 71, no. 14 (2022): 517–523, US Department of Health and Human Services, Centers for Disease Control and Prevention, https://www.cdc.gov/mmwr/volumes/71/wr/mm7114e1.htm.

308 Gilbert T. Chua et al., "Epidemiology of Acute Myocarditis/Pericarditis in Hong Kong Adolescents following Comirnaty Vaccination," *Clinical Infectious Diseases* 75, no. 4 (August 15, 2022): 673–681, doi: 10.1093/cid/ciab989.

309 Shuenn-Nan Chiu et al., "Changes of ECG parameters after BNT162b2 Vaccine in the Senior High School Students," *European Journal of Pediatrics* 182 (2023), doi: 10.1007/s00431-022-04786-0.

310 Suyanee Mansanguan et al., "Cardiovascular Manifestation of the BNT162b2 mRNA COVID-19 Vaccine in Adolescents," *Tropical Medicine & Infectious Disease* 7, no. 8 (2022): 196, doi: 10.3390/tropicalmed7080196.

311 Christian Müller, "Temporary Mild Damage to Heart Muscle Cells after Covid-19 Booster Vaccination," myScience, November 9, 2022, https://www.myscience.org/en/news/wire/temporary_mild_damage_to_heart_muscle_cells_after_covid_19_booster_vaccination-2022-unibas.

312 Jae Yeong Cho et al., "COVID-19 Vaccination-Related Myocarditis: A Korean Nationwide Study," *European Heart Journal* 44, no. 24 (June 21, 2023): 2234–2243, doi: 10.1093/eurheartj/ehad339; National Institutes of Health, *Q&A: COVID-19, Vaccines, and Myocarditis*, July 1, 2022, https://covid19.nih.gov/news-and-stories/

covid-19-vaccines-myocarditis; Frank Han and Jennifer H. Huang, "What Research Shows about Risks of Myocarditis from COVID Vaccines versus Risks of Heart Damage from COVID," CBS News, March 13, 2023, https://www.cbsnews.com/news/covid-19-vaccines-myocarditis-heart-damage-infection-children/.

313 Centers for Disease Control and Prevention, "Nationwide Commercial Lab Pediatric Antibody Seroprevalence," https://covid.cdc.gov/covid-data-tracker/#pediatric-seroprevalence; Dan-Yu Lin et al., "Effects of Vaccination and Previous Infection on Omicron Infections in Children," *New England Journal of Medicine* 387, no. 2 (1141–1143), doi: 10.1056/NEJMc2209371.

314 Ortal Tuvali et al., "The Incidence of Myocarditis and Pericarditis in Post COVID-19 Unvaccinated Patients—A Large Population-Based Study," *Journal of Clinical Medicine* 11, no. 8 (April 15, 2022): 2219, doi: 10.3390/jcm11082219.

315 Monique G. Davis et al., "COVID-19 Associated Myocarditis Clinical Outcomes among Hospitalized Patients in the United States: A Propensity Matched Analysis of National Inpatient Sample," *Viruses* 14, no. 12 (December 2022): 2791, doi: 10.3390/v14122791.

316 Allison Krug et al., "BNT162b2 Vaccine-Associated Myo/Pericarditis in Adolescents: A Stratified Risk-Benefit Analysis," *European Journal of Clinical Investigation* 52, no. 5 (May 2022): e13759, doi: 10.1111/eci.13759.

317 Centers for Disease Control and Prevention, "Nationwide Commercial Lab Pediatric Antibody Seroprevalence," https://covid.cdc.gov/covid-data-tracker/#pediatric-seroprevalence.

318 Nayva Voleti et al., "Myocarditis in SARS-CoV-2 infection vs. COVID-19 Vaccination: A Systematic Review and Meta-Analysis," *Frontiers in Cardiovascular Medicine* 9 (August 2022): 951314, doi: 10.3389/fcvm.2022.951314.

319 Emma K. Accorsi et al., "How to Detect and Reduce Potential Sources of Biases in Studies of SARS-CoV-2 and COVID-19," *European Journal of Epidemiology* 36, no. 2 (February 2021): 179–196, doi: 10.1007/s10654-021-00727-7; Monia Makhoul et al., "Analyzing Inherent Biases in SARS-CoV-2 PCR and Serological Epidemiologic Metrics," *BMC Infectious Diseases* 22 (2022): 458, doi: 10.1186/s12879-022-07425-z; Daniel Andrés Díaz-Pachón and J. Sunil Rao, "A Simple Correction for COVID-19 Sampling Bias," *Journal of Theoretical Biology* 512 (March 7, 2021): 110556, doi: 10.1016/j.jtbi.2020.110556.

320 Nationwide Children's Hospital, "Return to Play after COVID-19 Infection without Major Symptoms: For Physicians and Referral Sources," https://www.nationwidechildrens.org/-/media/nch/for-medical-professionals/practice-tools-new/return-to-play-covid-guidelines-asymptomatic.ashx.

321 Jamie Ducharme, "Almost 60% of Americans Have Had COVID-19, CDC Says," *Time*, April 26, 2022, https://time.com/6170735/how-many-people-have-had-covid-19/.

322 Renata J. M. Engler et al., "A Prospective Study of the Incidence of Myocarditis/ Pericarditis and New Onset Cardiac Symptoms following Smallpox and Influenza Vaccination," *PLOS One* 10, no. 3 (March 20, 2015): e0118283, doi: 10.1371/journal.pone.0118283.

323 "Temporary Mild Damage to Heart Muscle Cells after Covid-19 Booster Vaccination," myScience, November 9, 2022, https://www.myscience.org/en/news/wire/temporary_mild_damage_to_heart_muscle_cells_after_covid_19_booster_vaccination-2022-unibas.

324 Steven R. Gundry, "Abstract 10712: Observational Findings of PULS Cardiac Test Findings for Inflammatory Markers in Patients Receiving mRNA Vaccines," *Circulation* 144 (November 16, 2021): A10712, doi: 10.1161/circ.144.suppl_1.10712.

325 US Department of Health and Human Services, Centers for Disease Control and Prevention, "Myocarditis and Pericarditis after mRNA COVID-19 Vaccination," September 12, 2023, https://www.cdc.gov/coronavirus/2019-ncov/vaccines/safety/myocarditis.html.

326 Muzhda Ghanizada et al., "Long-Term Prognosis following Hospitalization for Acute Myocarditis—A Matched Nationwide Cohort Study," *Scandinavian Cardiovascular Journal* 55, no. 5 (2021), doi: 10.1080/14017431.2021.1900596.

327 Ian Kracalik et al., "Outcomes at Least 90 Days since Onset of Myocarditis after mRNA COVID-19 Vaccination in Adolescents and Young Adults in the USA: A Follow-Up Surveillance Study," *Lancet Child Adolescent Health* 6, no. 11 (2022): 788–98, doi: 10.1016/S2352-4642(22)00244-9.

328 Sylvia Krupickova et al., "Short-Term Outcome of Late Gadolinium Changes Detected on Cardiovascular Magnetic Resonance Imaging following Coronavirus Disease 2019 Pfizer/BioNTech Vaccine-Related Myocarditis in Adolescents," *Pediatric Radiology* 53 (January 9, 2023): 892–899, doi: 10.1007/s00247-022-05573-7; Carolyn M. Rosner et al., "Patients with Myocarditis Associated with COVID-19 Vaccination," *Journal of the American College of Cardiology* 79, no. 13 (April 2022): 1317–1319, doi: 10.1016/j.jacc.2022.02.004; Stephanie M. Hadley et al., "Follow-Up Cardiac Magnetic Resonance in Children with Vaccine-Associated Myocarditis," *European Journal of Pediatrics* 181, no. 7 (2022): 2879–2883, doi: 10.1007/s00431-022-04482-z.

329 Carsten Tschöpe et al., "Management of Myocarditis-Related Cardiomyopathy in Adults," *Circulation Research* 124, no. 11 (2019): 1568–1583, doi: 10.1161/CIRCRESAHA.118.313578.

330 Tianyang Li et al., "Platelets Mediate Inflammatory Monocyte Activation by SARS-CoV-2 Spike Protein," *Journal of Clinical Investigations* 132, no. 4 (February 15, 2022): e150101, doi: 10.1172/JCI150101.

331 Yi Zheng et al., "SARS-CoV-2 Spike Protein Causes Blood Coagulation and Thrombosis by Competitive Binding to Heparan Sulfate," *International Journal*

of *Biological Macromolecules* 193, pt. B, (December 15, 2021): 1124–1129, doi: 10.1016/j.ijbiomac.2021.10.112.

332 Lize M. Grobbelaar et al., "SARS-CoV-2 Spike Protein S1 Induces Fibrin(ogen) Resistant to Fibrinolysis: Implications for Microclot Formation in COVID-19," *Bioscience Reports* 41, no. 8 (August 27, 2021): BSR20210611, doi: 10.1042/BSR20210611.

333 Celine Boschi et al., "SARS-CoV-2 Spike Protein Induces Hemagglutination: Implications for COVID-19 Morbidities and Therapeutics and for Vaccine Adverse Effects," *International Journal of Molecular Science* 23, no. 24 (2022): 15480, doi: 10.3390/ijms232415480.

334 Pei-Shan Sung et al., "CLEC5A and TLR2 Are Critical in SARS-CoV-2-Induced NET Formation and Lung Inflammation," *Journal of Biomedical Science* 29, no. 52 (2022), doi: 10.1186/s12929-022-00832-z.

335 Roberto Carnevale et al., "Toll-Like Receptor 4-Dependent Platelet-Related Thrombosis in SARS-CoV-2 Infection," *Circulation Research* 132, no. 3 (2023): 290–305, doi: 10.1161/CIRCRESAHA.122.321541.

336 Manuela De Michele et al., "Evidence of SARS-CoV-2 Spike Protein on Retrieved Thrombi from COVID-19 Patients," *Journal of Hematology Oncology* 15, no. 108 (2022), doi: 10.1186/s13045-022-01329-w.

337 Jacob Dag Berild et al., "Analysis of Thromboembolic and Thrombocytopenic Events after the AZD1222, BNT162b2, and MRNA-1273 COVID-19 Vaccines in 3 Nordic Countries," *JAMA Network Open* 5, no. 6 (2022): e2217375, doi: 10.1001/jamanetworkopen.2022.17375.

338 Edward Burn et al., "Thrombosis and Thrombocytopenia after Vaccination against and Infection with SARS-CoV-2 in the United Kingdom," *Nature Communications* 13, no. 7167, doi: 10.1038/s41467-022-34668-w.

339 Martina Patone et al., "Neurological Complications after First Dose of COVID-19 Vaccines and SARS-CoV-2 Infection," *Nature Medicine* 27 (2021): 2144–2153, doi: 10.1038/s41591-021-01556-7.

340 Celine Sze Ling Chui et al., "Thromboembolic Events and Hemorrhagic Stroke after mRNA (BNT162b2) and Inactivated (CoronaVac) Covid-19 Vaccination: A Self-Controlled Case Series Study," *EClinicalMedicine* 50, no. 101504, doi: 10.1016/j.eclinm.2022.101504.

341 Julia Hippisley-Cox et al., "Risk of Thrombocytopenia and Thromboembolism after Covid-19 Vaccination and SARS-CoV-2 Positive Testing: Self-Controlled Case Series Study," *BMJ* 374 (2021): n1931, doi: 10.1136/bmj.n1931.

342 Jing-Xing Li et al., "Risk Assessment of Retinal Vascular Occlusion after COVID-19 Vaccination," *npj Vaccines* 8, no. 64 (May 2, 2023), doi: 10.1038/s41541-023-00661-7.

343 Marco Zaffanello et al., "Thrombotic Risk in Children with COVID-19 Infection: A Systematic Review of the Literature," *Thrombosis Research* 205 (September 2021): 92–98, doi: 10.1016/j.thromres.2021.07.011.

344 Hilary Whitworth et al., "Rate of Thrombosis in Children and Adolescents Hospitalized with COVID-19 or MIS-C," *Blood* 138, no. 2 (2021): 190–198, doi: 10.1182/blood.2020010218.

345 Stefan Pilz, John PA Ioannidis, "Does natural and hybrid immunity obviate the need for frequent vaccine boosters against SARS-CoV-2 in the endemic phase?" *Eur J Clin Invest*. February 2023, 53(2): e13906, doi: 10.1111/eci.13906

Chapter 9: Neurological Injuries from the modRNA "Vaccines"

346 Kathleen Stratton et al., eds., "Immunization Safety Review: Influenza Vaccines and Neurological Complications," Institute of Medicine, Board on Health Promotion and Disease Prevention, Immunization Safety Review Committee, 2004, https://nap.nationalacademies.org/catalog/10822/immunization-safety-review-influenza-vaccines-and-neurological-complications.

347 David J. Sencer and J. Donald Millar, "Reflections on the 1976 Swine Flu Vaccination Program," *Emerging Infectious Diseases* 12, no. 1 (January 2006): 29–33, doi: 10.3201/eid1201.051007.

348 Matt Bain, "Indiana Doctor Warns Legislators That Covid Vaccines Are Causing Neurological Issues," testimony to Indiana Senate's Health and Provider Services Committee, February 16, 2022, *Crossroads Report*, YouTube, https://www.youtube.com/watch?v=1BbQQTb06Kk.

349 Shreya Shah et al., "Development of Transverse Myelitis after Vaccination, A CDC/FDA Vaccine Adverse Event Reporting System (VAERS) Study, 1985–2017," *Neurology* 90, no. 15 supplement (April 2018): p5.099, https://n.neurology.org/content/90/15_Supplement/P5.099.

350 Timothy W. West et al., "Acute Transverse Myelitis: Demyelinating, Inflammatory, and Infectious Myelopathies," *Seminars in Neurology* 32, no. 2 (April 2012): 97–113, doi: 10.1055/s-0032-1322586; Fatima Naz Naeem et al., "The Association between SARS-CoV-2 Vaccines and Transverse Myelitis: A Review," *Annals of Medicine & Surgery* 79, no. 103870, doi: 10.1016/j.amsu.2022.103870.

351 Chitra Krishnan et al., "Demyelinating Disorders: Update on Transverse Myelitis," *Current Neurology & Neuroscience Reports* 6, no. 3 (May 2006): 236–43, doi: 10.1007/s11910-006-0011-1.

352 Ingrid Loma and Rock Heyman, "Multiple Sclerosis: Pathogenesis and Treatment," *Current Neuropharmacology* 9, no. 3 (September 2011): 409–16, doi: 10.2174/157015911796557911.

353 Erin Clough et al., "Mitochondrial Dynamics in SARS-COV2 Spike Protein Treated Human Microglia: Implications for Neuro-COVID," *Journal of*

Neuroimmune Pharmacology 16, no. 4 (December 2021): 770–784, doi: 10.1007/s11481-021-10015-6.

354 Kunyi Li et al., "Clinical Presentation and Outcomes of Acute Disseminated Encephalomyelitis in Adults Worldwide: Systematic Review and Meta-Analysis," *Frontiers in Immunology* 13 (June 9, 2022), Sec. Multiple Sclerosis and Neuroimmunology, doi: https://doi.org/10.3389/fimmu.2022.870867.

355 Shubham V. Nimkar et al., "Fatal Acute Disseminated Encephalomyelitis Post-COVID-19 Vaccination: A Rare Case Report," *Cureus* 14, no. 11 (November 22, 2022): e31810, doi: 10.7759/cureus.31810.

356 Ross Lazarus et al., "Electronic Support for Public Health: Validated Case Finding and Reporting for Notifiable Diseases Using Electronic Medical Data," *Journal of the American Medical Informatics Association* 16, no. 1 (January–February 2009): 18–24, doi: 10.1197/jamia.M2848.

357 Ray Wynford-Thomas et al., "Neurological Update: MOG Antibody Disease," *Journal of Neurology* 266, no. 5 (May 2019): 1280–1286, doi: 10.1007/s00415-018-9122-2.

358 Matthew G. Frank et al., "SARS-CoV-2 Spike S1 Subunit Induces Neuroinflammatory, Microglial and Behavioral Sickness Responses: Evidence of PAMP-Like Properties," *Brain, Behavior, and Immunity* 100 (February 2022): 267277, doi: 10.1016/j.bbi.2021.12.007.

359 Seneff et al., "Innate Immune Suppression by SARS-CoV-2 mRNA Vaccinations: The Role of G-Quadruplexes, Exosomes, and MicroRNAs," *Food and Chemical Toxicology* 164, no. 113008 (June 2022):, doi: 10.1016/j.fct.2022.113008.

360 Carol L. Vanderlugt and Stephen D. Miller, "Epitope Spreading in Immune-Mediated Diseases: implications for Immunotherapy," *Nature Reviews Immunology* 2 (2002): 85–95, doi: 10.1038/nri724.

361 Smyk DS, et al. "Acute disseminated encephalomyelitis progressing to multiple sclerosis: Are infectious triggers involved?" *Immunol Res*, 60, no. 1 (2014): 16-22, Doi: 10.1007/s12026-014-8499-y.

362 Lei, "SARS-CoV-2 Spike Protein Impairs Endothelial Function via Downregulation of ACE 2."

363 Si Zhang et al., "SARS-CoV-2 Binds Platelet ACE2 to Enhance Thrombosis in COVID-19," *Journal of Hematology & Oncology* 13, no. 120 (2020), doi: 10.1186/s13045-020-00954-7; Norma Maugeri et al., "Unconventional CD147-Dependent Platelet Activation Elicited by SARS-CoV-2 in COVID-19," *Journal of Thrombosis and Haemostasis* 20, no. 2 (February 2022): 434–448, doi: 10.1111/jth.15575; "Coronavirus Spike Protein Activated Natural Immune Response, Damaged Heart Muscle Cells," *DAIC*, July 27, 2022, https://www.dicardiology.com/content/coronavirus-spike-protein-activated-natural-immune-response-damaged-heart-muscle-cells; Pei-Shan Sung et al., "CLEC5A and TLR2 Are Critical in SARS-CoV-2-Induced NET Formation and Lung Inflammation," *Journal of Biomedical Science* 29, no. 52,

doi: 10.1186/s12929-022-00832-z; Roberto Carnevale et al., "Toll-Like Receptor 4-Dependent Platelet-Related Thrombosis in SARS-CoV-2 Infection," *Circulation Research* 132, no. 3 (2023): 290–305, doi: 10.1161/CIRCRESAHA.122.321541; Yi Zheng et al., "SARS-CoV-2 Spike Protein Causes Blood Coagulation and Thrombosis by Competitive Binding to Heparan Sulfate," *International Journal of Biological Macromolecules* 193, part B (December 15, 2021): 1124–1129, doi: 10.1016/j.ijbiomac.2021.10.112; Celine Boschi et al., "SARS-CoV-2 Spike Protein Induces Hemagglutination: Implications for COVID-19 Morbidities and Therapeutics and for Vaccine Adverse Effects," *International Journal of Molecular Science* 23 (2022): 15480 doi: 10.3390/ijms232415480.

364 Lize M. Grobbelaar et al., "SARS-CoV-2 Spike Protein S1 Induces Fibrin(ogen) Resistant to Fibrinolysis: Implications for Microclot Formation in COVID-19," *Bioscience Reports* 41, no. 8 (August 27, 2021): BSR20210611, doi: 10.1042/BSR20210611.

365 Alexander Smith et al., "Morbidity Prevalence Estimate at 6 Months Following a Stroke: Protocol for a Cohort Study," *JMIR Research Protocols* 9, no. 6 (June 17, 2020): e15851, doi: 10.2196/15851; Eric S. Donkor, "Stroke in the 21st Century: A Snapshot of the Burden, Epidemiology, and Quality of Life," *Stroke Research and Treatment* 2018, no. 3238165 (November 27, 2018):, doi: 10.1155/2018/3238165.

366 Waqar Waheed et al., "Post COVID-19 Vaccine Small Fiber Neuropathy," *Muscle & Nerve* 64, no. 1 (July 2021): e1–e2, doi: 10.1002/mus.27251.

367 Stephen A. Johnson et al., "Small Fiber Neuropathy Incidence, Prevalence, Longitudinal Impairments, and Disability," *Neurology* 97, no. 22 (November 2021): e2236–e2247, doi: 10.1212/WNL.0000000000012894.

368 Ankit Malik et al., "*Campylobacter Jejuni* Induces Autoimmune Peripheral Neuropathy via Sialoadhesin and Interleukin-4 Axes," *Gut Microbes* 14, no. 1 (January–December 2022): 2064706, doi: 10.1080/19490976.2022.2064706.

369 Penina Haber et al., "Vaccines and Guillain-Barré Syndrome," *Drug Safety* 32 (April 2009): 309–323, doi: 10.2165/00002018-200932040-00005; Centers for Disease Control and Prevention, "Guillain-Barré Syndrome and Vaccines," reviewed February 6, 2023, https://www.cdc.gov/vaccinesafety/concerns/guillain-barre-syndrome.html.

370 Josef Finsterer, "Triggers of Guillain-Barré Syndrome: *Campylobacter Jejuni* Predominates," *International Journal of Molecular Science* 23, no. 22 (November 17, 2022): 14222, doi: 10.3390/ijms232214222.

371 Faith H. N. Howard et al., "Understanding Immune Responses to Viruses—Do Underlying Th1/Th2 Cell Biases Predict Outcome?" *Viruses* 14, no. 7 (July 8, 2022):1493, doi: 10.3390/v14071493.

372 Seneff et al., "Innate Immune Suppression by SARS-CoV-2 mRNA Vaccinations: The Role of G-Quadruplexes, Exosomes, and MicroRNAs," *Food and Chemical Toxicology* 164, no. 113008 (June 2022), doi: 10.1016/j.fct.2022.113008.

373 Twinkle Ghosh, "Health Canada Adds Bell's Palsy Warning to Pfizer Labels, but Says Vaccine Is Safe," *Global News*, August 6, 2021, https://globalnews.ca/news/8092666/health-canada-bells-palsy-warning-pfizer-covid-vaccine/; Eric Yuk Fai Wan et al., "Bell's Palsy following Vaccination with mRNA (BNT162b2) and Inactivated (CoronaVac) SARS-CoV-2 Vaccines: A Case Series and Nested Case-Control Study," *Lancet* 22, no. 1 (January 2022): 64–72, doi: 10.1016/S1473-3099(21)00451-5.

374 Nicola Cirillo and Richard Doan, "Bell's Palsy and SARS-CoV-2 Vaccines—An Unfolding Story," *Lancet Infectious Diseases* 21, no. 9 (June 2021): 1210–1211, doi: 10.1016/S1473-3099(21)00273-5.

375 Anthony Zandian et al., "The Neurologist's Dilemma: A Comprehensive Clinical Review of Bell's Palsy, with Emphasis on Current Management Trends," *Medical Science Monitor* 20 (January 20, 2014): 83–90, doi: 10.12659/MSM.889876.

376 Jeong Yun Choi et al., "Brachial Plexopathy following Herpes Zoster Infection: Two Cases with MRI Findings," *Journal of the Neurological Sciences* 285, nos. 1–2 (October 15, 2009): 224–6, doi: 10.1016/j.jns.2009.05.016.

377 Seneff et al., "Innate Immune Suppression by SARS-CoV-2 mRNA Vaccinations: The Role of G-Quadruplexes, Exosomes, and MicroRNAs,"; Ganesh A. Kolumam, "Type I Interferons Act Directly on CD8 T Cells to Allow Clonal Expansion and Memory Formation in Response to Viral Infection," *Journal of Experimental Medicine* 202, no. 5 (2005): 637–650, doi: 10.1084/jem.20050821.

378 Nicola Principi and Susanna Esposito, "Do Vaccines Have a Role as a Cause of Autoimmune Neurological Syndromes?" *Frontiers in Public Health* 8, no. 361 (July 28, 2020), doi: 10.3389/fpubh.2020.00361.

379 Nirav Sanghani et al., "Myasthenia Gravis after Vaccination in Adults the United States: A Report from the CDC/FDA Vaccine Adverse Event Reporting System (1990–2017): p6.437," *Neurology* 90, no. 15 supplement (April 10 2018): p.6.437, https://www.neurology.org/doi/10.1212/WNL.90.15_supplement.P6.437.

380 William D. Phillips and Angela Vincent, "Pathogenesis of Myasthenia Gravis: Update on Disease Types, Models, and Mechanisms," *F1000Research* 5, no. F1000, Faculty Rev-1513 (June 27, 2016), https://f1000research.com/articles/5-1513/v1 doi: 10.12688/f1000research.8206.1.

381 Masakatsu Motomura and Tomoko Narita Masuda, "Autoantibodies in Myasthenia Gravis," *Brain and Nerve*, 65, no. 4 (April 2013): 433–9, Japanese, https://www.researchgate.net/publication/236140417_Autoantibodies_in_myasthenia_gravis; Ana Maria Yamamoto et al., "Anti-Titin Antibodies in Myasthenia Gravis: Tight Association with Thymoma and Heterogeneity of Nonthymoma Patients," *JAMA Neurology* 58, no. 6 (June 2001): 885–90, doi: 10.1001/archneur.58.6.885.

382 Keva Green et al., *Central Nervous System Lymphoma* (Treasure Island, FL: StatPearls Publishing, updated 2023, internet), https://www.ncbi.nlm.nih.gov/books/NBK545145/.

383 Arayamparambil C. Anilkumar et al., *Acute Disseminated Encephalomyelitis* (Treasure Island, FL: StatPearls, January, 2024), https://www.ncbi.nlm.nih.gov/books/NBK430934/.
384 Katherine A. McLaughlin and Kai W. Wucherpfennig, "Chapter 4 B Cells and Autoantibodies in the Pathogenesis of Multiple Sclerosis and Related Inflammatory Demyelinating Diseases," *Advances in Immunology* 98 (2008):121–49, doi: 10.1016/S0065-2776(08)00404-5.
385 Dennis C. Thunstedt et al., "Isolated Intracranial Hypertension following COVID-19 Vaccination: A Case Report," *Cephalalgia Reports* 4 (2021), doi:10.1177/25158163211044797.
386 Seneff et al., "Innate Immune Suppression by SARS-CoV-2 mRNA Vaccinations: The Role of G-Quadruplexes, Exosomes, and MicroRNAs."
387 Marcello Silvestro et al., "Headache Worsening after COVID-19 Vaccination: An Online Questionnaire-Based Study on 841 Patients with Migraine," *Journal of Clinical Medicine* 10, no. 24 (December 16, 2021): 5914, doi: 10.3390/jcm10245914.
388 Seneff et al., "Innate Immune Suppression by SARS-CoV-2 mRNA Vaccinations: The Role of G-Quadruplexes, Exosomes, and MicroRNAs."
389 Geetanjali Saini and Ritu Aneja, "Cancer as a Prospective Sequela of Long COVID-19," *Bioessays* 43, no. 6 (June 2021): e2000331, doi: 10.1002/bies.202000331.
390 Nishant Singh and Anuradha Bharara Singh, "S2 Subunit of SARS-nCoV-2 Interacts with Tumor Suppressor Protein p53 and BRCA: An in Silico Study," *Translational Oncology* 13, no. 10 (October 2020): 100814, doi: 10.1016/j.tranon.2020.100814.
391 Lee M. Greenberger et al., "Anti-Spike T-cell and Antibody Responses to SARS-CoV-2 mRNA Vaccines in Patients with Hematologic Malignancies," *Blood Cancer Discovery* 3, no. 6 (November 2, 2022): 481–489, doi: 10.1158/2643-3230.BCD-22-0077; Seneff et al., "Innate Immune Suppression by SARS-CoV-2 mRNA Vaccinations: The Role of G-Quadruplexes, Exosomes, and MicroRNAs."
392 Katalin Karikó et al., "Incorporation of Pseudouridine into mRNA Yields Superior Nonimmunogenic Vector with Increased Translational Capacity and Biological Stability," *Molecular Therapy* 16, no. 11 (November 2008): 1833–40, doi: 10.1038/mt.2008.200.
393 Aldén M, et al. "Intracellular Reverse Transcription of Pfizer BioNTech COVID-19 mRNA Vaccine BNT162b2 In Vitro in Human Liver Cell Line," *Curr Issues Mol Biol* 44, no. 3 (February 25, 2022): 1115-1126, doi: 10.3390/cimb44030073.
394 Liguo Zhang et al., "SARS-CoV-2 RNA Reverse-Transcribed and Integrated into the Human Genome," bioRxiv preprint, December 13, 2020, doi: 10.1101/2020.12.12.422516; Walter Doerfler, "Adenoviral Vector DNA- and SARS-CoV-2 mRNA-Based Covid-19 Vaccines: Possible Integration into the Human Genome—Are Adenoviral Genes Expressed in Vector-based Vaccines?" *Virus Research* 302, no. 198466 (September 2021), doi: 10.1016/j.virusres.2021.198466.

395 Xiao Zhang et al., "New Understanding of the Relevant Role of LINE-1 Retrotransposition in Human Disease and Immune Modulation," *Frontiers in Cell & Developmental Biology* 8 (August 2020): 657, doi: 10.3389/fcell.2020.00657.
396 Paul E. Fraser, "Prions and Prion-Like Proteins," *Journal of Biological Chemistry* 289, no. 29 (July 18, 2014): 19839–40, doi: 10.1074/jbc.R114.583492.
397 Danish Idrees and Vijay Kumar, "SARS-CoV-2 Spike Protein Interactions with Amyloidogenic Proteins: Potential Clues to Neurodegeneration," *Biochemical and Biophysical Research Communications* 554 : 94–98, doi: 10.1016/j.bbrc.2021.03.100.
398 Peter L. Parry et al., "'Spikeopathy': COVID-19 Spike Protein Is Pathogenic, from Both Virus and Vaccine mRNA," *Biomedicine* 11, no. 8 (August 17, 2023): 2287, doi: 10.3390/biomedicines11082287; Idrees and Kumar, "SARS-CoV-2 Spike Protein Interactions with Amyloidogenic Proteins: Potential Clues to Neurodegeneration,"; George Tetz and Victor Tetz, "Prion-Like Domains in Spike Protein of SARS-CoV-2 Differ across Its Variants and Enable Changes in Affinity to ACE2," *Microorganisms* 10, no. 2 (January 25, 2022): 280, doi: 10.3390/microorganisms10020280.
399 Tetz and Tetz, "Prion-Like Domains in Spike Protein of SARS-CoV-2 Differ across Its Variants and Enable Changes in Affinity to ACE2."
400 Seneff et al., "Innate Immune Suppression by SARS-CoV-2 mRNA Vaccinations: The Role of G-Quadruplexes, Exosomes, and MicroRNAs."
401 Xiaoling Cao et al., "Spike Protein of SARS-CoV-2 Activates Macrophages and Contributes to Induction of Acute Lung Inflammation in Male Mice," *FASEB Journal* 35, no. 9 (September 2021): 21801, doi: 10.1096/fj.202002742RR; T. C. Theoharides and P. Conti, "Be Aware of SARS-CoV-2 Spike Protein: There Is More Than Meets the Eye," *Journal of Biological Regulators and Homeostatic Agents* 35, no. 3 (May–June 2021): 833–838 doi: 10.23812/THEO_EDIT_3_21; Rita Rubin, "Large Cohort Study Finds Possible Association between Postural Orthostatic Tachycardia Syndrome and COVID-19 Vaccination but Far Stronger Link with SARS-CoV-2 Infection," *Medical News & Perspectives* 329, no. 6 (February 14, 2023): 454–456, doi: 10.1001/jama.2023.0050.
402 Tsukasa Uranaka et al., "Expression of ACE2, TMPRSS2, and Furin in Mouse Ear Tissue, and the Implications for SARS-CoV-2 Infection," *Laryngoscope* 131, no. 6 (June 2021): e2013–e2017, doi: 10.1002/lary.29324.
403 Adam Armada-Moreira et al., "Going the Extra (Synaptic) Mile: Excitotoxicity as the Road toward Neurodegenerative Diseases," *Frontiers in Cellular Neuroscience* 14 (April 24, 2020), Sec. Cellular Neurophysiology: 90, doi: 10.3389/fncel.2020.00090.
404 Jennifer Couzin-Frankel and Gretchen Vogel, "In Rare Cases, Coronavirus Vaccines May Cause Long Covid-Like Symptoms," *Science*, January 20, 2022, https://www.science.org/content/article/rare-cases-coronavirus-vaccines-may-cause-long-covid-symptoms.

405 Mina Psichogiou et al., "Reactivation of Varicella Zoster Virus after Vaccination for SARS-CoV-2," *Vaccines* (Basel) 9, no. 6 (June 2021): 572, doi: 10.3390/vaccines9060572.

406 Ibid.

407 Seneff et al., "Innate Immune Suppression by SARS-CoV-2 mRNA Vaccinations: The Role of G-Quadruplexes, Exosomes, and MicroRNAs."

408 Lazarus et al., "Electronic Support for Public Health–Vaccine Adverse Event Reporting System."

409 John R. Sims et al., "Donanemab in Early Symptomatic Alzheimer Disease: The TRAILBLAZER-ALZ 2 Randomized Clinical Trial," *Journal of the American Medical Association,* July 17, 2023, doi: 10.1001/jama.2023.13239.

410 Takashi Tanikawa et al., "Degradative Effect of Nattokinase on Spike Protein of SARS-CoV-2," *Molecules* 27, no.17 (August 24, 2022): 5405, doi: 10.3390/molecules27175405.

411 G. Colussi et al., "Impact of Omega-3 Polyunsaturated Fatty Acids on Vascular Function and Blood Pressure: Relevance for Cardiovascular Outcomes," *NMCD* 27, no. 3 (March 2017): 191–200, doi: 10.1016/j.numecd.2016.07.011.

412 M. Kyla Shea et al., "Vitamin K and Vitamin D Status: Associations with Inflammatory Markers in the Framingham Offspring Study," *American Journal of Epidemiology* 167, no. 3 (February 1, 2008): 313–20, doi: 10.1093/aje/kwm306.

413 Natalia Vallianou et al., "Alpha-Lipoic Acid and Diabetic Neuropathy," *Review of Diabetic Studies* 6, no. 4 (December 2009): 230–6, doi: 10.1900/RDS.2009.6.230.

414 Djamel Messaoudene et al., "*Ex Vivo* Effects of Flavonoïds Extracted from *Artemisia herba alba* on Cytokines and Nitric Oxide Production in Algerian Patients with Adamantiades-Behçet's Disease," *Journal of Inflammation* 8, no. 35 (November 2011), doi: 10.1186/1476-9255-8-35.

415 J. C. Bertoglio et al., "*Andrographis paniculata* Decreases Fatigue in Patients with Relapsing-Remitting Multiple Sclerosis: A 12-Month Double-Blind Placebo-Controlled Pilot Study," *BMC Neurology* 16, no. 77, doi: 10.1186/s12883-016-0595-2.

416 Huan Zhang et al., "A Review of the Pharmacological Effects of the Dried Root of *Polygonum cuspidatum* (Hu Zhang) and Its Constituents," *Evidence Based Complementary and Alternative Medicine* 2013, no. 208349 (September), doi: 10.1155/2013/208349.

417 Alan D. Snow et al., "The Amazon Rain Forest Plant *Uncaria tomentosa* (Cat's Claw) and Its Specific Proanthocyanidin Constituents Are Potent Inhibitors and Reducers of Both Brain Plaques and Tangles," *Scientific Reports* 9, no. 561 (February 6, 2019), doi: 10.1038/s41598-019-38645-0.

418 Kah-Hui Wong et al., "Neuroregenerative Potential of Lion's Mane Mushroom, *Hericium erinaceus* (Bull.: Fr.) Pers. (Higher Basidiomycetes), in the Treatment of Peripheral Nerve Injury (Review)," *International Journal of Medicinal Mushrooms* 14, no. 5 (2012): 427–46, doi: 10.1615/intjmedmushr.v14.i5.10.

419 Hewlings SJ, Kalman DS. Curcumin: A Review of Its Effects on Human Health. Foods. 2017 Oct 22;6(10):92. doi: 10.3390/foods6100092. PMID: 29065496; PMCID: PMC5664031.

Chapter 10: Cancer Risks of the COVID-19 "Vaccines"

420 Anna D. Barker and Hamilton Jordan, "Public Attitudes Concerning Cancer," in *Holland-Frei Cancer Medicine,* 6th ed., eds. Donald W. Kufe et al. (Hamilton: BC Decker, 2003), https://www.ncbi.nlm.nih.gov/books/NBK12354/; YouGov UK, "Cancer Britons Most Feared Disease," August 15, 2011, https://yougov.co.uk/topics/society/articles-reports/2011/08/15/cancer-britons-most-feared-disease.

421 International Agency for Research on Cancer, *World Cancer Report: Cancer Research for Cancer Prevention,* ed. C. P. Wild et al., 2020, https://publications.iarc.fr/Non-Series-Publications/World-Cancer-Reports/World-Cancer-Report-Cancer-Research-For-Cancer-Prevention-2020.

422 US Food and Drug Administration, Center for Drug Evaluation and Research, *Guidance for Industry S2(R1) Genotoxicity Testing and Data Interpretation for Pharmaceuticals Intended for Human Use,* 2021, https://www.fda.gov/media/71980/download.

423 US Food and Drug Administration, Center for Drug Evaluation and Research, *Guidance for Industry Carcinogenicity Study Protocol Submissions,* 2002, https://www.fda.gov/files/drugs/published/Carcinogenicity-Study-Protocol-Submissions.pdf; International Council for Harmonisation of Technical Requirements for Pharmaceuticals for Human Use, *Addendum to the Guideline on Testing for Carcinogenicity of Pharmaceuticals,* 2021, https://database.ich.org/sites/default/files/ICH_S1BR1_Step2_DraftGuideline_2021_0510.pdf; FDA, CDER, *Guidance for Industry S2R1*; European Medicines Agency, *ICH Guideline S2 (R1) on Genotoxicity Testing and Data Interpretation for Pharmaceuticals Intended for Human Use,* 2021, https://www.ema.europa.eu/en/documents/scientific-guideline/ich-guideline-s2-r1-genotoxicity-testing-data-interpretation-pharmaceuticals-intended-human-use-step_en.pdf.

424 US Food and Drug Administration, *Package Insert (for USA distribution)—COMIRNATY,* https://www.fda.gov/media/151707/download; Australian Department of Health, Therapeutic Goods Administration, *Package Insert (for Australia Distribution)—COMIRNATY,* https://www.tga.gov.au/sites/default/files/auspar-bnt162b2-mrna-210125-pi.pdf; Antonio F. Hernández et al., "Safety of COVID-19 Vaccines Administered in the EU: Should We Be Concerned?" *Toxicology Reports* 8 (2021): 871–879, doi: 10.1016/j.toxrep.2021.04.003; European Medicines Agency, Committee for Medicinal Products for Human Use, *Assessment Report Comirnaty Common Name: COVID-19 mRNA Vaccine,* 2021, https://www.ema.europa.eu/en/documents/assessment-report/comirnaty-epar-public-assessment-report_en.pdf; European Medicines Agency, Committee for Medicinal Products for Human Use, *Assessment Report COVID-19 Vaccine Moderna, INN-COVID-19 mRNA Vaccine,*

2021, https://www.ema.europa.eu/en/documents/assessment-report/spikevax-previously-covid-19-vaccine-moderna-epar-public-assessment-report_en.pdf; Australian Department of Health, Therapeutic Goods Administration, *Nonclinical Evaluation Report BNT162b2 [mRNA] COVID-19 vaccine (COMIRNATY TM)*, https://www.tga.gov.au/sites/default/files/foi-2389-06.pdf; Xiao Wang et al., US Food and Drug Administration, *COMIRNATY—FDA Summary Basis for Regulatory Action*, 2021, https://www.fda.gov/media/151733/download; Hong Yang et al., US Food and Drug Administration, *SPIKEVAX: FDA Summary Basis for Regulatory Action*, 2022, https://www.fda.gov/media/155931/download.

425 Nevio Cimolai, "Do RNA Vaccines Obviate the Need for Genotoxicity Studies?" *Mutagenesis* 35, no. 6 (December 31, 2020): 509–510, doi: 10.1093/mutage/geaa028; Helene Banoun, "mRNA: Vaccine or Gene Therapy? The Safety Regulatory Issues," *International Journal of Molecular Science* 24, no. 13 (2023): 10514, doi: 10.3390/IJMS241310514; Ronald H. B. Meyboom et al., "Principles of Signal Detection in Pharmacovigilance," *Drug Safety* 16, no. 6 (1997): 355–365, doi: 10.2165/00002018-199716060-00002; World Health Organization, Programme for International Drug Monitoring, Uppsala Monitoring Centre, "What Is a signal?" 2022, https://who-umc.org/signal-work/what-is-a-signal/.

426 European Medicines Agency, Committee for Medicinal Products for Human Use, *Assessment Report COVID-19 Vaccine Moderna, INN-COVID-19 mRNA Vaccine*, 2021, https://www.ema.europa.eu/en/documents/assessment-report/spikevax-previously-covid-19-vaccine-moderna-epar-public-assessment-report_en.pdf.

427 Ibid.

428 Cimolai, "Do RNA Vaccines Obviate the Need for Genotoxicity Studies?"; Banoun, "mRNA: Vaccine or Gene Therapy? The Safety Regulatory Issues."

429 Meyboom, "Principles of Signal Detection in Pharmacovigilance."

430 Manfred Hauben and Jeffrey K. Aronson, "Defining 'Signal' and Its Subtypes in Pharmacovigilance Based on a Systematic Review of Previous Definitions," *Drug Safety* 32, no. 2 (2009): 99–110, doi: 10.2165/00002018-200932020-00003; Uppsala Monitoring Centre, "What Is a signal?"

431 Jae-Young Lee et al., "The Use of Social Media in Detecting Drug Safety–Related New Black Box Warnings, Labeling Changes, or Withdrawals: Scoping Review," *JMIR Public Health and Surveillance* 7 no. 6 (2021), doi: 10.2196/30137.

432 Frederick Varricchio et al., "Understanding Vaccine Safety Information from the Vaccine Adverse Event Reporting System," *Pediatric Infectious Disease Journal* 23, no. 4 (April 2004): 287–294, doi: 10.1097/00006454-200404000-00002.

433 US Department of Health and Human Services, Vaccine Adverse Event Reporting System (VAERS), https://vaers.hhs.gov/.

434 Centers for Disease Control and Prevention, *V-Safe after Vaccination Health Checker Webpage*, https://www.cdc.gov/vaccinesafety/ensuringsafety/monitoring/v-safe/index.

html (no longer updated as of May 2023); Centers for Disease Control and Prevention, *V-Safe Active Surveillance for COVID-19 Vaccine Safety CDC Protocol*, 2021, https://www.cdc.gov/vaccinesafety/pdf/V-safe-Protocol-508.pdf.

435 Fidelia Cascini et al., "Social Media and Attitudes towards a COVID-19 Vaccination: A Systematic Review of the Literature," *eClinicalMedicine* 48, no. 101454 (June 2022), doi: 10.1016/J.ECLINM.2022.101454; Sihong Zhao et al., "The Prevalence, Features, Influencing Factors, and Solutions for COVID-19 Vaccine Misinformation: Systematic Review," *JMIR Public Health and Surveillance* 9 (January 2023): e40201, doi: 10.2196/40201.

436 Scott C. Ratzan, "The Plural of Anecdote Is Not Evidence," *Journal of Health Communication* 7, no. 3 (2002): 169–170, doi: 10.1080/10810730290088058.

437 Meredith Wadman, "Antivaccine Activists Use a Government Database on Side Effects to Scare the Public," *Science*, May 6, 2021, https://www.science.org/content/article/antivaccine-activists-use-government-database-side-effects-scare-public; Jonathan Jarry, "Don't Fall for the 'VAERS Scare' Tactic," McGill University, Office for Science and Society, 2021, https://www.mcgill.ca/oss/article/covid-19-critical-thinking-health/dont-fall-vaers-scare-tactic.

438 Jane M. Orient, "Negative Evidence: Antibody Dependent Enhancement," *Journal of American Physicians and Surgeons* 27, no. 1 (2022): 2–6, https://www.jpands.org/vol27no1/orient.pdf; Jane M. Orient, "Negative Evidence: Postmortem Examinations of Post- COVID-19 Vaccine Fatalities," *Journal of American Physicians and Surgeons*, 27, no. 2 (2022): 35–41, https://www.jpands.org/vol27no2/orient.pdf; Jane M. Orient, "Negative Evidence: COVID-19 Vaccines and Fertility," *Journal of American Physicians and Surgeons* 27, no. 3 (2022): 69–77, https://www.jpands.org/vol27no3/orient.pdf; Jane M. Orient, "Negative Evidence: COVID-19 Vaccines and Disorders of Hemostasis," *Journal of American Physicians and Surgeons* 27, no. 4 (2022): 98–107, https://www.jpands.org/vol27no4/orient.pdf.

439 National Institutes of Health, National Cancer Institute, "COVID-19 Vaccines and People with Cancer," updated August 1, 2023, https://www.cancer.gov/about-cancer/coronavirus/covid-19-vaccines-people-with-cancer.

440 Seneff, et al., "Innate Immune Suppression by SARS-CoV-2 mRNA Vaccinations: The Role of G-Quadruplexes, Exosomes, and MicroRNAs," *Food and Chemical Toxicology* 164, no. 113008 (June 2022), doi: 10.1016/j.fct.2022.113008; "Alarming Cancer Trend Suggests COVID-19 Vaccines Alter Natural Immune Response," *Epoch Times*, February 1, 2022, YouTube video, https://www.theepochtimes.com/epochtv/dr-ryan-cole-alarming-cancer-trend-suggests-covid-19-vaccines-alter-natural-immune-response-4250442; Charles Hoffe, "Cancer Link with Pfizer mRNA Boosters Dr. Charles Hoffe Explains," *The Other News Show*, 2022, Rumble video, https://rumble.com/v1qtt9k-dr.-charles-hoffe-explains-cancer-link-with-covid-19-jabs.html; Doctors for COVID Ethics (D4CE), "COVID Vaccination and Turbo

Cancer: Pathological Evidence," July 26, 2022, video, https://doctors4covidethics.org/covid-vaccination-and-turbo-cancer-pathological-evidence/.

441 Jeffrey Morris, "Does McCullough's Paper Really 'Establish a Mechanistic Framework' for mRNA Vaccine Harm?" COVID-19 Data Science, April 21, 2022, https://www.covid-datascience.com/post/does-mccullough-s-paper-really-establish-a-mechanistic-framework-for-mrna-vaccine-harm.

442 Sonia Paytubi et al., "Everything Causes Cancer? Beliefs and Attitudes towards Cancer Prevention among Anti-Vaxxers, Flat Earthers, and Reptilian Conspiracists: Online Cross Sectional Survey," *BMJ* 379 (2022): e072561, doi: 10.1136/BMJ-2022-072561.

443 InfoHealer, "Politicization, Polarization & Power Asymmetry," *Information Heals* (Substack), December 3, 2022, https://neutralresearcher.substack.com/p/politicization-polarization-and-power.

444 Vincent T. DeVita et al., *DeVita, Hellman, and Rosenberg's Cancer Principles and Practice of Oncology*, 12th ed., (Netherlands: LWW, 2022), https://www.wolterskluwer.com/en/know/cancer-principles-and-practice-of-oncology; Franco Dammacco and Franco Silvestris, eds., *Oncogenomics: From Basic Research to Precision Medicine*, 1st ed. (Philadelphia: Academic Press, 2018), https://shop.elsevier.com/books/oncogenomics/dammacco/978-0-12-811785-9; Lee Harrington et al., *The Basic Science of Oncology*, 6th ed. (Ontario: McGraw Hill, 2021), https://www.mhprofessional.com/the-basic-science-of-oncology-sixth-edition-9781259862076-usa; Lauren Pecorino, *Molecular Biology of Cancer: Mechanisms, Targets, and Therapeutics*, 5th ed. (New York: Oxford University Press, 2021), https://global.oup.com/ukhe/product/molecular-biology-of-cancer-9780198833024; Elspeth A. Bruford et al., "Guidelines for Human Gene Nomenclature," *Nature Genetics* 52, no. 8 (2020): 754, doi: 10.1038/s41588-020-0669-3; Stanley Maloy and Kelly Hughes, eds., *Brenner's Encyclopedia of Genetics*, 2nd ed. (Philadelphia: Academic Press, 2013), https://shop.elsevier.com/books/brenners-encyclopedia-of-genetics/maloy/978-0-12-374984-0.

445 Douglas Hanahan and Robert A. Weinberg, "The Hallmarks of Cancer," *Cell* 100, no. 1 (January 7, 2000): 57–70, doi: 10.1016/S0092-8674(00)81683-9.

446 Yousef Ahmed Fouad and Carmen Aanei, "Revisiting the Hallmarks of Cancer," *American Journal of Cancer Research*, 7, no. 5 (May 1, 2017): 1016–1036, http://www.ajcr.us/files/ajcr0053932.pdf.

447 Jocelyn Kaiser, "Making Trouble," *Science* 378, no. 6617 (October 21, 2022): 242–245, doi: 10.1126/science.adf3764.

448 Benjamin E. Housden et al., "Loss-of-Function Genetic Tools for Animal Models: Cross-Species and Cross-Platform Differences," *Nature Reviews Genetics*, 18, no. 1 (2017): 24–40, doi: 10.1038/NRG.2016.118.

449 Alfred G. Knudson, "Two Genetic Hits (More or Less) to Cancer," *Nature Reviews Cancer* 1, no. 2 (November 1, 2001): 157–162, doi: 10.1038/35101031.

450 Seul Ji Lee et al., "Distinguishing between Genotoxic and Non-genotoxic Hepatocarcinogens by Gene Expression Profiling and Bioinformatic Pathway Analysis," *Scientific Reports* 3, no. 1 (2013): 1–9, doi: 10.1038/srep02783.

451 Pippa F. Cosper et al., "Biology of HPV Mediated Carcinogenesis and Tumor Progression," *Seminars in Radiation Oncology* 31, no. 4 (October 2021): 265–273, doi: 10.1016/j.semradonc.2021.02.006.

452 François Jacob and Jacques Monod, "Genetic Regulatory Mechanisms in the Synthesis of Proteins," *Journal of Molecular Biology* 3, no. 3 (1961): 318–356, doi: 10.1016/S0022-2836(61)80072-7.

453 Susan Gottesman, "Micros for Microbes: Non-coding Regulatory RNAs in Bacteria," *Trends in Genetics* 21, no. 7 (July 2005): 399–404, doi: 10.1016/J.TIG.2005.05.008.

454 Kevin V. Morris and John S. Mattick, "The Rise of Regulatory RNA," *Nature Reviews Genetics* 15, no. 6 (June 2014): 423–437, doi: 10.1038/NRG3722.

455 Yi-Neng Han et al., "PIWI Proteins and PIWI-Interacting RNA: Emerging Roles in Cancer," *Cellular Physiology and Biochemistry* 44, no. 1 (2018): 1–20, doi: 10.1159/000484541.

456 Howard M. Temin and Satoshi Mizutani, "RNA-Dependent DNA Polymerase in Virions of Rous Sarcoma Virus," *Nature,* 226, no. 5252 (June 27, 1970): 1211–1213, doi: 10.1038/226121 1a0; S. Spiegelman et al., "Characterization of the Products of RNA-Directed DNA Polymerases in Oncogenic RNA Viruses," *Nature* 227, no. 5258 (August 8, 1970): 563–567, doi: 10.1038/227563a0.

457 Pottegård A, et al. "Considerations for Pharmacoepidemiological Studies of Drug-Cancer Associations." *Basic Clin Pharmacol Toxicol*, 122, no. 5 (May 2018): 451-459, doi: 10.1111/bcpt.12946

458 Sabrina Nour and Gilles Plourde, "Pharmacoepidemiology and Pharmacovigilance: Synergistic Tools to Better Investigate Drug Safety," (Philadelphia: Academic Press, 2018), 1–224, https://www.scribd.com/book/391163649/Pharmacoepidemiology-and-Pharmacovigilance-Synergistic-Tools-to-Better-Investigate-Drug-Safety; Pottegård, ibid.

459 EGRP, DCCPS, NCI, NIH, *Cancer Pharmacoepidemiology and Pharmacogenomics*, updated June 28, 2023, https://epi.grants.cancer.gov/pharm/.

Chapter 11: COVID-19 "Vaccine" Effects on Women of Reproductive Age and Pregnancy

460 Pfizer Documents Investigation Team and Amy Kelly, *War Room/DailyClout Pfizer Documents Analysis Volunteers' Reports eBook: Find Out What Pfizer, FDA Tried to Conceal*, ed. DailyClout LLC (B0BSK6LV5D: January 16, 2023), Kindle, https://www.amazon.com/DailyClout-Documents-Analysis-Volunteers-Reports-ebook/dp/B0BSK6LV5D/; *The Pfizer Papers: Pfizer's Crimes against Humanity*, ed. DailyClout LLC (October 15, 2024), Kindle, https://www.amazon.com/Pfizer-Papers-Pfizers-Against-Humanity/dp/1648210376/.

461 Judicial Watch, "JW v HHS Biodistribution Prod 4 02418 pgs 671–701," Document Archives, December 13, 2022, https://www.judicialwatch.org/documents/jw-v-hhs-biodistribution-prod-4-02418-pgs-671-701/.

462 Pfizer Documents Investigation Team and Amy Kelly, *War Room/DailyClout Pfizer Documents Analysis Volunteers' Reports eBook: Find Out What Pfizer, FDA Tried to Conceal*, ed. DailyClout LLC (B0BSK6LV5D: January 16, 2023), Kindle, https://www.amazon.com/DailyClout-Documents-Analysis-Volunteers-Reports-ebook/dp/B0BSK6LV5D/; *The Pfizer Papers: Pfizer's Crimes against Humanity*, ed. DailyClout LLC (October 15, 2024), Kindle, https://www.amazon.com/Pfizer-Papers-Pfizers-Against-Humanity/dp/1648210376/.

463 Beth L. Pineles et al., "In-Hospital Mortality in a Cohort of Hospitalized Pregnant and Nonpregnant Patients with COVID-19," *Annals of Internal Medicine* 174, no. 8 (August 2021): 1186–1188, doi: 10.7326/M21-0974.

464 Beth L. Pineles et al., "Pregnancy and the Risk of In-Hospital Coronavirus Disease 2019 (COVID-19) Mortality," *Obstetrics & Gynecology* 139, no. 5 (May 2022): 846–854, doi: 10.1097/AOG.0000000000004744.

465 Shari Roan, "Swine Flu 'Debacle' of 1976 Is Recalled," *Los Angeles Times*, April 27, 2009, https://www.latimes.com/archives/la-xpm-2009-apr-27-sci-swine-history27-story.html; National Library of Medicine, "Vaccine Development: Current Status and Future Needs," American Academy of Microbiology, March 4–6, 2005, https://www.ncbi.nlm.nih.gov/books/NBK561254/table/T4/.

466 James A. Thorp et al., "COVID-19 Vaccines: The Impact on Pregnancy Outcomes and Menstrual Function," *Journal of American Physicians & Surgeons* 28, no. 1 (Spring 2023): 28–34, https://www.jpands.org/vol28no1/thorp.pdf.

467 Pfizer Documents Investigation Team and Amy Kelly, *War Room/DailyClout Pfizer Documents Analysis Volunteers' Reports eBook: Find Out What Pfizer, FDA Tried to Conceal*, ed. DailyClout LLC (B0BSK6LV5D: January 16, 2023), Kindle, https://www.amazon.com/DailyClout-Documents-Analysis-Volunteers-Reports-ebook/dp/B0BSK6LV5D/; *The Pfizer Papers: Pfizer's Crimes against Humanity*, ed. DailyClout LLC (October 15, 2024), Kindle, https://www.amazon.com/Pfizer-Papers-Pfizers-Against-Humanity/dp/1648210376/.

468 Pfizer Documents Investigation Team and Amy Kelly, *War Room/DailyClout Pfizer Documents Analysis Volunteers' Reports eBook: Find Out What Pfizer, FDA Tried to Conceal*, ed. DailyClout LLC (B0BSK6LV5D: January 16, 2023), Kindle, https://www.amazon.com/DailyClout-Documents-Analysis-Volunteers-Reports-ebook/dp/B0BSK6LV5D/; *The Pfizer Papers: Pfizer's Crimes against Humanity*, ed. DailyClout LLC (October 15, 2024), Kindle, https://www.amazon.com/Pfizer-Papers-Pfizers-Against-Humanity/dp/1648210376/.

469 Heather S. Lipkind et al., "Receipt of COVID-19 Vaccine During Pregnancy and Preterm or Small-for-Gestational-Age at Birth—Eight Integrated Health Care

Organizations, United States, December 15, 2020–July 22, 2021," *Morbidity and Mortality Weekly Report (MMWR)* 71, no. 1 (2022): 26–30, doi: 10.15585/mmwr.mm7101e1, US Department of Health and Human Services, Centers for Disease Control and Prevention.

470 "The COVID-19 Vaccine and Pregnancy: What You Need to Know," Flo, updated March 22, 2022, https://flo.health/pregnancy/pregnancy-health/covid-19-vaccination-during-pregnancy; Petros Galanis et al., "Uptake of COVID-19 Vaccines among Pregnant Women: A Systematic Review and Meta-Analysis," *Vaccines* (Basel) 10, no. 5 (May 2022): 766, doi: 10.3390/vaccines10050766.

471 Pfizer Documents Investigation Team and Amy Kelly, *War Room/DailyClout Pfizer Documents Analysis Volunteers' Reports eBook: Find Out What Pfizer, FDA Tried to Conceal*, ed. DailyClout LLC (B0BSK6LV5D: January 16, 2023), Kindle, https://www.amazon.com/DailyClout-Documents-Analysis-Volunteers-Reports-ebook/dp/B0BSK6LV5D/; *The Pfizer Papers: Pfizer's Crimes against Humanity*, ed. DailyClout LLC (October 15, 2024), Kindle, https://www.amazon.com/Pfizer-Papers-Pfizers-Against-Humanity/dp/1648210376/.

472 "Decline of Live Births in Europe," Initiative-corona.info website, updated August 8, 2022, https://www.initiative-corona.info/fileadmin/dokumente/Geburtenrueckgang-Europe-EN.pdf.

473 Amanda Morris, "Women Said Coronavirus Shots Affect Periods. New Study Shows They're Right," *Washington Post*, September 27, 2022, https://www.washingtonpost.com/wellness/2022/09/27/covid-vaccine-period-late/.

474 Arwa Mahdawi, "Who Says It's No Big Deal if the Covid Vaccine Temporarily Disrupts Menstrual Cycles?" The *Guardian*, September 18, 2021, https://www.theguardian.com/commentisfree/2021/sep/18/covid-vaccine-changes-menstrual-cycles.

475 Kate Clancy, "Why Reports of Period Weirdness after Shots Were Ignored," *Washington Post*, April 18, 2023, https://www.washingtonpost.com/opinions/2023/04/18/period-kate-clancy-coronavirus-vaccines-menstruation/.

476 National Institutes of Health, "Study Confirms Link between COVID-19 Vaccination and Temporary Increase in Menstrual Cycle Length," September 27, 2022, https://www.nih.gov/news-events/news-releases/study-confirms-link-between-covid-19-vaccination-temporary-increase-menstrual-cycle-length.

477 Tiffany Parotto et al., "COVID-19 and the Surge in Decidual Cast Shedding," *TheGMS* 3, no. 1 (2022): 107–117, doi: 10.46766/thegms.pubheal.22041401.

478 Jennifer Couzin-Frankel, "Thousands Report Unusual Menstruation Patterns after COVID-19 Vaccination," *Science* July 15, 2022, https://www.science.org/content/article/thousands-report-unusual-menstruation-patterns-after-covid-19-vaccination.

479 James A. Thorp et al., "Unprecedented Menstrual Abnormalities Strongly Associated with Proximity to COVID-19 Vaccinated Individuals: A Survey Study in Unvaccinated

Women," submitted for publication; "Unprecedented Menstrual Abnormalities," https://mycyclestory.com/project/is-shedding-causing-menstrual-irregularities/.
480 Nazeeh Hanna et al., "Detection of Messenger RNA COVID-19 Vaccines in Human Breast Milk," *JAMA Pediatrics* 176, no. 12 (September 26, 2022): 12681270, doi: 10.1001/jamapediatrics.2022.3581; Kevin McKernan et al., "Sequencing of Bivalent Moderna and Pfizer mRNA Vaccines Reveals Nanogram to Microgram Quantities of Expression Vector dsDNA per Dose," *OSF* preprint, updated April 11, 2023, doi: 10.31219/osf.io/b9t7m.
481 BioNTech-Pfizer, "A Phase 1/2/3 Placebo-Controlled, Randomized, Observer-Blind, Dose-Finding Study to Evaluate the Safety, Tolerability, Immunogenicity, and Efficacy of SARS-CoV-2 RNA Vaccine Candidates against COVID-19 in Healthy Individuals," Study Intervention No. PF-07302048, Protocol No. C4591001, November 2020, https://cdn.pfizer.com/pfizercom/2020-11/C4591001_Clinical_Protocol_Nov2020.pdf.
482 Roberto Romero et al., "Inflammation in Pregnancy: Its Roles in Reproductive Physiology, Obstetrical Complications, and Fetal Injury," *Nutrition Reviews* 65, no. 12 pt 2 (December 2007): S194–202, doi: 10.1111/j.1753-4887.2007.tb00362.x; Roberto Romero et al.; "Inflammation in Preterm and Term Labour and Delivery," *Seminars in Fetal & Neonatal Medicine* 11, no. 5 (October 2006): 317–26, doi: 10.1016/j.siny.2006.05.001; Roberto Romero et al., "Toward a New Taxonomy of Obstetrical Disease: Improved Performance of Maternal Blood Biomarkers for the Great Obstetrical Syndromes When Classified According to Placental Pathology," *AJOG* 227, no. 4 (October 2022): p615.e1–615.e25, doi: 10.1016/j.ajog.2022.04.015.
483 Eunjung Jung et al., "The Fetal Inflammatory Response Syndrome: The Origins of a Concept, Pathophysiology, Diagnosis, and Obstetrical Implications," *Seminars in Fetal & Neonatal Medicine* 25, no. 4 (August 2020): 101146, doi: 10.1016/j.siny.2020.101146.
484 Amaro N. Duarte-Neto et al., "Testicular Pathology in Fatal COVID-19: A Descriptive Autopsy Study," *Andrology* 10, no. 1 (January 2022): 13–23, doi: 10.1111/andr.13073.
485 Nadja Auerbach, Gunjan Gupta, and Kunal Mahajan, *Cystic Hygroma* (Treasure Island, FL: StatPearls, 2023, last updated February 20, 2023), https://www.ncbi.nlm.nih.gov/books/NBK560672/; Miroslava Koleva and Orlando De Jesus, *Hydrocephalus* (Treasure Island, FL: StatPearls, last updated July 20, 2023), https://www.ncbi.nlm.nih.gov/books/NBK560875/; Jenish Bhandari and Pawan K. Thada, *Neural Tube Disorders*, (Treasure Island, FL: StatPearls, last updated March 6, 2023), https://www.ncbi.nlm.nih.gov/books/NBK555903/; Vikramaditya Dumpa and Praveen Chandrasekharan, *Congenital Diaphragmatic Hernia* (Treasure Island, FL: StatPearls, last updated August 8, 2023), https://www.ncbi.nlm.nih.gov/books/NBK556076/.
486 Hae Young Lee, et al., "Role of Inflammation in Arterial Calcification," *Korean Circulation Journal* 51, no. 2 (February 2021): 114–125, doi: 10.4070/kcj.2020.0517;

Raquel López-Mejías and Miguel A. González-Gay, "IL-6: Linking Chronic Inflammation and Vascular Calcification," *Nature Reviews Rheumatology* 15, no. 8 (August 2019): 457–459, doi: 10.1038/s41584-019-0259-x; Netta Vidavsky et al., "Multiple Pathways for Pathological Calcification in the Human Body," *Advanced Healthcare Materials* 10, no. 4 (February 2021): e2001271, doi: 10.1002/adhm.202001271.

487 K. E. Thorp et al., "Energy Dynamics in Dementia & the Neurodegenerative Diseases: A New Causal Paradigm" (submitted for publication), June 2023, Researchgate, doi:10.46766/thegms.neuro.22062901.

488 Pfizer Documents Investigation Team and Amy Kelly, *War Room/DailyClout Pfizer Documents Analysis Volunteers' Reports eBook: Find Out What Pfizer, FDA Tried to Conceal*, ed. DailyClout LLC (B0BSK6LV5D: January 16, 2023), Kindle, https://www.amazon.com/DailyClout-Documents-Analysis-Volunteers-Reports-ebook/dp/B0BSK6LV5D/; *The Pfizer Papers: Pfizer's Crimes against Humanity*, ed. DailyClout LLC (October 15, 2024), Kindle, https://www.amazon.com/Pfizer-Papers-Pfizers-Against-Humanity/dp/1648210376/.

489 James Thorp MD, (@jathorpmfm), "Read this leaked email out of CRMC and Clovis Community Hospital in California. Instead of warning expecting mothers not to receive the covid vaccine, they are concerned about how to place a dead baby in a bucket," jpegs of documents in Tweet, September 2021, https://twitter.com/jathorpmfm/status/1663771732224753664/photo/1; Dan Fournier, "Canadian Doctors Still Under Attack for Exposing Stillbirths Caused by C19 Vaccines," Substack, November 27, 2022, https://fournier.substack.com/p/bc-doctors-still-under-attack-for.

490 Itai Gat et al., "Covid-19 Vaccination BNT162b2 Temporarily Impairs Semen Concentration and Total Motile Count among Semen Donors," *Andrology* 10, no. 6 (September 2022): 1016–1022, doi: 10.1111/andr.13209.

491 Initiative Corona. "Decline of live births in Europe." https://www.initiative-corona.info/fileadmin/dokumente/Geburtenrueckgang-Europe-EN.pdf, updated Aug 8, 2022.

492 Melissa S. Kearney and Phillip Levine, "US Births Are Down Again, after the COVID Baby Bust and Rebound," Brookings Institution, May 31, 2023, https://www.brookings.edu/2023/05/31/us-births-are-down-again-after-the-covid-baby-bust-and-rebound/.

493 Daniel Crown et al., "The Demographic Outlook: 2022 to 2052," Congressional Budget Office, July 2022, https://www.cbo.gov/publication/58347#_idTextAnchor013.

494 Initiative Corona, ibid.

495 Martin Bujard and Gunnar Andersson, "Fertility Declines Near the End of the COVID-19 Pandemic: Evidence of the 2022 Birth Declines in Germany and Sweden," German Federal Office for Population Research, June 2022, https://www.bib.bund.de/Publikation/2022/Fertility-declines-near-the-end-of-the-COVID-19-pandemic-Evidence-of-the-2022-birth-declines-in-Germany-and-Sweden.html?nn=1219558.

496 German Federal Office of Statistics, "Live Births per Month—Provisional Results," Destatis website, updated June 14, 2023, https://www.destatis.de/EN/Themes/Society-Environment/Population/Births/Tables/live-birth-provisional.html; "Germany Plays Down Scale of Vaccine Boost in April," Reuters, March 10, 2021, https://www.reuters.com/business/healthcare-pharmaceuticals/germany-plays-down-scale-vaccine-boost-april-2021-03-10/.

497 German Federal Office of Statistics, "Births," Destatis website, updated June 14, 2023, https://www.destatis.de/EN/Themes/Society-Environment/Population/Births/_node.html#267500.

498 Bujard and Andersson, "Fertility Declines Near the End of the COVID-19 Pandemic: Evidence of the 2022 Birth Declines in Germany and Sweden."

499 Sandra Mounier-Jack et al., "Covid-19 Vaccine Roll-Out in England: A Qualitative Evaluation," *PLOS One,* 18, no. 6 (2023): e0286529, doi: 10.1371/journal.pone.0286529.

500 UK Office of National Statistics, "Live Births by Month of Occurrence, Sex and Area of Usual Residence of Mother, England and Wales, September 2021 to August 2022, Provisional," updated April 20, 2023, https://www.ons.gov.uk/peoplepopulationandcommunity/birthsdeathsandmarriages/livebirths/adhocs/1078livebirthsbymonthofoccurrencesexandareaofusualresidenceofmotherenglandandwalesseptember2021toaugust2022provisional.

501 Sylvain Papon, *Demographic Report 2022,* Institut National de la Statistique et des Études Économiques, January 1, 2023, https://www.insee.fr/en/statistiques/6797730.

502 Gilles Pison, "France 2022: A Narrowing Gap between Births and Deaths," *Population Societies* 609, no. 3 (March 2023):1–4. Doi: 10.3917/popsoc.609.0001; L. Cambon et al., "Increasing Acceptance of a Vaccination Program for Coronavirus Disease 2019 in France: A Challenge for One of the World's Most Vaccine-Hesitant Countries," *Vaccine* 40, no. 2 (January 21, 2022): 178–182, doi: 10.1016/j.vaccine.2021.11.023.

503 Hannah Thompson, "Fertility Crisis? France's Birth Rate Hits Near 30-Year Low," *Connexion France,* May 12, 2023, https://www.connexionfrance.com/article/French-news/Health/Fertility-crisis-France-s-birth-rate-hits-near-30-year-low.

504 Mari Yamaguchi, "Japan Birth Rate Hits Record Low Amid Concerns over Shrinking and Aging Population," Associated Press, June 2, 2023, https://apnews.com/article/japan-birth-rate-record-low-population-aging-ade0c8a5bb52442f4365d-b1597530ee4; Justin McMurry, "South Korea's Birthrate Sinks to Fresh Record Low as Population Crisis Deepens," *The Guardian,* February 22, 2023, https://www.theguardian.com/world/2023/feb/22/south-koreas-birthrate-sinks-to-fresh-record-low-as-population-crisis-deepens; Mayuko Tani, "Singapore Fertility Rate Hits New Low, Putting Focus on Housing Prices," *Nikkei,* February 23, 2023, https://asia.nikkei.com/Spotlight/Society/Singapore-fertility-rate-hits-new-low-putting-focus-on-housing-prices.

505 Clara Calvert et al., "Changes in Preterm Birth and Stillbirth during COVID-19 Lockdowns in 26 Countries," *Nature Human Behavior* 7 (February 23, 2023): 529–533, doi: 10.1038/s41562-023-01522-y.

506 Brady E. Hamilton et al., "Births: Provisional Data for 2021," NVSS Vital Statistics Rapid Release, May 2022, no. 20, US Department of Health and Human Services, Centers for Disease Control and Prevention, https://www.cdc.gov/nchs/data/vsrr/vsrr020.pdf.

507 Joyce A. Martin and Michelle J.K. Osterman, "Exploring the Decline in the Singleton Preterm Birth Rate in the United States, 2019–2020, NCHS," Data Brief No. 430, January 2022, US Department of Health and Human Services, Centers for Disease Control and Prevention, https://www.cdc.gov/nchs/products/databriefs/db430.htm.

508 Ju Hyun Jin et al., "Medical Utilization and Costs in Preterm Infants in the First 6 Years of Life after Discharge from Neonatal Intensive Care Unit: A Nationwide Population-Based Study in Korea," *Journal of Korean Medical Science* 37, no. 12 (March 28, 2022): e93, doi: 10.3346/jkms.2022.37.e93.

509 Lee Jaeeun, "More Premature Births amid Low Birthrates: Report," *Korea Herald*, March 26, 2023, https://www.koreaherald.com/view.php?ud=20230326000085.

510 Aharon Dick et al., "Safety of SARS-CoV-2 Vaccination during Pregnancy—Obstetric Outcomes from a Large Cohort Study," *BMC Pregnancy and Childbirth* 22, no.166 (2022), doi: 10.1186/s12884-022-04505-5.

511 Mika Gissler et al., "Clarity and Consistency in Stillbirth Reporting in Europe: Why Is It So Hard to Get This Right?" *European Journal of Public Health* 32, no. 2 (April 2022): 200–206, doi: 10.1093/eurpub/ckac001.

512 Calvert et al., "Changes in Preterm Birth and Stillbirth during COVID-19 Lockdowns in 26 Countries."

513 Anthony King, "Doctors Investigate Several Stillbirths among Moms with COVID-19," *The Scientist*, April 23, 2021, https://www.the-scientist.com/news-opinion/doctors-investigate-several-stillbirths-among-moms-with-covid-19-68703; Joshua Cohen, "Dutch Study Confirms That Covid-19 in Pregnant Women Can Lead to Stillbirths," *Forbes*, December 2, 2021, https://www.forbes.com/sites/joshuacohen/2021/12/02/dutch-study-confirms-that-covid-19-in-pregnant-women-can-lead-to-stillbirths/?sh=405e6531dcd1; Lee Jae-ho, "S. Korea Reports First Stillbirth after Mother Tests Positive for COVID-19," *Hankyoreh*, November 25, 2021, https://english.hani.co.kr/arti/english_edition/e_national/1020831.html.

514 Carla L. DeSisto et al., "Risk for Stillbirth among Women with and without COVID-19 at Delivery Hospitalization—United States, March 2020–September 2021," *Morbidity and Mortality Weekly Report (MMWR)*, 70, no. 47 (2021): 1640–1645, US Department of Health and Human Services, Centers for Disease Control and Prevention, doi: 10.15585/mmwr.mm7047e1.

515 Christof Kuhbandner and Matthias Reitzner, "Estimation of Excess Mortality in Germany during 2020–2022," *Cureus* 15, no. 5 (May 23, 2023): e39371, doi: 10.7759/cureus.39371.

516 UK Office of National Statistics, "Births in England and Wales: 2021," August 9, 2023, https://www.ons.gov.uk/peoplepopulationandcommunity/birthsdeathsandmarriages/livebirths/bulletins/birthsummarytablesenglandandwales/2021.

517 Swiss Confederation Federal Statistical Office, "Infant Mortality, Stillbirths," 2022, https://www.bfs.admin.ch/bfs/en/home/statistics/health/state-health/mortality-causes-death/infant-stillbirths.html.

518 Statistics Netherlands, "Birth; Key Figures," updated July 27, 2022, https://www.cbs.nl/en-gb/figures/detail/37422eng.

519 Selena Simmons-Duffin and Carmel Wroth, "Maternal Deaths in the U.S. Spiked in 2021, CDC Reports," NPR, March 16, 2023, https://www.npr.org/sections/health-shots/2023/03/16/1163786037/maternal-deaths-in-the-u-s-spiked-in-2021-cdc-reports.

520 Sabrina Moreno, "COVID Played a Role in 1 in 4 Maternal Deaths, Federal Watchdog Says," Axios, October 19, 2022, https://www.axios.com/2022/10/19/covid-maternal-deaths-gao-report.

521 NPEU, MBRRACE-UK, "Maternal Mortality 2019–2021," updated May 2023, https://www.npeu.ox.ac.uk/mbrrace-uk/data-brief/maternal-mortality-2019-2021; Gareth Iacobucci, "UK and Ireland See Sharp Rise in Maternal Deaths," *BMJ* 379 (2022): o2732, doi: 10.1136/bmj.o2732.

522 Ah Khan Syed, "Debunking Viki Male: Part 1," *Arkmedic's blog*, June 3, 2023, https://arkmedic.substack.com/p/debunking-viki-male-part-1; Pierre Kory and Jenna McCarthy, *The War on Ivermectin* (New York: Skyhorse Publishing, 2023), https://www.amazon.com/War-Ivermectin-Medicine-Millions-Pandemic/dp/151077386X; Robert F. Kennedy Jr., *The Real Anthony Fauci* (New York: Skyhorse Publishing, 2022), https://www.amazon.com/Real-Anthony-Fauci-Democracy-Childrens/dp/1510766804/; Peter A. McCullough and John Leake, *The Courage to Face COVID-19* (Dallas: Counterplay Books, 2022), https://www.amazon.com/COURAGE-FACE-COVID-19-Hospitalization-Bio-Pharmaceutical/dp/B09ZLVWMD9.

523 Abigail Zuger, "A Drumbeat on Profit Takers," *New York Times*, March 20, 2012, https://www.nytimes.com/2012/03/20/science/a-drumbeat-on-profit-takers.html.

524 Pfizer Documents Investigation Team and Amy Kelly, *War Room/DailyClout Pfizer Documents Analysis Volunteers' Reports eBook: Find Out What Pfizer, FDA Tried to Conceal*, ed. DailyClout LLC (B0BSK6LV5D: January 16, 2023), Kindle, https://www.amazon.com/DailyClout-Documents-Analysis-Volunteers-Reports-ebook/dp/B0BSK6LV5D/; *The Pfizer Papers: Pfizer's Crimes against Humanity*,

ed. DailyClout LLC (October 15, 2024), Kindle, https://www.amazon.com/Pfizer-Papers-Pfizers-Against-Humanity/dp/1648210376/

525 US Department of Health and Human Services, "COVID-19 Community Corps," COVID-19 Public Education Campaign, April 1, 2021, https://wecandothis.hhs.gov/covidcommunitycorps.

526 US Department of Health and Human Services, "U.S. Department of Health and Human Services Launches Nationwide Network of Trusted Voices to Encourage Vaccination in Next Phase of COVID-19 Public Education Campaign," HHS Office on Women's Health website, April 1, 2021, https://www.womenshealth.gov/blog/us-department-health-and-human-services-launches-nationwide-network-trusted-voices-encourage.

527 Graham Kates, "Inside the $250 Million Effort to Convince Americans the Coronavirus Vaccines Are Safe," CBS News, December 23, 2020, https://www.cbsnews.com/news/covid-vaccine-safety-250-million-dollar-marketing-campaign/.

528 US Department of Health and Human Services, "U.S. Department of Health and Human Services Launches Nationwide Network of Trusted Voices to Encourage Vaccination in Next Phase of COVID-19 Public Education Campaign. Full List of COVID-19 Community Corps Founding Members: Public Health & Medical Organizations," news release, April 1, 2021, screen snapshot captured by Internet Archive Wayback Machine, https://web.archive.org/web/20210401225102/https:/www.hhs.gov/about/news/2021/04/01/hhs-launches-nationwide-network-trusted-voices-encourage-vaccination-next-phase-covid-19-public-education-campaign.html; USASPENDING.gov, "Spending by Prime Award," 2023, https://www.usaspending.gov/search/?hash=2b9bbf7349e6c520a55164cbe34c6321.

529 Kates, "Inside the $250 Million Effort to Convince Americans the Coronavirus Vaccines Are Safe."

530 Mark A. Weber et al., "Creating the HHS COVID-19 Public Education Media Campaign: Applying Systems Change Learnings," *Journal of Health Communication* 27, no. 3 (April 25, 2022): 201–207, doi: 10.1080/10810730.2022.2067272.

531 USASPENDING.gov, "Spending by Prime Award."

532 Centers for Disease Control and Prevention, *Documents Responsive to FOIA Request, 2023:* 569–575, https://earlycovidcare.org/wp-content/uploads/2024/05/ACOG-FOIA_responsive-records.pdf.

533 Ibid, 436–441, 439.

534 Ibid, 439.

535 Ibid, 440.

536 Ibid.

537 Ibid, 441.

538 Ibid, 1000.

539 Justine Coleman, "CDC Recommends Pregnant People Get COVID-19 Vaccine," *The Hill*, April 23, 2021, https://thehill.com/policy/healthcare/549965-cdc-declares-it-recommends-pregnant-people-get-covid-19-vaccine/.

540 Shimabukuro et al., "Safety Monitoring in the Vaccine Adverse Event Reporting System (VAERS),"; CDC V-SAFE COVID-19 Pregnancy Registry Team, "Preliminary Findings of mRNA Covid-19 Vaccine Safety in Pregnant Persons," *New England Journal of Medicine* 384, no. 24 (June 17, 2021): 2273–2282, doi: 10.1056/NEJMoa2104983; erratum in: *New England Journal of Medicine* 385, no. 16 (October 14, 2021): 1536, doi: 10.1056/NEJMx210016.

541 Pfizer Documents Investigation Team and Amy Kelly, *War Room/DailyClout Pfizer Documents Analysis Volunteers' Reports eBook: Find Out What Pfizer, FDA Tried to Conceal*, ed. DailyClout LLC (B0BSK6LV5D: January 16, 2023), Kindle, https://www.amazon.com/DailyClout-Documents-Analysis-Volunteers-Reports-ebook/dp/B0BSK6LV5D/; *The Pfizer Papers: Pfizer's Crimes against Humanity*, ed. DailyClout LLC (October 15, 2024), Kindle, https://www.amazon.com/Pfizer-Papers-Pfizers-Against-Humanity/dp/1648210376/

542 Sudeshna Mukherjee et al., "Risk of Miscarriage among Black Women and White Women in a US Prospective Cohort Study," *American Journal of Epidemiology* 177, no. 11 (June 1, 2013): 1271–1278, doi: 10.1093/aje/kws393.

543 Nathalie Kapp et al., "Medical Abortion in the Late First Trimester: A Systematic Review," *Contraception* 99, no. 2 (February 2019): 77–86, doi: 10.1016/j.contraception.2018.11.002.

544 The American College of Obstetricians and Gynecologists, "ACOG and SMFM Recommend COVID-19 Vaccination for Pregnant Individuals," July 30, 2021, https://www.acog.org/news/news-releases/2021/07/acog-smfm-recommend-covid-19-vaccination-for-pregnant-individuals.

545 See ACOG recommendations dated December 31, 2020, https://web.archive.org/web/20201231213634/https:/www.acog.org/covid-19/covid-19-vaccines-and-pregnancy-conversation-guide-for-clinicians; February 28, 2021, https://web.archive.org/web/20210228211947/https:/www.acog.org/covid-19/covid-19-vaccines-and-pregnancy-conversation-guide-for-clinicians; March 31, 2021, https://web.archive.org/web/20210331111624/https:/www.acog.org/covid-19/covid-19-vaccines-and-pregnancy-conversation-guide-for-clinicians; and April 26, 2021, https://web.archive.org/web/20210426181952/https:/www.acog.org/covid-19/covid-19-vaccines-and-pregnancy-conversation-guide-for-clinicians. ACOG's advice remained consistent throughout this period: "In the interest of patient autonomy, ACOG recommends that pregnant individuals be free to make their own decision regarding COVID-19 vaccination."

546 Pineles et al., "In-Hospital Mortality in a Cohort of Hospitalized Pregnant and Nonpregnant Patients with COVID-19."

547 American Board of Obstetrics and Gynecology, "Statement Regarding Dissemination of COVID-19 Misinformation," January 27, 2021, https://www.abog.org/about-abog/news-announcements/2021/09/27/statement-regarding-dissemination-of-covid-19misinformation.

548 Pfizer Documents Investigation Team and Amy Kelly, *War Room/DailyClout Pfizer Documents Analysis Volunteers' Reports eBook: Find Out What Pfizer, FDA Tried to Conceal*, ed. DailyClout LLC (B0BSK6LV5D: January 16, 2023), Kindle, https://www.amazon.com/DailyClout-Documents-Analysis-Volunteers-Reports-ebook/dp/B0BSK6LV5D/; *The Pfizer Papers: Pfizer's Crimes against Humanity*, ed. DailyClout LLC (October 15, 2024), Kindle, https://www.amazon.com/Pfizer-Papers-Pfizers-Against-Humanity/dp/1648210376/

Chapter 12: Risks to Children

549 Deidre McPhillips, "CDC Sounds Alarm about Low Vaccination Rates amid Rising Respiratory Virus Activity," CNN, December 14, 2023, https://www.cnn.com/2023/12/14/health/low-vaccination-rates-flu-covid-rsv/index.html.

550 Johns Hopkins University Coronavirus Research Center, "Vaccine Research & Development: Typical Timeline," https://coronavirus.jhu.edu/vaccines/timeline.

551 "Diarrhea Vaccine Pulled from Market," *Tampa Bay Tribune*, October 16, 1999, https://www.tampabay.com/archive/1999/10/16/diarrhea-vaccine-pulled-from-market/; Gilles Delage, "Rotavirus Vaccine Withdrawal in the United States: The Role of Postmarketing Surveillance," *Canadian Journal of Infectious Diseases and Medical Microbiology* 11, no. 414396 (January–February 2000): 10–12, doi: 10.1155/2000/414396.

552 Pfizer. "Pfizer-BioNTech COVID-19 Vaccine Demonstrates Strong Immune Response, High Efficacy and Favorable Safety in Children 6 Months to Under 5 Years of Age Following Third Dose." May 23, 2022, https://www.pfizer.com/news/press-release/press-release-detail/pfizer-biontech-covid-19-vaccine-demonstrates-strong-immune

553 Meike Meyer et al., "Morbidity of Respiratory Syncytial Virus (RSV) Infections: RSV Compared with Severe Acute Respiratory Syndrome Coronavirus 2 Infections in Children Aged 0–4 Years in Cologne, Germany," *Journal of Infectious Disease* 226, no. 12 (December 13, 2022): 2050–2053, doi: 10.1093/infdis/jiac052.

554 Yuanyuan Dong et al., "Epidemiology of COVID-19 among Children in China," *Pediatrics* 145, no. 6 (June 2020): e20200702, doi: 10.1542/peds.2020-0702.

555 Istituto Superiore di Sanità (ISS), "Epidemia COVID-19. Aggiornamento Nazionale," March 23, 2020, https://www.epicentro.iss.it/coronavirus/bollettino/Bollettino-sorveglianza-integrata-COVID-19_23-marzo%202020.pdf; Sunil S. Bhopal et al., "Children and Young People Remain at Low Risk of COVID-19 Mortality," *Lancet Child & Adolescent Health* 5, no. 5 (May 2021): e12–e13, doi: 10.1016/S2352-4642(21)00066-3.

556 Andrew T. Levin et al., "Assessing the Age Specificity of Infection Fatality Rates for COVID-19: Systematic Review, Meta-Analysis, and Public Policy Implications," *European Journal of Epidemiology* 35, no. 12 (December 2020): 1123–1138, doi: 10.1007/s10654-020-00698-1.

557 Johns Hopkins University School of Medicine, "Risk Factors for COVID-19 Mortality among Privately Insured Patients: A Claims Data Analysis," FAIR Health White Paper in Collaboration with the West Health Institute and Marty Makary, MD, MPH, November 11, 2020, https://s3.amazonaws.com/media2.fairhealth.org/whitepaper/asset/Risk Factors for COVID-19 Mortality among Privately Insured Patients—A Claims Data Analysis—A FAIR Health White Paper.pdf.

558 National COVID-19 School Response Dashboard, "Consistent State Data," via Statsiq, https://statsiq.co1.qualtrics.com/public-dashboard/v0/dashboard/web/5f78e5d-4de521a001036f78e/pages/Page_abe56848-c8f1-4308-b6d1-bd2d2b855adf/view.

559 Jayme Fraser et al., "Florida Schools Reopened En Masse, but a Surge in Coronavirus Didn't Follow, a *USA Today* Analysis Finds," *USA Today*, September 28, 2020, https://www.usatoday.com/story/news/investigations/2020/09/28/florida-schools-reopened-en-mass-feared-covid-surge-hasnt-followed/3557417001/.

560 Kanecia O. Zimmerman et al., "Incidence and Secondary Transmission of SARS-CoV-2 Infections in Schools," *Pediatrics* 147, no. 4 (April 2021): e2020048090, doi: 10.1542/peds.2020-048090.

561 Jonas F. Ludvigsson et al., "Open Schools, Covid-19, and Child and Teacher Morbidity in Sweden," *New England Journal of Medicine* 384, no. 7 (February 18, 2021): 669–671, doi: 10.1056/NEJMc2026670.

562 Sivan Gazit et al., "Severe Acute Respiratory Syndrome Coronavirus 2 (SARS-CoV-2) Naturally Acquired Immunity versus Vaccine-induced Immunity, Reinfections versus Breakthrough Infections: A Retrospective Cohort Study," *Clinical Infectious Diseases* 75, no. 1 (August 24, 2022): e545–e551, doi: 10.1093/cid/ciac262.

563 Nabin K. Shrestha et al., "Necessity of Coronavirus Disease 2019 (COVID-19) Vaccination in Persons Who Have Already Had COVID-19," *Clinical Infectious Diseases* 75, no. 1 (July 1, 2022): e662–e671, doi: 10.1093/cid/ciac022.

564 COVID-19 Forecasting Team, "Past SARS-CoV-2 Infection Protection against Re-infection: a systematic review and meta-analysis," *Lancet*, 401, no. 10379 (March 11, 2023): 833-842, doi: 10.1016/S0140-6736(22)02465-5.

565 Guy Witberg et al., "Myocarditis after Covid-19 Vaccination in a Large Health Care Organization," *New England Journal of Medicine* 385 (December 2021): 2132–2139, doi: 10.1056/NEJMoa2110737.

566 "JCVI Statement on Vaccination of Children aged 5 to 11 Years Old,"; Alistair Smout, "UK Panel Does Not Recommend COVID Vaccines for Healthy 12- to 15-Year-Olds," Reuters, September 3, 2021, https://www.reuters.com/world/uk/uk-advisers-

decide-against-covid-vaccines-healthy-12-15-year-olds-2021-09-03/; Stephen Griffin, "COVID Vaccines: Why the UK Needs to Rethink Its Decision to Stop Boosters for Young and Healthy People," The Conversation, February 10 2023, https://theconversation.com/covid-vaccines-why-the-uk-needs-to-rethink-its-decision-to-stop-boosters-for-young-and-healthy-people-199044.

567 Matthew E. Oster et al., "Myocarditis Cases Reported after mRNA-Based COVID-19 Vaccination in the US from December 2020 to August 2021," *Journal of the American Medical Association* 327, no. 4 (2022): 331–340, doi:10.1001/jama.2021.24110.

568 Rujittika Mungmunpuntipantip and Viroj Wiwanitkit, "Autopsy Histopathologic Cardiac Findings following the Second COVID-19 Vaccine Dose," *Archives of Pathology and Laboratory Medicine* 146, no. 12 (December 2022): 1432, doi: 10.5858/arpa.2022-0171-LE.

569 Tuvali et al., "The Incidence of Myocarditis and Pericarditis in Post COVID-19 Unvaccinated Patients—A Large Population-Based Study."

570 Krug et al., "BNT162b2 Vaccine-Associated Myo/Pericarditis in Adolescents: A Stratified Risk-Benefit Analysis."

571 "One Week Deadline for Under-50s in England to Get Covid Booster Jab," *The Guardian,* February 4, 2023, https://www.theguardian.com/world/2023/feb/04/people-in-england-aged-49-and-younger-urged-to-get-free-covid-booster.

572 Arati Sharma et al., "Toxicological Considerations When Creating Nanoparticle Based Drugs and Drug Delivery Systems?" *Expert Opinion on Drug Metabolism & Toxicology* 8 no. 1 (January 2012): 47–69, doi: 10.1517/17425255.2012.637916.

573 Amy Peykoff Hardin et al., "Age Limit of Pediatrics," *Pediatrics* 140, no. 3 (2017): e20172151, doi: 10.1542/peds.2017-2151.

574 Mariam Arain et al., "Maturation of the Adolescent Brain," *Neuropsychiatric Disease and Treatment* 9 (2013): 449–461, doi: 10.2147/NDT.S39776.

575 Josef Finsterer, "Neurological Side Effects of SARS-CoV-2 Vaccinations," *Acta Neurologica Scandinavica* 145, no. 1 (January 2022): 5–9, doi: 10.1111/ane.13550.

576 Aparajita Chatterjee and Ambar Chakravarty, "Neurological Complications following COVID-19 Vaccination," *Current Neurology and Neuroscience Reports* 23, no. 1 (2023): 1–14., doi: 10.1007/s11910-022-01247-x.

577 Jagannadha Avasarala et al., "VAERS-Reported New-Onset Seizures following Use of COVID-19 Vaccinations as Compared to Influenza Vaccinations," *British Journal of Clinical Pharmacology* 88, no. 11 (November 2022): 4784-4788, doi: 10.1111/bcp.15415.

578 Bernard Bannwarth, "Drug-Induced Musculoskeletal Disorders," *Drug Safety* 30, no. 1 (2007): 27–46, doi: 10.2165/00002018-200730010-00004.

579 Francesco Ursini et al., "Spectrum of Short-Term Inflammatory Musculoskeletal Manifestations after COVID-19 Vaccine Administration: A Report of 66 Cases,"

Annals of the Rheumatic Diseases 81, no. 3 (March 2022): 440–441, doi: 10.1136/annrheumdis-2021-221587.

580 Jiaxin Chen et al., "Nervous and Muscular Adverse Events after COVID-19 Vaccination: A Systematic Review and Meta-Analysis of Clinical Trials," *Vaccines* (Basel) 9, no. 8 (August 23, 2021): 939, doi: 10.3390/vaccines9080939.

581 Ruolan Wang et al., "Potential Adverse Effects of Nanoparticles on the Reproductive System," *International Journal of Nanomedicine* 13 (2018): 8487–8506, doi: 10.2147/IJN.S170723.

582 Atsuyuki Watanabe et al., "Assessment of Efficacy and Safety of mRNA COVID-19 Vaccines in Children Aged 5 to 11 Years. A Systematic Review and Meta-Analysis," *JAMA Pediatrics* 177, no. 4 (January 23, 2023): 384–394, doi: 10.1001/jamapediatrics.2022.6243.

Chapter 13: "Vaccine" Mortality Insights from Autopsy Reports

583 Barbara J. Kuter et al., "The Development of COVID-19 Vaccines in the United States: Why and How So Fast?" *National Library of Medicine* 39, no. 18 (April 28, 2021): 2491–2495, doi: 10.1016/j.vaccine.2021.03.077.

584 World Health Organization, *Coronavirus (COVID-19) Dashboard*, accessed May 17, 2023, https://covid19.who.int/.

585 Ioannis P. Trougakos et al., "Adverse Effects of COVID-19 mRNA Vaccines: The Spike Hypothesis," *Trends in Molecular Medicine* 28, no. 7 (July 2022): 542–554, doi: 10.1016/j.molmed.2022.04.007; Seneff et al., "Innate Immune Suppression by SARS-CoV-2 mRNA Vaccinations: The Role of G-Quadruplexes, Exosomes, and MicroRNAs," *Food & Chemical Toxicology* 164, no. 113008 (June 2022), doi: 10.1016/j.fct.2022.113008; T. C. Theoharides, "Could SARS-CoV-2 Spike Protein Be Responsible for Long-COVID Syndrome?" *Molecular Neurobiology* 59, no. 3 (March 2022): 1850–1861, doi: 10.1007/s12035-021-02696-0; T. C. Theoharides and P. Conti, "Be Aware of SARS-CoV-2 Spike Protein: There Is More Than Meets the Eye," *Journal of Biological Regulators & Homeostatic Agents* 35, no. 3 (May–June 2021): 833–838, doi: 10.23812/THEO_EDIT_3_21; Biykim Bozkurt et al., "Myocarditis with COVID-19 mRNA Vaccines," *Circulation* 144, no. 6 (August 10, 2021): 471–484, doi: 10.1161/CIRCULATIONAHA.121.056135; Lael M. Yonker et al., "Circulating Spike Protein Detected in Post-COVID-19 mRNA Vaccine Myocarditis," *Circulation* 147, no. 11 (March 14, 2023): 867–876, doi: 10.1161/CIRCULATIONAHA.122.061025.

586 Carolina Graña et al., "Efficacy and Safety of COVID-19 Vaccines," *Cochrane Database of Systematic Reviews*, 12, no. 12 (December 7, 2022): CD015477, doi: 10.1002/14651858.CD015477.

587 Trougakos et al., "Adverse Effects of COVID-19 mRNA Vaccines: The Spike Hypothesis."

588 Yuyang Lei et al., "SARS-CoV-2 Spike Protein Impairs Endothelial Function via Downregulation of ACE 2," *Circulation Research* 128 (2021): 1323–1326, doi: 10.1161/CIRCRESAHA.121.318902; Elisa Avolio et al., "The SARS-CoV-2 Spike Protein Disrupts Human Cardiac Pericytes Function through CD147 Receptor-Mediated Signalling: A Potential Non-infective Mechanism of COVID-19 Microvascular Disease," *Clinical Science* 135, no. 24 (December 22, 2021): 2667–2689, doi: 10.1042/CS20210735; "Coronavirus Spike Protein Activated Natural Immune Response, Damaged Heart Muscle Cells," *DAIC*, July 27, 2022, https://www.dicardiology.com/content/coronavirus-spike-protein-activated-natural-immune-response-damaged-heart-muscle-cells.

589 Seneff et al., "Innate Immune Suppression by SARS-CoV-2 mRNA Vaccinations: The Role of G-Quadruplexes, Exosomes, and MicroRNAs."

590 Vladimir N. Uversky et al., "IgG4 Antibodies Induced by Repeated Vaccination May Generate Immune Tolerance to the SARS-CoV-2 Spike Protein," *Vaccines* (Basel) 11, no. 5 (May 17, 2023): 991, doi: 10.3390/vaccines11050991.

591 Theoharides, "Could SARS-CoV-2 Spike Protein Be Responsible for Long-COVID Syndrome?"

592 Abdul Aleem and Ahmed Nadeem, *Coronavirus (COVID-19) Vaccine-Induced Immune Thrombotic Thrombocytopenia (VITT)* (Treasure Island, FL: StatPearls, January, 2023); Bozkurt et al., "Myocarditis with COVID-19 mRNA Vaccines."

593 Bozkurt et al., "Myocarditis with COVID-19 mRNA Vaccines,"; Jose Alfredo Samaniego Castruita et al., "SARS-CoV-2 Spike mRNA Vaccine Sequences Circulate in Blood Pp to 28 Days after COVID-19 Vaccination," *APMI* 131, no. 3 (March 2023): 128–132, doi: 10.1111/apm.13294.

594 Rachel Scarl et al., "The Hospital Autopsy: The Importance in Keeping Autopsy an Option," *Autopsy Case Report* 12 (February 17, 2022):e2021333, doi: 10.4322/acr.2021.333.

595 Yvonne Hojberg et al., "Generalized Eosinophilia Following Moderna COVID-19 Vaccine Administration: A Case Report," *Academic Forensic Pathology* 13, no. 1 (March 2023): 9–15, doi: 10.1177/19253621231157933; Hideyuki Nushida et al., "A Case of Fatal Multi-Organ Inflammation following COVID-19 Vaccination," *Legal Medicine* (Tokyo), 63 (March 20, 2023): 102244, doi: 10.1016/j.legalmed.2023.102244; Yo Han Jeon et al., "Sudden Death Associated with Possible Flare-Ups of Multiple Sclerosis after COVID-19 Vaccination and Infection: A Case Report and Literature Review," *Journal of Korean Medical Science* 38, no. 10 (March 13, 2023): e78, doi: 10.3346/jkms.2023.38.e78; Massimiliano Esposito et al., "Death from COVID-19 in a Fully Vaccinated Subject: A Complete Autopsy Report," *Vaccines* (Basel) 11, no. 1 (January 9, 2023): 142, doi: 10.3390/vaccines11010142; Juan José Chaves et al., "A Postmortem Study of Patients Vaccinated for SARS-CoV-2 in Colombia," *Revista Española de Patología* 56, no. 1 (January–March 2023): 4–9, doi: 10.1016/j.

patol.2022.09.003; Michael Mörz, "A Case Report: Multifocal Necrotizing Encephalitis and Myocarditis after BNT162b2 mRNA Vaccination against COVID-19," *Vaccines* (Basel) 10, no. 10 (October 1, 2022): 1651, doi: 10.3390/vaccines10101651; V. Alunni et al., "Postmortem PF4 Antibodies Confirm a Rare Case of Thrombosis Thrombocytopenia Syndrome Associated with ChAdOx1 nCoV-19 anti-COVID Vaccination," *International Journal of Legal Medicine* 137, no. 2 (March 2023): 487–492, doi: 10.1007/s00414-022-02910-1; Motonori Takahashi et al., "An Autopsy Case Report of Aortic Dissection with Histiolymphocytic Pericarditis and Aortic Inflammation after mRNA COVID-19 Vaccination," *Legal Medicine* (Tokyo) 59, no. 102154 (November 2022), doi: 10.1016/j.legalmed.2022.102154; Kazuhiro Murata et al., "Four Cases of Cytokine Storm after COVID-19 Vaccination: Case Report," *Frontiers in Immunology* 13: 967226 (August 15, 2022), doi: 10.3389/fimmu.2022.967226; Hidetoshi Satomi et al., "An Autopsy Case of Fulminant Myocarditis after Severe Acute Respiratory Syndrome Coronavirus 2 Vaccine Inoculation," *Pathology International* 72, no. 10 (October 2022): 519–524, doi: 10.1111/pin.13267; Hideto Suzuki et al., "Autopsy Findings of Post-COVID-19 Vaccination Deaths in Tokyo Metropolis, Japan, 2021," *Legal Medicine* (Tokyo) 59, no. 102134 (November 2022), doi: 10.1016/j.legalmed.2022.102134; Federica Mele et al., "Cerebral Venous Sinus Thrombosis after COVID-19 Vaccination and Congenital Deficiency of Coagulation Factors: Is There a Correlation?" *Human Vaccines & Immunotherapeutic* 18, no. 6 (November 30, 2022): 2095166, doi: 10.1080/21645515.2022.2095166; Yukihiro Yoshimura et al., "An Autopsy Case of COVID-19-Like Acute Respiratory Distress Syndrome after mRNA-1273 SARS-CoV-2 Vaccination," *International Journal of Infectious Diseases* 121 (August 2022): 98–101, doi: 10.1016/j.ijid.2022.04.057; Luca Roncati et al., "A Three-Case Series of Thrombotic Deaths in Patients over 50 with Comorbidities Temporally after modRNA COVID-19 Vaccination," *Pathogens* 11, no. 4 (April 3, 2022): 435, doi: 10.3390/pathogens11040435; Dong-Hoon Kang et al., "Fulminant Giant Cell Myocarditis following Heterologous Vaccination of ChAdOx1 nCoV-19 and Pfizer-BioNTech COVID-19," *Medicina* (Kaunas) 58, no. 3 (March 20, 2022): 449, doi: 10.3390/medicina58030449; Yuya Kamura et al., "Fatal Thrombotic Microangiopathy with Rhabdomyolysis as an Initial Symptom after the First Dose of mRNA-1273 Vaccine: A Case Report," *International Journal of Infectious Diseases* 117 (April 2022): 322–325, doi: 10.1016/j.ijid.2022.02.031; Yoshiko Ishioka et al., "Acute Exacerbation of Interstitial Lung Disease after SARS-CoV-2 Vaccination: A Case Series," *Chest* 162, no. 6 (December 2022): e311–e316, doi: 10.1016/j.chest.2022.08.2213; James R. Gill et al., "Autopsy Histopathologic Cardiac Findings in 2 Adolescents Following the Second COVID-19 Vaccine Dose," *Archives of Pathology & Laboratory Medicine* 146, no. 8 (August 1, 2022): 925–929, doi: 10.5858/arpa.2021- 0435-SA; Christofora Pomara et al., "Histological and Immunohistochemical Findings in a Fatal Case of

Thrombotic Thrombocytopenia after ChAdOx1 nCov-19 Vaccination," *Pathology— Research and Practice* 231, no. 153796 (March 2022), doi: 10.1016/j.prp.2022.153796; Audrey Yeo et al., "Post COVID-19 Vaccine Deaths—Singapore's Early Experience," *Forensic Science International* 332, no. 111199 (March 2022), doi: 10.1016/j.forsciint.2022.111199; Rohan Ameratunga et al., "Identified Case of Fatal Fulminant Necrotizing Eosinophilic Myocarditis following the Initial Dose of the Pfizer-BioNTech mRNA COVID-19 Vaccine (BNT162b2, Comirnaty): An Extremely Rare Idiosyncratic Hypersensitivity Reaction," *Journal of Clinical Immunology* 42, no. 3 (April 2022): 441–447, doi: 10.1007/s10875-021-01187-0; Albrecht Günther et al., "Complicated Long Term Vaccine Induced Thrombotic Immune Thrombocytopenia—A Case Report," *Vaccines* (Basel) 9, no. 11 (November 17, 2021): 1344, doi: 10.3390/vaccines9111344; Fiona Permezel et al., "Acute Disseminated Encephalomyelitis (ADEM) following Recent Oxford/AstraZeneca COVID- 19 Vaccination," *Forensic Science, Medicine and Pathology* 18, no. 1 (March 2022): 74–79, doi: 10.1007/s12024-021-00440-7; Sangyoon Choi et al., "Myocarditis-Induced Sudden Death after BNT162b2 mRNA COVID-19 Vaccination in Korea: Case Report Focusing on Histopathological Findings," *Journal of Korean Medical Science* 36, no. 40 (October 18, 2021): e286, doi: 10.3346/jkms.2021.36.e286; Julia Schneider et al., "Postmortem Investigation of Fatalities following Vaccination with COVID-19 Vaccines," *International Journal of Legal Medicine* 135, no. 6 (November 2021): 2335–2345, doi: 10.1007/s00414-021-02706-9; Amanda K. Verma et al., "Myocarditis after Covid-19 mRNA Vaccination," *New England Journal of Medicine* 385, no. 14 (September 30, 2021): 1332–1334, doi: 10.1056/NEJMc2109975; Markus Wiedmann et al., "Vaccine Induced Immune Thrombotic Thrombocytopenia Causing a Severe Form of Cerebral Venous Thrombosis with High Fatality Rate: A Case Series," *Frontiers in Neurology* 12, no. 721146 (July 30, 2021), doi: 10.3389/fneur.2021.721146; Cristoforo Pomara et al., "COVID-19 Vaccine and Death: Causality Algorithm According to the WHO Eligibility Diagnosis," *Diagnostics* (Basel) 11, no. 6 (May 26, 2021): 955, doi: 10.3390/diagnostics11060955; Karina Althaus et al., "Antibody-Mediated Procoagulant platelets in SARS- CoV-2-Vaccination Associated Immune Thrombotic Thrombocytopenia," *Haematologica* 106, no. 8 (August 1, 2021): 2170–2179, doi: 10.3324/haematol.2021.279000; Carolin Edler et al., "Deaths Associated with Newly Launched SARS-CoV-2 Vaccination (Comirnaty®)," *Legal Medicine* (Tokyo) 51, no. 101895 (July 2021), https://www.sciencedirect.com/science/article/pii/S1344622321000596; Torsten Hansen et al., "First Case of Postmortem Study in a Patient Vaccinated against SARS-CoV-2," *International Journal of Infectious Diseases* 107 (June 2021): 172–175, doi: 10.1016/j.ijid.2021.04.053; Arianna Baronti et al., "Myocardial Infarction following COVID-19 Vaccine Administration: Post Hoc, Ergo Propter Hoc?," *Viruses* 14, no. 8 (July 27, 2022): 1644, doi: 10.3390/v14081644; Chupong Ittiwut et al., "Genetic Basis of Sudden Death after COVID-19 Vaccination in Thailand," *Heart Rhythm* 19, no. 11 (August 5, 2022): 1874–9, doi: 10.1016/j.hrthm.2022.07.019; Andreas Greinacher et al., "Thrombotic Thrombocytopenia after ChAdOx1 nCov-19 Vaccination," *New England Journal of Medicine* 384, no. 22 (June 3, 2021): 2092–2101, doi: 10.1056/NEJMoa2104840; Alessandro Mauriello et al., "Thromboembolism after COVID-19 Vaccine in Patients with Preexisting Thrombocytopenia," *Cell Death & Disease* 12, no. 8 (August 3, 2021): 762, doi: 10.1038/s41419-021-04058-z; Tor Halvor Bjørnstad-Tuveng et al., "Fatal Cerebral Haemorrhage after COVID-19 Vaccine," *Tidsskr Nor Laegeforen* 141 (April 29, 2021), doi:10.4045/tidsskr.21.0312; Marie Scully et al., "Pathologic Antibodies to Platelet Factor 4 after ChAdOx1 nCoV-19 Vaccination," *New England Journal of Medicine* 384, no. 23 (June 10, 2021): 2202–2211, doi: 10.1056/NEJMoa2105385; Gwang-Jun Choi et al., "Fatal Systemic Capillary Leak Syndrome after SARS-CoV-2 Vaccination in Patient with Multiple Myeloma," *Emerging Infectious Diseases* 27, no. 11 (November 2021): 2973– 2975, doi: 10.3201/eid2711.211723; Constantin Schwab et al., "Autopsy-Based Histopathological Characterization of Myocarditis after Anti-SARS-CoV-2-Vaccination," *Clinical Research in Cardiology* 112, no. 3 (March 2023): 431–440, doi: 10.1007/s00392-022-02129-5; Klaus Hirschbühl et al., "High Viral Loads: What Drives Fatal Cases of COVID- 19 in Vaccines?—An Autopsy Study," *Modern Pathology* 35, no. 8 (August 2022): 1013–1021, doi: 10.1038/s41379-022-01069-9; Naoki Hoshino et al., "An Autopsy Case Report of Fulminant Myocarditis: Following mRNA COVID-19 Vaccination," *Journal of Cardiology Cases* 26, no. 6 (December 2022): 391–394, doi: 10.1016/j.jccase.2022.06.006; Daniele Colombo et al., "Autopsies Revealed Pathological Features of COVID-19 in Unvaccinated vs. Vaccinated Patients," *Biomedicines* 11, no. 2 (February 14, 2023): 551, doi: 10.3390/biomedicines11020551; Kristina Mosna et al., "Guillain- Barré Syndrome with Lethal Outcome following Covid 19 Vaccination—Case Report Supported by Autopsy Examination," *The Open Neurology Journal* 16, no. 1 (March 10, 2022), doi: 10.2174/1874205x-v16-e2207270; Ryo Kaimori et al., "Histopathologically TMA- Like Distribution of Multiple Organ Thromboses following the Initial Dose of the BNT162b2 mRNA Vaccine (Comirnaty, Pfizer/BioNTech): An Autopsy Case Report," *Thrombosis Journal* 20, no. 1 (October 6, 2022): 61, doi: 10.1186/s12959-022-00418-7.

596 Bozkurt et al., "Myocarditis with COVID-19 mRNA Vaccines,"; Yonker et al., "Circulating Spike Protein Detected in Post–COVID-19 mRNA Vaccine Myocarditis."

597 Zoon Wangu et al., "Multisystem Inflammatory Syndrome in Children (MIS-C) Possibly Secondary to COVID-19 mRNA Vaccination," *BMJ Case Reports* 15, no. (3): e247176, doi: 10.1136/bcr-2021-247176; Kelvin Ehikhametalor et al., "Multisystem Inflammatory Syndrome in Adults (MIS-A) After COVID-19 Infection and Recent Vaccination with Recombinant Adenoviral Vector Encoding the Spike Protein Antigen

of SARS-CoV-2 (ChAdOx1 nCoV-19, Vaxzevria)," *Journal of Intensive Care Medicine* 38, no. 2 (February 2023): 232–237, doi: 10.1177/08850666221121589.

598 Australian Government Department of Health, Therapeutic Goods Administration, "Nonclinical Evaluation of BNT162b2 [mRNA] COVID-19 vaccine (COMIRNATY)," accessed May 23, 2023, https://www.tga.gov.au/sites/default/files/foi-2389-06.pdf.

599 Ali Zidan et al., "COVID-19 Vaccine-Associated Immune Thrombosis and Thrombocytopenia (VITT): Diagnostic Discrepancies and Global Implications," *Seminars in Thrombosis and Hemostasis* 49, no. 1 (February 2023): 9–14, doi: 10.1055/s-0042-1759684; Nwosu Ifeanyi et al., "Isolated Pulmonary Embolism following COVID Vaccination: 2 Case Reports and a Review of Post-Acute Pulmonary Embolism Complications and Follow-Up," *Journal of Community Hospital Internal Medicine Perspectives* 11, no. 6 (November 15, 2021): 877–879, doi: 10.1080/20009666.2021.1990825.

600 Betsy Abraham et al., "Acute Respiratory Distress Syndrome Secondary to COVID-19 mRNA Vaccine Administration in a Pregnant Woman: A Case Report," *Qatar Medical Journal* 2022, no. 3 (August 9, 2022): 40, doi: 10.5339/qmj.2022.40; Ayumi Yoshifuji et al., "COVID-19 Vaccine Induced Interstitial Lung Disease," *Journal of Infection and Chemotherapy* 28, no. 1 (January 2022): 95–98, doi: 10.1016/j.jiac.2021.09.010.

601 Yue Chen et al., "New-Onset Autoimmune Phenomena Post-COVID-19 Vaccination," *Immunology* 165, no. 4 (April 2022): 386–401, doi: 10.1111/imm.13443; Roya Hosseini and Nayere Askari, "A Review of Neurological Side Effects of COVID-19 Vaccination," *European Journal of Medical Research* 28, no. 1 (February 25, 2023): 102, doi: 10.1186/s40001- 023-00992-0; Kunal Ajmera et al., "Gastrointestinal Complications of COVID-19 Vaccines, *Cureus* 14, no, 4 (April 12, 2022): e24070, doi: 10.7759/cureus.24070.

602 Spiro Pantazatos and Herve Seligmann, "COVID Vaccination and Age-Stratified All-Cause Mortality Risk," Research Gate, October 26, 2021, doi: 10.13140/RG.2.2.28257.43366.

603 Jarle Aarstad and Olav Andreas Kvitastein, "Is There a Link between the 2021 COVID-19 Vaccination Uptake in Europe and 2022 Excess All-Cause Mortality?" Preprints.org, February 21, 2023, doi: 10.20944/preprints202302.0350.v1.

604 Sanjay Beesoon et al., "Excess Deaths during the COVID-19 Pandemic in Alberta, Canada," *IJID Regions,* 5 (December 2022): 62–67, doi: 10.1016/j.ijregi.2022.08.011; Megan Todd and Annaka Scheeres, "Excess Mortality from Non-COVID-19 Causes during the COVID-19 Pandemic in Philadelphia, Pennsylvania, 2020–2021," *American Journal of Public Health* 112, no. 12 (December 2022): 1800–1803, doi: 10.2105/AJPH.2022.307096; Ariel Karlinsky and Dmitry Kobak, "The World Mortality Dataset: Tracking Excess Mortality across Countries during the COVID-19 Pandemic," medRxiv [preprint], June 4, 2021: 2021.01.27.21250604, doi:

10.1101/2021.01.27.21250604; COVID-19 Excess Mortality Collaborators, "Estimating Excess Mortality due to the COVID-19 Pandemic: A Systematic Analysis of COVID-19-Related Mortality, 2020–21," *Lancet* 399, no. 10334 (April 16, 2022): 1513–1536, doi: 10.1016/S0140-6736(21)02796-3; William Msemburi et al., "The WHO Estimates of Excess Mortality Associated with the COVID-19 Pandemic," *Nature* 613, no. 7942 (January 2023): 130–137, doi: 10.1038/s41586-022-05522-2; Weijing Shang et al., "Global Excess Mortality during COVID-19 Pandemic: A Systematic Review and Meta-Analysis," *Vaccines* (Basel) 10, no. 10 (October 12, 2022):1702, doi: 10.3390/vaccines10101702.

605 Pantazatos and Herve Seligmann, "COVID Vaccination and Age-Stratified All-Cause Mortality Risk."

606 From Vaccine Adverse Event Reporting System (VAERS), https://vaers.hhs.gov.

Chapter 14: "All Hands on Deck" The Catastrophe of US Longevity, and What We Can Do about It

607 Dr. Robert M. Califf (@DrCaliff_FDA), "We are facing extraordinary headwinds in our public health with a major decline in life expectancy. The major decline in the U.S. is not just a trend. I'd describe it as catastrophic," Twitter (X), November 30, 2023, https://twitter.com/DrCaliff_FDA/status/1730298837950927246; Califf, "I believe that we need to seriously examine our level of accountability and changes that we can make to help what needs to be an 'all hands on deck' effort to continue and amplify the improvement in life expectancy discussed in CDCs latest report," https://twitter.com/DrCaliff_FDA/status/1730298858792689829; Califf, "The government, industry, and the public all have a role to play in improving life expectancy. Let's get to it," https://twitter.com/DrCaliff_FDA/status/1730298863485960206.

608 Elizabeth Arias, Ph.D. et al., *Vital Statistics Surveillance Report: Provisional Life Expectancy Estimates for 2022*, US Department of Health and Human Services, Centers for Disease Control and Prevention, November 29, 2023, https://www.cdc.gov/nchs/data/vsrr/vsrr031.pdf.

609 Data accessed December 10, 2023, including deaths which occurred up to September 30, 2023, if reported by December 3, 2023.

610 "Data Table for Figure 5," *Data Brief 456: Mortality in the United States, 2021*, US Department of Health and Human Services, Centers for Disease Control, December 2022, https://www.cdc.gov/nchs/data/databriefs/db456-tables.pdf#5; "Children are Dying at the Highest Rate in 13 Years," USAFacts, June 13, 2023, https://usafacts.org/data-projects/child-death.

611 Daniel Crown et al., *The Demographic Outlook: 2022 to 2052*, Congressional Budget Office website, July 2022, https://www.cbo.gov/publication/58347#_idTextAnchor013.

612 Eurostat, "Excess Mortality Rose Sharply to 19% in December 2022," February 17, 2023, https://ec.europa.eu/eurostat/web/products-eurostat-news/w/DDN-20230217-

1; Jarle Aarstad and Olav Andreas Kvitastein, "Is There a Link between the 2021 COVID-19 Vaccination Uptake in Europe and 2022 Excess All-Cause Mortality?" Preprints.org, February 21, 2023, doi: 10.20944/preprints202302.0350.v1.

613 Robert Cuffe and Rachel Schraer, "Excess Deaths in 2022 among Worst in 50 Years," BBC News, January 10, 2023, https://www.bbc.com/news/health-64209221.

614 IFO Institute, "180,000 More People Died Than Normally Expected in Germany during the Covid Years," press release, January 20, 2023, https://www.ifo.de/en/press-release/2023-01-20/180000-more-people-died-normally-expected-germany-during-covid-years.

615 Sarah Dumeau, "Excess Mortality in France Was Higher in 2022 Than during COVID," *Les Echos*, June 6, 2023, https://www.lesechos.fr/politique-societe/societe/en-2022-la-surmortalite-en-france-a-ete-plus-elevee-que-pendant-la-pandemie-1949597.

616 Kentaro Iwamoto, "Deaths Jumped 8.9% in Japan in 2022 to Almost Double Birth Total," *Nikkei*, February 28, 2023, https://asia.nikkei.com/Spotlight/Society/Deaths-jumped-8.9-in-Japan-in-2022-to-almost-double-birth-total; Song Soo-youn, "Korea Alone Has Seen an Increase in Excess Death amid the Omicron Wave. Why?" *Korea Biomedical Review*, September 6, 2022, https://www.koreabiomed.com/news/articleView.html?idxno=14542; Chloe Whelan, "Thousands More Aussies Dying as 'Excess Deaths' Rise," News.com.au, April 7, 2023, https://www.news.com.au/lifestyle/health/health-problems/thousands-more-aussies-dying-as-excess-deaths-rise/news-story/2e6d46659884d19d9a8d27c52808cf61.

617 "Table A-6. Employment Status of the Civilian Population by Sex, Age, and Disability Status, not Seasonally Adjusted," US Bureau of Labor Statistics, last modified June 2, 2023, https://www.bls.gov/news.release/empsit.t06.htm.

618 US Bureau of Labor Statistics, *Labor Force Statistics from the Current Population Survey. Series ID: LNU00074597*, accessed September 23, 2023, https://data.bls.gov/pdq/SurveyOutputServlet.

619 Robert Joyce, Sam Ray-Chaudhuri, and Tom Waters, "The Number of New Disability Benefit Claimants Has Doubled in a Year," Institute for Fiscal Studies, December 7, 2022, https://ifs.org.uk/news/number-new-disability-benefit-claimants-has-doubled-year.

620 Statistics Canada, "Mental Health-Related Disability Rises among Employed Canadians during Pandemic, 2021," March 4, 2022, https://www150.statcan.gc.ca/n1/daily-quotidien/220304/dq220304b-eng.htm; National Disability Insurance Agency, *NDIA Annual Report*, June 30, 2019, https://www.ndis.gov.au/media/1860/download?attachment; Australian Government Productivity Commission, *Report on Government Services 2023—Part F, Section 15, Services for People with Disability*, January 24, 2023, https://www.pc.gov.au/ongoing/report-on-government-services/2023/community-services/services-for-people-with-disability.

About the Authors

621 Alex Pierson, "On Point with Alex Pierson: New Peer Reviewed Study on COVID-19 Vaccines Suggests Why Heart Inflammation, Blood Clots and Other Dangerous Side Effects Occur," May 27, 2021, *The Alex Pierson Show* (podcast), https://podcasts.apple.com/ca/podcast/new-peer-reviewed-study-on-covid-19-vaccines-suggests/id1318830191.

622 Dr. Steven Hatfill, Robert J. Coullahan, and Dr. John J. Walsh Jr., *Three Seconds Until Midnight* (self-pub, November 1, 2019), https://www.amazon.com/Three-Seconds-Midnight-Steven-Hatfill/dp/1700120298/r.

623 Peter A. McCullough, MD, Harvey Risch, et al., "Pathophysiological Basis and Rationale for Early Outpatient Treatment of SARS-CoV-2 (COVID-19) Infection," *American Journal of Medicine* 134 no. 1 (January 2021): 16–22, doi: 10.1016/j.amjmed.2020.07.003; Peter A. McCullough, MD, et al., "Multifaceted Highly Targeted Sequential Multidrug Treatment of Early Ambulatory High-Risk SARS-CoV-2 Infection (COVID-19)," *Reviews in Cardiovascular Medicine* 21, no. 4 (, 2020): 517–530, doi: 10.31083/j.rcm.2020.04.264.

624 Peter A. McCullough, MD, MPH; Brian C. Procter, MD; and Cade Wynn, "Clinical Rationale for SARS-Co-V-2 Base Spike Protein Detoxification in Post COVID-19 and Vaccine Injury Syndromes," *Journal of American Physicians and Surgeons,* 28, no. 3 (2023): 91–93, https://jpands.org/vol28no3/mccullough.pdf.

625 Jane Orient, *YOUR Doctor Is Not In: Health Skepticism about National Health Care* (New York: Crown, 1994), https://www.amazon.com/Your-Doctor-Not-Skepticism-National/dp/0517590115.

626 Harvey Risch, "Early Outpatient Treatment of Symptomatic, High-Risk COVID-19 Patients That Should Be Ramped Up Immediately as Key to the Pandemic Crisis," *American Journal of Epidemiology* 189, no. 11 (November 2020): 1218–1226, doi: 10.1093/aje/kwaa093.

627 "Harvey Risch," Brownstone Institute, https://brownstone.org/author/harvey-rische/.

628 "Dr. Harvey Risch," *America Out Loud News,* https://www.americaoutloud.news/author/dr-harvey-risch/.

ACKNOWLEDGMENTS

This book is a collective effort of the medical freedom movement: all those advocating for patient sovereignty, physician autonomy, and scientific integrity. It would not be possible without the field of inquiry created by this movement as its scientific milieu—the largely unpaid work of thousands of committed clinicians and scientists.

While we cannot acknowledge everyone by name, we wish to honor medical professionals, scientists, activists, authors, and legal advocates who have publicly questioned the mass "vaccination" campaign or other aspects of the public health response to COVID-19, often paying a steep professional price for their principled dissent. Omitting titles and degrees, we are grateful to Paul Alexander, Richard Amerling, Bryan Ardis, Alan Bain, Steve Bannon, Maxime Bernier, Jay Bhattacharya, Alexander Boissonneau-Lehner, Geert Vanden Bossche, Mary Talley Bowden, Peter and Ginger Breggin, Joseph Brewer, Andrew Bridgen, Carole Browner, Adam Brufsky, Flavio Cadegiani, Todd Callender, John Campbell, Tucker Carlson, Hector Carosso, Deborah Catalano, Shankara Chetty, Igor Chudov, Ryan Cole, Jeff Colyer, Jonathan Jay Couey, Bobbie Ann Cox, Angus Dalgleish, Mary Davenport, Maryanne Demasi, Peter Doshi, Ed Dowd, George Fareed, Norman Fenton, Joseph Fraiman, Heather Gessling, Simone Gold, Maria Gutschi, Sabine Hazan, Roger Hodkinson, Tracy Beth Høeg, Charles Hoffe, C. J. Hopkins, Abraxas Hudson, Nicolas Hulscher, Laura Ingraham, Amy Kelly, Robert F. Kennedy Jr., Aaron Kheriaty, Steve Kirsch, Pierre Kory, Martin Kulldorff, Joseph Ladapo, Sasha Latypova, Tess Lawrie, John Leake, Retsef Levi, Katarina Lindley, John Littell, Lt. Col. Theresa Long, Ralph Lorigo, Tony Lyons, William Makis, Aseem Malhotra, Robert Malone, Paul Marik, David Martin, Warner Mendenhall, Kirk and Kimberly Milhoan, Mark Crispin Miller, Daniel Nagase, Meryl Nass, Drew Pinsky, Filipe Rafaeli, Didier Raoult, Joe Rogan, Toby Rogers, Gad Saad, Stephanie Seneff, Aaron Siri, Stephen M. Smith, Jeremy Snavely, Dan Stock, Liam Sturgess, Howard Tenenbaum, Paul Thacker, James Todaro, Mark Trozzi,

Jeffrey Tucker, Brian Tyson, Richard Urso, Joel Wallskog, the WarRoom/ DailyClout Pfizer Documents Research Team, Elizabeth Woodworth, and Michael Yeadon. Again, we regret this list is only partial and offer heartfelt apologies to the many not named.

Among the authors, we wish to extend our warm gratitude and appreciation to Dr. Kelly Victory for her tireless service as de facto managing editor. We are also indebted to the many talented writers and editors who have given so much time and attention to this lengthy, complex project. This book would naturally have been impossible without the unflagging support, patience, and wise counsel of family, friends, colleagues, and collaborators from all walks of life.

Finally, we recognize the countless doctors, scientists, and laymen fighting for medical freedom who must remain anonymous to protect their families and livelihoods.

ABOUT THE AUTHORS

Matt Bain, MD. Having recently founded an independent, direct-pay practice in central Indiana, Dr. Bain is dedicated to providing transparent neurologic care in a setting that allows him to work with his patients untethered from corporate interests. Dr. Bain has consistently been praised by his students for taking time to help them learn practical neurologic skills, to serve them regardless of their future specialties, and to mentor them into their roles as clinicians. With a worldview grounded in biblical truth and a hope firmly rooted in the power of the Gospel, he is passionate about the pursuit of truth. He urges his patients, students, and all caring individuals to remember that apparent consensus doesn't necessarily predicate fact, and that the promises of predictability and security offered by so-called "gold-standard" clinical studies may well prove illusory, for a range of reasons, unfortunately including unethical practices.

Though the process has been painful and deeply contemplative, Dr. Bain is grateful for the perspective that he has gained in the context of the pandemic. He remains passionate about pursuing all reasonable options, traditional and alternative, for helping his patients achieve true health. Dr. Bain encourages other providers to consider how this principle impacts their ability to maximize their skills for the benefit of their patients, and their own well-being in the post-COVID landscape.

Byram Bridle, PhD. Dr. Bridle holds a BS in biomedical sciences, an MS in immunology, and a PhD in immunology, and completed a postdoctoral fellowship in viral immunology. He serves as an associate professor of viral immunology at the University of Guelph in Ontario, Canada, specializing in vaccinology, immunology, virology, and cancer biology, including teaching students at the undergraduate, professional undergraduate, and graduate levels. Dr. Bridle is a cofounder and the chief operating officer of ImmunoCeutica, a company dedicated to the research and development of immunoceuticals—natural health products to ensure optimal functioning of the immune system. ImmunoCeutica had no role in funding, analysis, or publication of this book. Dr. Bridle is a member of the Canadian COVID Care Alliance and serves on their Scientific and Medical Advisory Committee, is a scientific advisor for the organization Taking Back Our Freedoms, and has served as an expert witness in COVID-19-related cases.

Dr. Bridle has published numerous peer-reviewed papers, mostly focusing on novel vaccine technologies, and holds several patents related to viruses and vaccines. He developed a vaccine technology that advanced into four human clinical trials. He has received millions of dollars in research funding, including two grants to develop new COVID-19 "vaccines," which are no longer being pursued due to Dr. Bridle's safety concerns about the COVID-19 spike protein.

On March 16, 2021, along with two other senior immunologists, Dr. Bridle wrote an open letter to Canadians, and the world, warning against Health Canada's authorization of AstraZeneca's COVID-19 "vaccine," noting possible association with blood clots. In a podcast published May 27, 2021, Dr. Bridle informed the world of major concerns about Pfizer's modRNA "vaccine" biodistribution study submitted to Japan's health regulatory agency—all of which were later verified by scientific evidence.[621] Within forty-eight hours of this interview, a well-organized global smear campaign was launched against Dr. Bridle, who was repeatedly accused of providing misinformation; the onslaught of public attacks has continued unrelentingly ever since.

Dr. Bridle has tried to engage in scientific discussions with those who have accused him of disseminating misinformation, but not one of these accusers has been willing to engage in a discussion to date, despite an offer from a concerned philanthropist of up to $2 million US dollars to engage in a civil, public debate moderated by an objective third party.

Steven Hatfill MD, MSc, MSc, MMed. Dr. Steven Hatfill is a physician, virologist, and public health consultant who has performed fellowships at Oxford University, the National Institutes of Health, and the National Research Council, when he studied the Ebola virus at the US Army Institute for Infectious Diseases at Fort Detrick, Maryland. For over a decade he served as an adjunct assistant professor in both the Department of Clinical Research and the Department of Microbiology, Immunology, and Tropical Medicine at the George Washington University Medical Center and School.

In 2015, Dr. Hatfill trained the first Rapid Hemorrhagic Fever Response Team for the National Medical Disaster Unit in Kenya, Africa. He is a Senior Fellow at the London Center for Policy Analysis and the lead author of *Three Seconds Until Midnight*, prophetically published two months before the US COVID-19 outbreak.[622] He has numerous peer-reviewed scientific publications. From February 3, 2020, until the 2021 transition, he served as a daily medical and scientific advisor to the Executive Office of the President of the United States, where he fought for the doctrine of early outpatient drug treatment for COVID-19.

Peter A. McCullough, MD, MPH. After receiving a bachelor's degree from Baylor University, Dr. McCullough completed his medical degree as an Alpha Omega Alpha graduate from the University of Texas Southwestern Medical School. He went on to complete his internal medicine residency at the University of Washington, cardiology fellowship including service as chief fellow at William Beaumont Hospital, and master's degree in public health at the University of Michigan. Dr. McCullough is an independent, practicing internist and cardiologist in Dallas, Texas.

Dr. McCullough has broadly published on a range of topics in medicine, with over 1,000 publications and 685 citations in the National Library of Medicine. His works include the "Interface between Renal Disease and Cardiovascular Illness" in *Braunwald's Heart Disease Textbook*. Dr. McCullough is a recipient of the Simon Dack Award from the American College of Cardiology and has received multiple humanitarian awards for his pandemic service. His publications have appeared in the *New England Journal of Medicine, Journal of the American Medical Association, Lancet, British Medical Journal*, and other top-tier journals worldwide. He is the former editor in chief of *Cardiorenal Medicine, Reviews in Cardiovascular Medicine*, and senior associate editor of the *American Journal of Cardiology*. Dr. McCullough has made presentations on the advancement of medicine across the world and has been an invited lecturer at the New York Academy of Sciences, the National Institutes of Health, US Food and Drug Administration, and the European Medicines Agency. He has served as member or chair of dozens of data safety monitoring boards for randomized clinical trials.

Since the outset of the pandemic, Dr. McCullough has been a leader in the medical response to the COVID-19 disaster, including publication of "Pathophysiological Basis and Rationale for Early Outpatient Treatment of SARS-CoV-2 (COVID-19) Infection," the first synthesis of sequenced multidrug treatment of ambulatory patients infected with SARS-CoV-2 in the *American Journal of Medicine*, subsequently updated in *Reviews in Cardiovascular Medicine*.[623] Subsequently he published the first detoxification approach, titled "Clinical Rationale for SARS-CoV-2 Base Spike Protein Detoxification in Post COVID-19 and Vaccine Injury Syndromes," in the *Journal of American Physicians and Surgeons*.[624] He has dozens of peer-reviewed publications on the viral infection and has commented extensively in the media on the COVID-19 crisis. Dr. McCullough testified in the US Senate, Colorado General Assembly, and the state senates of Arizona, Texas, New Hampshire, Mississippi, Pennsylvania, and South Carolina concerning many aspects of the pandemic response. He is considered among the world's experts on COVID-19.

Jane M. Orient, MD. Dr. Jane Orient obtained her undergraduate degrees in chemistry and mathematics from the University of Arizona in Tucson, and her MD from Columbia University College of Physicians and Surgeons in 1974. She completed an internal medicine residency at Parkland Memorial Hospital and University of Arizona Affiliated Hospitals, then served as an instructor and assistant professor at the University of Arizona College of Medicine, as well as a staff physician at the Tucson Veterans Administration Hospital. She has been in solo private practice since 1981.

Dr. Orient has served as executive director of the Association of American Physicians and Surgeons (AAPS) since 1989. She is currently president of Doctors for Disaster Preparedness. She is the author of *YOUR Doctor Is Not In: Healthy Skepticism about National Healthcare*; *Sutton's Law* (a novel about where the money is in medicine today); and the second through fifth (current) editions of Sapira's *Art and Science of Bedside Diagnosis*, published by Wolters Kluwer.[625] More than two hundred of her papers and op-ed pieces have been published in the scientific and popular literature on a variety of subjects, including risk assessment, natural and technological hazards (and nonhazards), and medical economics and ethics. She is the editor of *AAPS News* (www.aapsonline.org), the *Doctors for Disaster Preparedness Newsletter* (www.ddponline.org), and *Civil Defense Perspectives* (www.physiciansforcivildefense.org), and is the managing editor of the *Journal of American Physicians and Surgeons* (www.jpands.org). Her contribution to this book (chapter 10) is repurposed, with gratitude, from an article originally published under the *J. Am. Physicians Surg.* imprint.

Harvey Risch, MD, PhD, FACE. Dr. Harvey Risch is professor emeritus of epidemiology at Yale School of Public Health, elected fellow of the

American College of Epidemiology, and elected member of the Connecticut Academy of Science and Engineering. He is a practicing epidemiologist with more than forty years of research and teaching experience, including graduate and postgraduate students and fellows in epidemiology. Dr. Risch received a bachelor of science degree in mathematics and biology from the California Institute of Technology in 1972 and completed medical training at University of California San Diego School of Medicine in 1976. He then completed a PhD in biomathematics in 1980 at the University of Chicago, where his dissertation work involved studies of the general stochastic epidemic model, on which he has published in the peer-reviewed scientific literature.

From 1980 to 1983, Dr. Risch held a postdoctoral fellowship in epidemiology at the University of Washington. In 1983 he was appointed assistant professor at the University of Toronto, later serving as associate professor, before his appointment as professor of public health at Yale School of Public Health in 1991. He was later additionally appointed professor of epidemiology at Yale in 2001, and professor emeritus in July 2022.

Dr. Risch has published more than 400 peer-reviewed original research papers in highly regarded scientific journals, and has an h-index of 111, with more than 51,500 publication citations to date. Dr. Risch has been associate editor of the *Journal of the National Cancer Institute* since 2000, member of the Board of Editors of the *American Journal of Epidemiology* from 2014–2020, and editor of the *International Journal of Cancer* since 2008. In May 2020, Dr. Risch published a foundational paper on early treatment of high-risk COVID-19 outpatients in the *American Journal of Epidemiology*, which has been downloaded more than 91,000 times and viewed over 166,000 times.[626] As noted, with Dr. Peter McCullough, Dr. Risch coauthored two papers that form the now-standard understanding of early outpatient COVID-19 management in the pre-Omicron era.

During the pandemic, Dr. Risch has been a leading scientific voice, with more than two hundred appearances in major TV and radio media. These appearances include *CNN*, *Newsmax*, Laura Ingraham, Tucker Carlson, Mark Levin, Sean Hannity, John Solomon, Dennis Prager, as well as journalists from Italy, France, Germany, Brazil, South Africa, Israel, Australia, Canada, Belgium, Romania, and many others.

Dr. Risch has testified three times in US Senate hearings on the COVID-19 pandemic and its public health management. He has written commentaries about the pandemic in *Newsweek, Wall Street Journal, France*

Soir, Washington Examiner, The Federalist, and at the Brownstone Institute, where he is a senior scholar.[627] Dr. Risch's weekly audio podcast may be heard at "America Out Loud."[628]

Jessica Rose, PhD. Dr. Rose is a Canadian researcher with advanced degrees in applied mathematics and immunology from Memorial University of Newfoundland, computational biology from Bar Ilan University and the Weizmann Institute, molecular biology from the Hebrew University of Jerusalem, and biochemistry from the Technion Institute of Technology. For the past three years, Dr. Rose has been independently analyzing the Vaccine Adverse Event Reporting System (VAERS) database in the context of the COVID-19 products, to bring understanding to the public of the magnitude and range of the safety signals emitted from VAERS in the context of these products.

Dr. Rose has become a prolific writer (https://jessicar.substack.com/), presenter (jessicasuniverse.com), and spokesperson for individuals suffering adverse events in the context of what are technologically and biologically novel products. She has presented her work to the European Parliament in Brussels, at three FDA Vaccines and Related Biological Products Advisory Committee meetings, and at many international conferences. She was also invited twice to provide testimony at United States Senate hearings, but on both occasions was not permitted to attend due to COVID-19 travel restrictions imposed on uninjected non-US citizens. Dr. Rose has contributed chapters to upcoming books on COVID-19 and participated in numerous video documentaries, podcasts, and interviews, in order to bring scientific information to the public.

Josh Stirling, MBA. Josh Stirling is founder and president of the Insurance Collaboration to Save Lives, a not-for-profit formed in spring 2023 by insurance leaders to help global insurers reduce the widespread tragedy of excess mortality and morbidity, through proactive, insurance-led, voluntary health screening, blood testing and triage to care for at-risk, in-force policyholders. The collaboration believes that insurers, employers, and governments that proactively screen, test, and triage those most at risk can use well-established medical science to widely and cost-effectively improve health, and likely save the lives of millions, if globally deployed. The collaboration had no role in funding this book.

Josh has more than twenty-five years of proven leadership in insurance, spanning underwriting and pricing, reinsurance and risk management, finance and investments, as well as technology, strategy, and mergers and acquisitions. Before founding the collaboration, Josh worked for five years in insurtech, in roles including board member, chief insurance officer, SVP of Strategy and Corporate Development, founder advisor, and angel investor. Prior to going into insurtech, Josh was a Wall Street analyst, and the managing director for U.S. insurance at Sanford C. Bernstein & Co., where he led its Institutional Investor #1 ranked sell-side research team for six years. Josh began his insurance career in product management at Progressive, and then worked in strategy, finance, and M&A for several other notable insurers, including OneBeacon, The Hanover, and Advantage Life.

Josh earned his BS from Cornell University and his MBA from the Stanford Graduate School of Business, where he was named an Arjay Miller Scholar, and is currently working to finish a JD at the Baylor University School of Law.

James Thorp, MD. Dr. Jim Thorp is a board-certified obstetrician gynecologist and maternal fetal medicine physician with forty-four years of obstetrical experience. He served in the United States Air Force as an obstetrician-gynecologist, having been awarded a Health Professions Scholarship for his medical school education. While serving as a busy clinician his entire career, he has also been active in clinical research with over 250 publications. He has served as a reviewer for major medical journals and served on the Board of Directors for the Society of Maternal Fetal Medicine for four years and served as an examiner for the American Board of ObGyn and a board of director for the Society for Maternal Fetal Medicine. Dr. Thorp testified in the US Senate in 2003, sharing his expertise in treating the fetus as a patient with in-utero therapies.

Dr. Thorp has seen about 27,500 high risk pregnancies in the last 4.5 years, spanning the COVID-19 pandemic and modRNA mass "vaccination" campaign. On December 7, 2022, he participated in an event at the US Capitol, organized by Senator Ron Johnson and others, to raise awareness of COVID-19 modRNA "vaccine" injuries. He has been interviewed on hundreds of media platforms. Most recently, Dr. Thorp has focused his research efforts on the COVID-19 pandemic, publishing over 70 publications, including two books, documenting the dangers of the "vaccine" in women of reproductive age and pregnancy.

Kelly Victory, MD. Dr. Kelly Victory is a residency-trained and board-certified emergency and trauma specialist with over thirty years of clinical experience. She is an expert in disaster preparedness and response, and the medical management of mass casualties. She has an extensive background in public health, having served as chief medical officer of the company providing on-site health-care services for dozens of Fortune 500 companies, including Continental Airlines, Nissan Automotive, Harrah's Entertainment, Sprint Wireless, USA Today-Gannett, and Scott's Miracle-Gro, as well as multiple federal agencies.

Dr. Victory is an alumnus of the National Preparedness Leadership Initiative—a combined effort of Harvard School of Public Health and the Kennedy School of Government to develop "meta-leaders" for national disaster preparedness and response. She has worked closely with officials from Homeland Security, HHS, FEMA, and multiple branches of the military. She also served as a member of the Leadership Council at Harvard School of Public Health.

Dr. Victory has worked with a broad range of organizations, including both public and private sector companies, hospitals, schools, churches, and municipalities on issues regarding public health, including disaster and pandemic preparedness and response planning, and contingency strategies for large disasters. She teaches "Active Shooter Rapid Response and Extraction" and "Leadership in Times of Crisis" for first responders, community leaders, and organizations, aimed at limiting casualties, improving outcomes, enhancing resiliency, and coordinating response efforts with law enforcement and EMS/fire agencies.

Dr. Victory makes frequent radio and television appearances to discuss issues of public health, disasters, and mass casualty preparedness and response efforts. She appears regularly on multiple news outlets, podcasts, and radio programs. She has advocated tirelessly for a more measured, risk-stratified approach to the COVID-19 pandemic response. She has been a consistent and vocal proponent of aggressive early outpatient treatment for COVID-19, as well as a cautious and informed, risk-benefit based approach to COVID "vaccination."

Dr. Victory holds a BS from Duke University, earned her MD from the University of North Carolina, and completed her residency at Carolinas Medical Center.

Naomi Wolf, PhD. Dr. Naomi Wolf received a D Phil Degree in English Literature from the University of Oxford in 2015. Dr Wolf taught Victorian Studies as a Visiting Professor at SUNY Stony Brook, received a Barnard College Research Fellowship at the Center for Women and Gender, was recipient of a Rothermere American Institute Research Fellowship for her work on John Addington Symonds at the University of Oxford, and taught English Literature at George Washington University as a visiting lecturer. She's lectured widely on the themes in Outrages: Sex, Censorship and the Criminalization of Love, presenting lectures on Symonds and the themes in Outrages at the Ashmolean Museum in Oxford, at Balliol College, Oxford, and to the undergraduates in the English Faculty at the University of Oxford. She lectured about Symonds and Outrages for the first LGBTQ Colloquium at Rhodes House. Dr Wolf was a Rhodes Scholar and a Yale graduate. She's written eight nonfiction bestsellers, about women's issues and civil liberties, and is the CEO of DailyClout.io, a news site and legislative database in which actual US state and Federal legislation is shared digitally and read and explained weekly. She holds an honorary doctorate from Sweet Briar College. She lives with her husband, private detective Brian O'Shea, in the Hudson Valley.

Martin Wucher, B.Sc, B.Ch.D, M.Dent. (*eq.* **DDS**). Dr. Martin Wucher was born in 1957 in Okahandja, Namibia. His school years were spent in Namibia, and he graduated from the DHPS German private school in Windhoek. In 1980 he earned his bachelor of science degree in zoology and microbiology from Rhodes University in South Africa, followed in 1985 by his bachelor of dental surgery degree in dentistry at the University of Pretoria (equivalent to DDS). Wucher further studied dentistry and cutting-edge prosthodontics in Germany from 1987 to 1989. In 1993 he earned his postgraduate diploma in periodontology from the University of Pretoria, with a further postgraduate diploma in aesthetic dentistry, University of Stellenbosch, cum laude, in 1997. In 2001 he earned his Master of Science in Dentistry in dental science at the University of Stellenbosch, cum laude. During 2019, Dr. Wucher acted as a founding member, part-time lecturer and cochair for the postgraduate master's program for preventive and functional medicine at the Dresden International University.

Dr. Martin Wucher is a member of the Namibian Dental Association and an associate member of the South African Dental Association. From 1989 to the present, he has served in private dental practice, with a focus on restorative and biological dentistry, including periodontology, implantology, and laser dentistry. Since 2008 he has integrated biological dentistry with a part-time practice in functional medicine. Dr. Wucher has lectured to expert audiences internationally on topics including implantology, psychological aspects of dentistry, bonding and shrinkage in tooth-colored restorations, biological dentistry, functional medicine, chronic disease, mechanism of cancer, and autoimmune diseases. His scientific interests also include cellular mechanisms in chronic disease, the impact of man-made environmental factors and man-made frequencies on biological systems, and mitochondrial medicine. In his free time, Dr. Wucher enjoys piloting gyrocopters.

Made in United States
North Haven, CT
18 November 2024

60502914R00173